Functional Brain Imaging

Functional Brain Imaging

Edited by

Gert Pfurtscheller
Technical University of Graz
and
F. H. Lopes da Silva
University of Amsterdam

Hans Huber Publishers
Toronto · Lewiston, NY · Bern · Stuttgart

Library of Congress Cataloging-in-Publication Data

Functional brain imaging / Gert Pfurtscheller, F. H. Lopes da Silva.

p. cm.
Bibliography: p.
Includes index.

1. Brain – Imaging – Congresses. 2. Electroencephalography – Congresses. 3. Cerebral circulation – Measurement – Congresses. I. Pfurtscheller, Gert, 1939–   . II. Lopes da Silva, F. H. 1935–   . III. Title.
QP376.P47   1988   612'.82-do19   88-19071

Canadian Cataloging in Publication Data

Main entry under title:

Functional brain imaging

Based on a symposium held in Graz, Austria, 1987.
Bibliography: p.
Includes index.

1. Brain – Imaging – Congresses. 2. Brain – Diseases – Diagnosis – Congresses. 3. Brain – Localization of functions – Congresses. I. Pfurtscheller, Gert. II Lopes da Silva, F. H., 1935–

RC386.5.F86   1988   616.8'04754   C88-094368-8

Copyright © 1988 by Hans Huber Publishers, Inc.

P.O. Box 51
Lewiston, NY 14092

12–14 Bruce Park Ave.
Toronto, Ontario M4P 2S3

Printed in Germany

ISBN 0-920887-28-7
Hans Huber Publishers · Toronto · Lewiston, NY · Bern · Stuttgart
ISBN 3-456-81655-3
Hans Huber Publishers · Bern · Stuttgart · Toronto · Lewiston, NY

Preface

In August 1987 a group of scientists and medical doctors met together in Graz with the aim of exchanging information on a topic of common interest: *Functional Brain Imaging*. Brain imaging implies not only the topographical analysis of the distribution of activity within the brain but also the construction of brain images providing comprehensive displays of such distributions. The term "functional" indicates clearly that the main interest lies on the analysis of the (patho)physiological states of the brain.

The concern of all participants was to optimize the processes of assessment of the functional state of different brain areas in relation not only to pathology, but also to psychological variables. In this respect three main approaches were discussed at the symposium: (i) the localization of sources of activity within the brain based on electrical and magnetic recordings from the scalp; (ii) the computer aided analysis of functional relationships between surface EEG or event related potentials recorded from different brain areas; (iii) the determination of the regional cerebral blood flow and metabolic state of the brain using SPECT and PET scans and the relations between these and electrophysiological measurements.

Each of these approaches has advantages and limitations. Electric potential and magnetic field measurements represent a two-dimensional continuum changing with time; these have a limited spatial resolution but allow the study of brain functions within milliseconds. Metabolic and cerebral blood flow measurements provide valuable spatial information, but have a poor temporal resolution.

Blood flow, metabolic, electric potential and magnetic field measurements can result in a topographical display known as a brain image or map. Since the pioneering work of Grey Walter, Rémond and Petsche modern computer algorithms have very strongly facilitated the analysis and display of topographic electric and magnetic field data. At the same time the development of tomographic techniques of displaying cerebral blood flow, metabolic and other neurochemical data has reached a high level of sophistication. One of the main aims of this book is to evaluate the value of the different functional brain imaging techniques, their advantages, drawbacks and limitations, and to provide links between different approaches.

The topics of the book range from magnetic and electric field source localization, electrical potential and magnetic field mapping to quantitative measurements of brain metabolism, cognitive activity and epilepsy. The different sections deal with a number of these problems.

Section I

Source localization using electrical potential and magnetic field measurements gives new insights in the functioning of the brain and allows a better understanding of the functional organization of the brain. Topographic mapping of evoked magnetic fields provides complementary information to that of electric potentials.

Section II

A main feature of electric and magnetic signals from the brain is their high temporal resolution, allowing the study of the dynamics of brain activity. Therefore, special attention is being paid to dynamic techniques such as short-term cross correlation or quantification of event-related desynchronization. Dynamic mapping can be used to study changes of cortical activation pattern within milliseconds.

Section III

EEG and EP mapping are non-invasive techniques for the evaluation of normal brain functions and can be helpful in the assessment of psychiatric and neurological patients. Two main problems are how such maps should be statistically handled and how different types of derivations may influence the topographical data.

Section IV

Regional blood flow and metabolic imaging using PET and SPECT are excellent for obtaining images of the brain and for revealing local variations in metabolism or rCBF, although not on a continuous time scale. The relationship between such measurements and topographic data based on electrophysiological data is an important issue both theoretically and practically.

This symposium would not have taken place without the generous support of the "Fonds zur Förderung der wissenschaftlichen Forschung in Österreich," the Ministry of Science and Research in Vienna, the Styrian Government in Graz and other institutions and firms. We wish to express our gratitude to all of them.

G. Pfurtscheller, Graz,
Austria
F. H. Lopes da Silva, Amsterdam,
The Netherlands

Contents

Preface   v

List of Contributors   ix

List of Contributors

O. Bertrand, INSERM–UNITE 280, Lyon, France.

S. L. Bressler, EEG Systems Laboratory, San Francisco, CA, USA.

P. Brickett, Department of Psychology and Brain Behaviour Laboratory, Simon Fraser University, Burnaby, BC, Canada.

D. Cheyne, Department of Psychology and Brain Behaviour Laboratory, Simon Fraser University, Burnaby, BC, Canada.

L. G. Cohen, National Institute of Neurological and Communicative Disorders and Stroke, National Institutes of Health, Bethesda, MD, USA.

L. Davis, Department of Psychiatry, Charing Cross & Westminster Medical School, London, UK.

L. Deecke, Department of Neurology, University of Vienna, Vienna, Austria.

P. Deniker, Centre Hospitalier Saint-Anne, Paris, France.

T. Dierks, Department of Psychiatry, University of Würzburg, Würzburg, FRG.

F. H. Duffy, Developmental Neurophysiology, Harvard Medical School, Boston, MA, USA.

J. F. Echallier, INSERM–UNITE 280, Lyon, France.

J. Engel, Jr., Departments of Neurology and Anatomy, Reed Neurological Research Center, UCLA School of Medicine, Los Angeles, CA, USA.

P. Etevenon, Centre Esquirol, Caen, France.

A. S. Gevins, EEG Systems Laboratory, San Francisco, CA, USA.

G. Goldenberg, Department of Neurology, University of Vienna, Vienna, Austria.

R. Gordon, Department of Psychology, Brain Behaviour Laboratory, Simon Fraser University, Burnaby, BC, Canada.

J. Gruzelier, Department of Psychiatry, Charing Cross & Westminster Medical School, London, UK.

B. Gueguen, Centre Hospitalier Sainte-Anne, Paris, France.

S. Guillou, Centre Hospitalier Sainte-Anne, Paris, France.

M. Hallett, National Institute of Neurological and Communicative Disorders and Stroke, National Institutes of Health, Bethesda, MD, USA.

R. Harrop, Department of Psychology, Brain Behaviour Laboratory, Simon Fraser University, Burnaby, BC, Canada.

S. Hiroi, Department of Neurology, Research Institute for Brain and Blood Vessels, Akita, Japan.

S. Homma, Department of Physiology, School of Medicine, Chiba University, Chiba, Japan.

J. Huttunen, Low Temperature Laboratory, Helsinki University of Technology, Espoo, Finland.

R. Ihl, Department of Psychiatry, University of Würzburg, Würzburg, FRG.

H. Kamoshita, Department of Physiology, School of Medicine, Chiba University, Chiba, Japan.

L. Kaufman, Neuromagnetism Laboratory, Department of Psychology, New York University, New York, USA.

Y. Kawashima, Department of Physiology, School of Medicine, Chiba University, Chiba, Japan.

W. Klimesch, Department of Physiological Psychology, Institute of Psychology, University of Salzburg, Salzburg, Austria.

M. Lang, Department of Neurology, University of Vienna, Vienna, Austria.

W. Lang, Department of Neurology, University of Vienna, Vienna, Austria.

K. L. Leenders, MRC Cyclotron Unit, Hammersmith Hospital, London, UK.

D. Liddiard, Department of Psychiatry, Charing Cross & Westminster Medical School, London, UK.

H. Loo, Centre Hospitalier Sainte-Anne, Paris, France.

F. H. Lopes da Silva, Biological Centre, University of Amsterdam, Amsterdam, The Netherlands.

H. Maresch, Department of Medical Informatics, Institute of Biomedical Engineering, Technical University of Graz, Graz, Austria.

K. Maurer, Department of Psychiatry, University of Würzburg, Würzburg, FRG.

J. W. H. Meijs, Twente University, Enschede, The Netherlands.

W. Mohl, Department of Medical Informatics, Institute of Biomedical Engineering, Technical University of Graz, Graz, Austria.

K. Nagata, Department of Neurology, EEG Laboratory and Department of Radiology and Nuclear Medicine, Research Institute for Brain and Blood Vessels, Akita, Japan.

Y. Nakajima, Department of Physiology, School of Medicine, Chiba University, Chiba, Japan.

M. Nara, EEG Laboratory, Research Institute for Brain and Blood Vessels, Akita, Japan.

P. L. Nunez, Department of Biomedical Engineering, Tulane University, New Orleans, LA, USA.

J. Pernier, INSERM–UNITE 280, Lyon, France.

P. Peron-Magnan, Centre Hospitalier Sainte-Anne, Paris, France.

F. Perrin, INSERM–UNITE 280, Lyon, France.

M. J. Peters, Department of .Technical Physics, Twente University, Enschede, The Netherlands.

H. Petsche, Institute of Brain Research, Austrian Academy of Sciences and Institute of Neurophysiology, University of Vienna, Vienna, Austria.

G. Pfurtscheller, Ludwig Boltzmann-Institute of Medical Informatics and Department of Medical Informatics, Institute of Biomedical Engineering, Technical University of Graz, Graz, Austria.

H. Pockberger, Institute of Brain Research, Austrian Academy of Sciences and Institute of Neurophysiology, University of Vienna, Vienna, Austria.

I. Podreka, Department of Neurology, University of Vienna, Vienna, Austria.

P. Rappelsberger, Institute of Brain Research, Austrian Academy of Sciences and Institute of Neurophysiology, University of Vienna, Vienna, Austria.

P. E. Roland, Department of Clinical Neurophysiology, Karolinska Hospital, Stockholm, Sweden.

G. L. Romani, Istituto di Elettronica dello Stato Solido–CNR, Rome, Italy.

F. Shishido, Department of Radiology and Nuclear Medicine, Research Institute for Brain and Blood Vessels, Akita, Japan.

J. Steffan, Institute of Fundamentals and Theory in Electrical Engineering, Technical University of Graz, Graz, Austria.

C. J. Stok, P.T.T. Telematics Laboratory, Groningen, The Netherlands.

K. Tagawa, Department of Neurology, Research Institute for Brain and Blood Vessels, Akita, Japan.

J. Tatsuno, Department of Physiology, National Defense Medical College, Saitama, Japan.

B. J. ten Voorde, Twente University, Enschede, The Netherlands.

M. Toussaint, Centre Hospitalier Saint-Anne, Paris, France.

K. Uemura, Department of Radiology and Nuclear Medicine, Research Institute for Brain and Blood Vessels, Akita, Japan.

S. Watanabe, Chiba College of Health Science, Chiba, Japan.

H. Weinberg, Department of Psychology and Brain Behaviour Laboratory, Simon Fraser University, Burnaby, BC, Canada.

L. Widen, Department of Clinical Neurophysiology, Karolinska Hospital, Stockholm, Sweden.

S. J. Williamson, Neuromagnetism Laboratory, Department of Physics, New York University, New York, NY, USA.

L. Wilson, Department of Psychiatry, Charing Cross & Westminster Medical School, London, UK.

P. K. H. Wong, Department of Paediatrics, University of British Columbia and EEG Department, Children's Hospital, Vancouver, Canada.

E. Zarifian, Centre Esquirol, Caen, France.

Section I

Magnetic and Electric Field
Source Localization

Methods to Estimate Spatial Properties of Dynamic Cortical Source Activity

P. L. Nunez

The general problem of extracting useful information from spatial EEG patterns is addressed. While the plotting of isopotential or isomagnetic field maps is an important first step, especially for the location of isolated cortical sources, more quantitative methods are required if *dynamic* brain processes are to be illuminated. It is suggested here that the development of such spatial pattern recognition methods be considered in the context of four categories of cortical sources: Type I (localized and statistically stationary), Type II (localized and nonstationary), Type III (distributed and stationary), and Type IV (distributed and nonstationary). Pattern recognition methods may be based on amplitude, phase, or correlation measures of EEG, but specific strategies should be evaluated for different neural source categories. For example, methods based on the assumption of isolated (dipole) sources can be expected to have very limited application.

Information about neural sources of EEG can be increased by various methods to improve spatial resolution like the radial current estimate (also called Laplacian or current source density) or spatial deconvolution method. The latter approach combines multichannel scalp EEG data with estimated resistive and geometric properties of tissue to predict cortical surface potentials. Neither of these methods require assumptions about sources; thus they can be used in conjunction with general pattern recognition methods.

Spatial-Temporal Information in EEG and Evoked Potentials

Studies of spatial-temporal properties of spontaneous EEG and evoked potentials have ranged from simple intuitive approaches to the subtle use of statistical methods. For example, early temporal studies were concerned with the near sinusoidal character of alpha rhythm which tends to be blocked by eye opening and often by mental calculations. The earliest spatial studies were concerned only with amplitude distribution of potential, for which statistically stationary signals can be estimated with a single EEG channel. For example, shortly after the first recording of human scalp potentials, a simple but critical experiment was devised involving patients with surgical holes in their skulls (Adrian & Mathews, 1934). Although alpha rhythm was first suspected to originate from eye muscles, this study showed its place of origin to be inside the cranium and mostly from posterior regions.

As the field of EEG progressed, hemispheric asymmetry of amplitude of raw EEG data came to be recognized as an important indicator of pathology, as in the case of cortical tumors. This approach was later refined with the use of temporal spectral analysis so that power in specific frequency bands might be compared between surface locations (Bickford, 1973). The routine use of multichannel recordings and automated computer analysis has made practical the plotting of instantaneous isopotential contours (Lehmann, 1972). Amplitude distributions of surface potential were combined with estimated volume conductive properties of the head to locate equivalent dipole sources (Kavanagh et al., 1978).

The above mentioned straightforward and intuitively appealing approaches are very effective in revealing large differences in spa-

Dept. of Biomedical Engineering, Tulane University, New Orleans, LA 70118, USA.

tial-temporal properties and are natural choices for any EEG research laboratory. However, it was long suspected that multichannel EEG records contain vast amounts of important but subtle information not revealed by the more obvious approaches listed above. Thus, more abstract statistical methods, some based on postulates about the underlying physiological mechanisms and/or borrowed from various branches of the physical sciences were suggested (reviews by John, 1977; Nunez, 1981a; Gevins 1984). Many of these methods are based on calculation of a covariance matrix, the elements of which contain cross channel correlation information. The covariance matrix yields estimates of coherency (correlation coefficient expressed as a function of frequency for spontaneous EEG), correlation function coefficient (expressed as a function of time lag for evoked potentials), wavenumber spectra (to estimate the direction of traveling waves), empirical orthogonal functions (the spatial factors of factor analysis), and, of course, the usual amplitude distribution of potential. These or other variables can, in turn, be incorporated into various spatial-temporal pattern recognition methods designed to distinguish subtle differences between physiological or clinical states (reviews by McGillen et al., 1981; Gevins, 1980, 1984). The problem of which variables (or "features") to chose and how they should be weighted in the pattern recognition algorithm is a formidable one. The criteria for such choices may involve the use of expert opinion, various statistical criteria based on some (often unstated) assumptions about the properties of signal and noise, or "classifier-directed methods," in which feedback from hypothesis testing is used in feature selection methods (Gevins & Morgan, 1986).

One might guess that future pattern recognition methods may be more closely linked to underlying physiological mechanisms, thereby making the study of EEG far more quantified as in examples from the physical sciences provided by the fields of radar signal detection or seismology. With this goal in mind, it is of interest to view a multichannel EEG record $\overline{V}$ ($\vec{r}$, t) as the sample function from an ensemble of statistically similar functions which form a stochastic process. Of course, surface poten-

tial is, in one sense, not random, but deterministic in the sense of being a solution to the "forward problem" in EEG, that is, surface potential occurs as a solution to Poisson's equation (Nunez, 1981a),

$$\nabla \cdot \overline{\sigma}(\vec{r}, t) \nabla \overline{V}(\vec{r}, t) = \overline{s}(\vec{r}, t), \qquad (1)$$

where $\overline{\sigma}(\vec{r}, t)$ and $\overline{s}(\vec{r}, t)$ are electrical conductivity and current source functions, respectively. The bars indicate macroscopic functions, that is, functions which are space averaged over more microscopic functions as in the example,

$$\overline{V}(\vec{r}, t) = \frac{1}{L^3} \int_{\text{vol}} V(\vec{r}, t) d^3 r. \qquad (2)$$

Here the integral of the more microscopic field $V(\vec{r}, t)$ is over a volume of characteristic size L, which must be consistent for all functions and operators in Poisson's equation. Data are recorded from inside the cranium at various hierarchical levels. That is, recorded potentials are space averaged over volumes having linear scales at least as large as the diameter of the electrode tip, which typically varies from 10^{-3} to 10^{-2} cm for "micro-EEG" recordings (Petsche et al., 1984). Such experiments are, of course, one step up in the hierarchy from studies of transmembrane potentials with microelectrodes of tip diameter 10^{-4} cm. Scalp potentials involve space averages over "micro-EEG" potentials with added complication due to the imposition of the poorly conducting skull. The relationship between the statistical properties of the macroscopic sources $\overline{s}(\vec{r}, t)$ and macroscopic surface potential $\overline{V}(\vec{r}, t)$ is by no means a simple one, but can be estimated by means of Poisson's equation (Katznelson, 1982).

The microscopic source function $s(\vec{r}, t)$ may itself be considered as a solution to some general set of nonlinear equations of the form

$$G[s(\vec{r}, t), V(\vec{r}, t)] = 0, \qquad (3)$$

where the symbol G denotes a general operator, most probably a set of integrodifferential equations. Such equations may be expressed at several levels of neural hierarchy ranging from the single neuron (Hodgkin & Huxley,

1952) to minicolumns or mesocolumns (Wilson & Cowan, 1973; Lopes da Silva et al., 1974; Freeman, 1975; van Rotterdam et al., 1982; Zhadin, 1984) to macrocolumns (Nunez, 1974 a, b, 1981 a, b, c, 1988 a, b; Katznelson, 1982). General methods to derive the "rules" of neural interactions at one hierarchical level from rules at other levels have been studied using modern methods of nonlinear, nonequilibrium statistical mechanics (Ingber, 1982). It should be emphasized that nonlinearity of Eq. (3) at one hierarchical level does not preclude linearity at higher levels (Nunez, 1981 a, 1988 b; Wright & Kydd, 1984). Also, Eq. (3) allows for the fact that extracellular fields may act explicitly to modify neural firing rates, although this mechanism is not well understood. A major challenge of electrophysiology is to derive reasonably realistic approximations to Eq. (3), hopefully containing only physiologic parameters (no free parameters, i.e., parameters that cannot be measured). Changes in physiologic or clinical state would then be reflected by changes in parameters as determined by experimental data, an approach already underway for potentials recorded in the olfactory bulb (Freeman & Skarda, 1985; Baird, 1986; Freeman, 1987) and to a limited extent for human scalp potentials (Nunez, 1988 b).

General Classification of Current Sources

Regardless of the specific form of Eq. (3) which determines the current source function s(r,t), most scalp potentials are believed due to neocortical current sources which form dipole layers of various sizes (Nunez, 1981 a, b, c, 1988 c). The origins of the time dependencies of EEG phenomena have been linked to post synaptic potentials (PSP), rise/decay times with local theories of minicolumn or mesocolumn (between mini and macro) interaction or to delays in corticocortical fibers with a global theory of neocortical dynamics. More recently, local and global theories have been combined to show that both intracortical and corticocortical delays may contribute to EEG (Nunez, 1988 b). For example, the two pictures of alpha rhythm as composed of either

(1) epicenters of activity from which short waves propagate along the cortical surface with velocities in the tens of cm/s range (Lopes da Silva et al., 1974; van Rotterdam et al., 1982; Ingber, 1985) or (2) long waves (both traveling and standing) with propagation velocities in the 5—10 m/s range (Nunez, 1974 a, b, 1981 a, b, c, 1988 a, b) are not mutually exclusive. Both kinds of phenomena can occur simultaneously with oscillations in the same frequency range. The physiologist with his small cortical electrode will tend to observe only the short wavelength potentials, while only relatively long wavelength activity is observed on the scalp, as discussed further in the next section. Evoked potential wave forms may also be dependent on both local and global effects.

Whatever the underlying mechanisms involved in the generation of spontaneous EEG and evoked potential phenomena, it is suggested here that the corresponding current sources be categorized as follows for the purpose of helping in the development of experimental paradigms.

Type I: Localized and Stationary

The sources are sufficiently localized so that the scalp potential distribution approximates that of a single dipole. Sources in the cortex must be confined to less than approximately 1 cm² of cortical surface. Deeper sources can perhaps occupy somewhat larger regions and still produce dipole-like scalp potentials. Furthermore, the dipole does not change location with the passage of time, that is, it remains fixed from stimulus to stimulus in evoked potential studies. The somatosensory evoked potential over some (perhaps narrow) latency range is perhaps an example of a Type I source.

Type II: Localized and Nonstationary

At any fixed instant in time, the scalp potential distribution is close to that of a single dipole; however the location of the dipole changes with time. Epileptic activity with multiple foci might roughly fit this definition, depending on how many foci were simultaneously active.

Type III: Distributed and Stationary

The current sources are distributed over a relatively large area of neocortex so that a dipole approximation is not possible; however, a characteristic spatial pattern of potential amplitude (or perhaps coherence) is observed to be relatively constant in time. This picture possibly matches time averaged properties of alpha and sleep rhythms (so that the test of stationarity is applied to much longer time scales); however it would not be consistent with instantaneous spontaneous EEG which displays considerable variation on a short time scale (Remond et al, 1969, Lehmann, 1972; Nunez, 1981 a, c).

Type IV: Distributed and Nonstationary

Most EEG and evoked potential phenomena are suspected to fall into this category. Certainly, *all* the models of EEG phenomena cited in the previous sections generally predict this kind of behavior. One approach to the study of spatial properties is then to study cases of Type IV sources which may, in some limiting cases, be approximated as Types I, II or III.

Some methods of spatial analysis are dependent on assumptions about the nature of the sources and some are not. Clearly, all methods based on averaging of amplitudes in evoked potential or MEG studies presuppose stationary sources (of Type I or III). If nonstationary sources are also active, it may be expected that their potentials will be averaged out, perhaps leading to highly oversimplified conclusions about brain function.

Methods to Improve Spatial Resolution

Limitations of Spatial Resolution

Whereas source localization methods presuppose source Types I or II, methods to improve spatial resolution are much more general since they can apply to all kinds of sources. The goal of improved spatial resolution is simply that of making the potential recorded from a single or small group of closely spaced electrods more closely represent the activity of the underlying sources, independent of the effects of volume conduction or reference electrode location. Studies of volume conduction, that is Poisson's Eq. (1), can provide information on the limitations of spatial information as well as suggest methods to improve resolution. For example, it has been shown that large cortical dipole layers (several tens of cm² or more) produce scalp potentials which are attenuated by factors of roughly two to four between cortex and scalp, a theoretical prediction that matches much of the available spontaneous EEG data. By contrast, small dipole layers have scalp attenuation factors of perhaps 100 or more (Nunez, 1981 a, 1988 c).

This "smearing" effect due to both the low conductivity of the skull and the separation between sources and recording electrode may also be expressed in terms of the spatial-temporal Fourier transform of the magnitude of cortical surface potential $V(\vec{k}, \omega)$. Here ω is the angular frequency, $\vec{k}$ is the two dimensional wavenumber, or spatial frequency, vector parallel to the cortical surface, and $V(\vec{r}, t)$ is space averaged over the depth of cortex. The effect of skull and spatial separation is to selectively attenuate large wavenumber (short wavelength) activity. The three-concentric sphere model of the head has shown that cortical surface potentials of wavenumber k are attenuated by approximately 90% for k > 1.5 cm^{-1} or 0.25 cycle/cm (Nunez, 1981 a). The two samples/cycle rule in the spatial domain then indicates that most of the available information in cortical potentials is obtained with an average electrode spacing of roughly 2 cm in a multichannel EEG recording, corresponding to several hundred electrodes required to cover the human scalp, a theoretical prediction in apparent agreement with experiments (Gevins et al., 1985). However, attenuation does not fall all that rapidly for larger wavenumbers, leaving open the possibility that future EEG studies may involve the use of hundreds or even a few thousand recording channels.

Three methods have been proposed to improve spatial resolution of brain signals: the radial current estimate (or "current source density" or "Laplacian"), spatial deconvolution, and measurement of the radial component of the brain's magnetic field (MEG). Each approach is under active development. A short overview of the strengths and shortcomings of each method follows.

Radial Current Estimate

The most straightforward and easiest to interpret of these methods is the radial current estimate. Both conventional reference and bipolar recordings of EEG provide a measure of tangential current flow in the scalp, a variable which is often only weakly related to the underlying source activity due to reference and volume conduction effects (Nunez, 1981 a, 1988 c). The radial current estimate, based on a combination of Ohm's law and current conservation, is obtained by an appropriate linear combination of potentials to provide a local estimate of the radial current flow through the skull into the scalp (Hjorth, 1975; Nunez, 1981 a). Radial current estimates have been obtained for alpha, sleep and evoked potentials using linear combinations of four (MacKay, 1984), five (Hjorth, 1975, Nunez, 1981 a) or more (Doyle & Gevins, unpublished) surface potentials, the latter approach being applicable to arbitrary placement of the electrodes. All other things being equal, large local radial skull currents should indicate the presence of local sources. Unfortunately, all other things are not equal. Skull thickness varies by a factor of about three over the surface (Todd, 1924) and skull conductivity variations are unknown (Nunez, 1981 a, 1988 d). Since radial skull current is directly proportional to the product of local thickness and local conductivity (the local resistance per unit area of the skull), radial current is only partly related to local sources. However, cross channel correlation measures (correlation function coefficient as a function of time lag in the case of evoked potentials and coherency estimates as a function of frequency for spontaneous EEG) are normalized so as to be amplitude independent. The radial current estimate appears to provide significant improvement in such measures of correlation function coefficient (Gevins et al., 1985) and interhemispheric coherency (Nunez, unpublished). Further improvement in the applica-

tion of the radial current estimate is dependent on a more accurate volume conductor model of the living human head.

Spatial Deconvolution

Spatial deconvolution combines information about the estimated volume conductive properties of the head with multichannel surface potential data to obtain estimates of either cortical source activity or cortical surface potential. Spatial deconvolution methods based on a planar, homogeneous model of the head were proposed in EEG (Nicholas & DeLoche, 1976) and applied to potentials recorded on the surface of a cat olfactory bulb (Freeman, 1980; review by Katznelson, 1981). More recently, the methods have been modified by use of the three-concentric sphere model of the head (Doyle & Gevins, unpublished, Nunez, 1986 a) and applied to EEG and evoked potential data (Gevins et al., 1985). It is well known from EEG research that there is no unique source distribution for any given surface potential distribution. However, it is less widely appreciated that a unique relationship does exist between scalp potential (assumed to be known over the entire outer surface) and cortical surface potential, provided only that there are no sources between the surfaces. Spatial deconvolution, in its most general formulation, is based on this principle. One version of spatial deconvolution is based on the additional assumption that EEG activity is due to a large number of radially oriented dipoles at fixed depth in the cortex and the three concentric sphere model of the head (Nunez, 1986 a). The theoretical potential difference between two locations on the surface of the three sphere model due to N radial dipole sources in the inner sphere (cortex) is given by (Rush & Driscoll, 1969, Nunez, 1981 a),

$$\overline{V}_k(t_i) = \sum_{n=1}^{N} H_{kn} s_n(t_i) \quad \begin{array}{l} k = 1, K \\ i = 1, I. \end{array} \quad (4)$$

Here, $\overline{V}(t_i)$ is the macroscopic scalp potential at time t_i at the k th surface location, measured with respect to a reference location. $s_n(t_i)$ is the current flowing between poles of the nth dipole source at time t_i. I is the total number of times to be sampled in the digitation of evoked potential waveforms, and K is the number of surface locations at which evoked potentials are recorded. The coefficients H_{kn} in the above sum are themselves given by a sum over Legendre polynomials P_m,

$$H_{kn} = \sum_{m=1}^{\infty} A_m [P_m(\cos\theta_{kn}) - P_m(\cos\theta_{rn})], \quad (5)$$

where θ_{kn} and θ_{rn} are the angular separations between the nth source and electrode k or reference electrode r, respectively. The coefficients A_m depend on the electric and geometric properties of the head and are given for the case of a radial dipole in (Nunez, 1981a).

If one source were located under each electrode, the number of sources (N) would equal the number of electrodes (K) and the system of algebraic equations (4) would have a unique solution for each time t_i. That is, given the measured evoked potentials $\overline{V}_k(t_i)$, the underlying source currents $s_n(t_i)$ could be found in terms of the $\overline{V}_k(t_i)$ and the physical properties of the head, which along with the electrode locations determine the coefficients H_{kn}. Since, in practice, it is expected that N $\gg$ K, an approximation is introduced in order to obtain an estimate of source activity valid when the average spacing between electrodes is sufficiently small. The source functions $s_n(t_i)$ are then replaced by their space averages values $\overline{s}_n(t_i)$ (averaged over the cortical surface surrounding each electrode), so that Eq. (4) is replaced by,

$$\overline{V}_k(t_i) = \sum_{l=1}^{K} H_{kl} \overline{s}_l(t_i) \quad \begin{array}{l} k = 1, K \\ i = 1, I \end{array} \quad (6)$$

with solution obtained from the matrix H (formed by the elements H_{kl}),

$$\overline{s}_l(t_i) = \sum_{k=1}^{K} h_{kl} \overline{V}_k(t_i) \quad \begin{array}{l} l = 1, K \\ i = 1, I, \end{array} \quad (7)$$

where the h_{kl} are the elements of the matrix H^{-1}. Thus, given the geometric and electric properties of the head, the coefficients H_{kl} can be calculated from Eq. (5). The H matrix is inverted to obtain the coefficients h_{kl}, and the space averaged source functions $\overline{s}_l(t_i)$ are then calculated from the evoked potentials, $\overline{V}_k(t_i)$.

While several computer simulations and studies of evoked potentials support the use of spatial deconvolution, the critical question of the sensitivity of the method to uncertainty in the volume conductor model of the head (especially local variations in skull thickness and conductivity) remains largely unanswered. This issue is currently under active study by the author and others. For example, the replacement of the three-concentric sphere model of the head with a finite element model, together with laboratory experiments involving known sources in skull-tank models and use of methods to estimate local skull resistance per unit area (the product of thickness and resistivity) in living subjects has been proposed (Nunez, 1988d).

Magnetic Field Measurements

Like the EEG the brain's magnetic field (MEG) is generated by current sources within the brain. MEG recordings may, however, avoid some of the volume conduction problems which hinder the interpretation of EEG (review by Williamson & Kaufman, 1987). The primary advantage of MEG is due to the skull's transparency to magnetic fields; the principal distortion of brain signals which occurs in EEG thus does not occur with MEG. Other volume conduction as well as sensor geometry effects do, however, cause MEG interpretation problems, especially for sources of Types II–IV (Nunez, 1968b).

At the time of this writing, nearly all of the published data in MEG have been obtained with single channel systems. The most common procedure is to map the average magnitude of the radial component of the magnetic field by successive movement of the sensor over the surface. The resulting map can yield estimates of the tangential location and depth of an equivalent dipole source. Such methods have been limited to a subclass of Type I sources which are not only stationary from trial to trial (stimulus stationary) but also stationary over the time (several hours) required to move the sensor over the surface. If other kinds of sources occur (as they most certainly do) their effects will not be observed due to the limitations of this procedure.

The recent introduction of multichannel sensors allows for estimation of cross correlation as well as amplitude measure of MEG.

This approach should allow for quantitative measures of map variance (Nunez, 1981 a, c) and other measures of brain dynamic function previously reserved to EEG; however in the short term at least, MEG will continue to suffer the serious disadvantage inherent in a system limited to a relatively small number of channels. Of course, EEG and MEG may be used in combination to further illuminate brain dynamic function. In such studies the role of MEG may be to "fine tune" the conclusions of EEG studies.

References

Adrian ED, Mathews BHC (1934) The Berger rhythm: Potential changes from the occipital lobes in man. *Brain, 57,* 355–385.

Baird B (1986) Nonlinear dynamics of pattern formation and pattern recognition in the rabbit olfactory bulb. *Physica 22 D,* 150–175.

Bickford RG (1973) *Clinical electroencephalography,* Medcom, New York.

Freeman WJ (1975) *Mass action in the nervous system.* Academic Press, New York.

Freeman WJ (1980) Use of spatial deconvolution to compensate for distortion of EEG by volume conduction. *IEEE Trans Biomed Eng, 27,* 421–429.

Freeman WJ (1987) Simulation of chaotic EEG patterns with a dynamic model of the olfactory system. *Biol Cybern, 55,* 139–150.

Freeman WJ, Skarda CA (1985) Spatial patterns, nonlinear dynamics, and perception: The Neo-Sherringtonian view. *Brain Res Reviews, 10,* 147–175.

Gevins AS (1980) Pattern recognition of human brain electrical potentials. *IEEE Trans Pattern Anal Machine Intell, 2,* 383–404.

Gevins AS (1984) Analysis of the electromagnetic signals of the human brain: Milestones, obstacles and goals. *IEEE Trans Biomed Eng, 31,* 833–850.

Gevins AS, Morgan NH (1986) Classifier-directed signal processing in brain research. *IEEE Trans Biomed Eng, 33,* 1054–1068.

Gevins AS, Doyle J, Cutillo BM, Schaffer R, Tannehill, RS, Bressler SL (1985) Neurocognitive pattern analysis of visuospatial task: Rapidly shifting foci of evoked correlations between electrodes. *Psychophysiology, 22,* 32–43.

Hjorth B (1975) An on-line transformation of EEG scalp potentials into orthogonal source derivations. *Electroenceph clin Neurophysiol, 39,* 526–530.

Hodgkin AL, Huxley AF (1952) A quantitative description of membrane current and its application to conductance and excitation in nerve. *J Physiol, 117,* 500–544.

Ingber L (1982) Statistical mechanics of neocortical interactions. Basic formulation. *Physica, 5D,* 83–107.

Ingber L (1985) Statistical mechanics of neocortical interactions. EEG dispersion relations. *IEEE Trans Biomed Eng, 32,* 91–94.

John ER (1977) *Functional neuroscience, Vol 2.* Wiley, New York.

Katznelson RD (1981) EEG recording, electrode placement, and aspects of generator localization. In Nunez PL (Ed.), *Electric fields of the brain: The neurophysics of EEG.* Oxford University Press, New York, 176–213.

Katznelson RD (1982) Deterministic and stochastic field theoretic models in the neurophysics of EEG. Thesis University of California San Diego.

Kavanagh RN, Darcy TM, Lehmann D, Fender DH. (1978) Evaluation of methods for three-dimensional localization of electrical sources in the human brain, *IEEE Trans Biomed Eng, 25,* 421–429.

Lehmann D (1972) Human scalp EEG fields: Evoked, alpha, sleep, and spike-wave patterns. In Petsche H, Brazier MAB (Eds.) *Synchronization of EEG activity in epilepsies.* Springer, New York, 301–325.

Lopes da Silva FH, Hoeks H, Smits H, Zetterberg LH (1974) Model of brain rhythmic activity. *Kybernetik, 15,* 27–37.

McGillem CD, Aunon JI, Childers D (1981) Signal processing in evoked potential research: Applications of filtering and pattern recognition. *CRC Crit Rev Bioeng, 6,* 225–265.

McKay DM (1984) Source density analysis of scalp potentials during evaluated action. I. Coronal distribution. *Exp Brain Res, 54,* 73–85.

Nicholas P, DeLoche G (1976) Convolution computer processing of brain electrical image transmission. *Inter J Biomed Comp, 7,* 143–159.

Nunez PL (1974a) The brain wave equation: A model for the EEG. *Math Biosciences, 21,* 279–297.

Nunez PL (1974b) Wave-like properties of the alpha rhythm. *IEEE Trans Biomed Eng, 21,* 473–482.

Nunez PL (1981a) *Electric fields of the brain: The neurophysics of EEG.* Oxford University Press, New York.

Nunez PL (1981b) A study of origins of the time dependencies of scalp EEG: I. Theoretical basis. *IEEE Trans Biomed Eng, 28,* 271–280.

Nunez PL (1981c) A study of the origins of the time dependencies of scalp EEG: II. Experimental support of theory. *IEEE Trans Biomed Eng, 28,* 281–288.

Nunez PL (1986a) *Removal of reference electrode and volume conduction effects form evoked potentials. I. Derivation of method and computer simulation.* Technical Note, Navy Personnel Research and Development Center, San Diego, LTN 71—85—13.

Nunez PL (1986b) The brain's magnetic field: Some effects of multiple sources on localization methods, *Electroencephal clin Neurophysiol, 63,* 75—82.

Nunez PL (1988a) Global contributions to cortical dynamics: theoretical and experimental evidence for standing wave phenomena. In Basar E (Ed.) *Dynamics of sensory and cognitive processing of the brain.* Springer-Verlag, Berlin, 172—182.

Nunez PL (1988b, in press) *Neocortical dynamics: Physiological bases for human electroencephalographic rhythms.* Oxford University Press, New York.

Nunez PL (1988c, in press) *Physical principals and neurophysiological mechanisms underlying event related potentials.* EPIC VIII Proc., Oxford University Press.

Nunez PL (1988d) A method to estimate local skull resistance in living subjects. *IEEE Trans Biomed Eng, 34,* 902-904.

Petsche H, Pockberger H, Rappelsberger P (1984) On the search for the sources of the electroencephalogram. *Neuroscience, 11,* 1—27.

Remond A, Leseure N, Joseph JP, Rieger H, Lairy GC (1969) The alpha average. I Methodology and description. *Electroenceph clin Neurophysiol, 26,* 245—265.

Rush S, Driscoll DA (1969) EEG electrode sensitivity: An application of reciprocity. *IEEE Trans Biomed Eng, 16,* 15—22.

Todd TW (1924) Thickness of the male white cranium. *Anatomical Record, 27,* 245—256.

van Rotterdam A, Lopes da Silva FH, Ende van der J, Viergever MA, Hermans AJ (1982) A model of the spatial-temporal characteristics of the alpha rhythm. *Bull Math Biology, 44,* 283—305.

Williamson SJ, Kaufmann L (1987) Analysis of neuromagnetic signals. In Gevins AS, Remond A (Eds.) *Methods of analysis of brain electrical and magnetic signals.* (Handbook of Electroencephalography and Clinical Neurophysiology, Vol. 1). Elsevier, Amsterdam, 405—448.

Wilson HR, Cowan JD (1973) A mathematical theory of the functional dynamics of cortical and thalamic nervous tissue. *Kybernetik, 13,* 55—80.

Wright JJ, Kydd RR (1984) A linear theory for global electrocortical activity and its control by the lateral hypothalamus. *Biol Cybern, 50,* 75—82.

Zhadin MN (1984) Rhythmic processes in the cerebral cortex. *J Theor Biol, 108,* 565—595.

Recent Developments in Neuromagnetism: Implications for Imaging

L. Kaufman and S. J. Williamson

This paper reviews some of the most recent developments in Neuromagnetism at New York University (NYU). It focuses on three general areas—advances in instrumentation, recent developments in analytical methods and, finally, the application of neuromagnetic methods to the study of higher order cognitive processes. These themes are representative of the central lines of research now being advanced by the several dozen neuromagnetism groups throughout the world and are basic to the development of a new kind of imagery—spatio-temporal images of brain function. Earlier reviews of neuromagnetism, such as those of Williamson and Kaufman (1981, 1987), Kaufman and Williamson (1982, 1986), Romani and Narizil (1986), and Hari and Ilmoniemi (1986), as well as a textbook (Williamson et al., 1983), treat many of the topics discussed here in greater depth.

Instrumentation

Some Basic Concepts

An instrument incorporating a single superconducting sensor was employed in a magnetically shielded environment to detect the first magnetoencephalogram (MEG) (Cohen, 1972). Since a single sensor was employed, it was capable of detecting the field at only one position outside the head. Since the neuromagnetic field of the brain is many orders of magnitude weaker than the field of the earth and that of other objects and devices in an urban environment, enormous sensitivity was required to detect it. This was provided by a cryogenic device known as the SQUID (Superconducting QUantum Interference Device). The SQUID is isolated from its environment by enclosing it inside a superconducting shield, and it senses the field of interest indirectly. The field it senses is that associated with the flow of current in the "input coil" which is wound in series with another coil, the so-called "detection coil"; these are depicted schematically in Figure 1. These coils are composed of a superconducting material. Current flows in the detection and input coils in response to an applied magnetic field applied at the detection coil, so that the amount of flux trapped in the coil remains constant—a phenomenon known as the Meisner effect. Since this shielding current also flows in the input coil, it is sensed by the SQUID to which the input coil is magnetically coupled. The detection coil and SQUID are kept at superconducting temperatures by bathing them in liquid helium (4.2 °K). The helium and the superconducting electronics are contained in a vacuum-insulated container called a "dewar."

The first advance made in our laboratory allowed us to measure the brain's magnetic field in a normal unshielded laboratory environment. This was accomplished by using a

Neuromagnetism Laboratory, Departments of Psychology and Physics, New York University, USA.
We thank Dr. Risto J. Ilmoniemi for stimulating discussions and comments on portions of the manuscript. The Neuromagnetism Laboratory is supported in part by Air Force Office of Scientific Research Grant F49620-85-K-004.

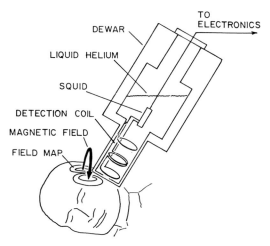

Figure 1. Schematic showing a SQUID enclosed within a superconducting chamber inside a cryogenic dewar. The coil near the SQUID is the "input coil," and it is wound in series with the detection coil which, in this case, is wound in the configuration of a second order gradiometer. The bottommost loop of the detection coil (the "pickup coil") is nearest the source of the neuromagnetic field, which links the detection coil. If the source is father away than the distance separating the pickup coil and its nearest neighbor (which is wound in the opposite direction) then it will have equal and opposed effects on both loops, resulting in no net current flow in the gradiometer. Furthermore, a field having a uniform spatial gradient will also have no effect on this gradiometer because of the presence of the upper two loops. However, sources close-by as compared to the distance separating the two bottommost loops will produce fields having high spatial derivatives, and the differential effects of these fields on the loops of the gradiometer results in a net current flow that affects the SQUID. The SQUID electronics produce a voltage output that is proportional to the field linking the detection coil.

detection coil having the geometry of a second-order gradiometer, which is also illustrated in Figure 1. This type of detection coil discriminates against distant noise sources because they produce spatially uniform fields, to which the gradiometer is insensitive. To improve the rejection of such fields, small superconducting tabs placed near the coil were adjusted by rods extending through the top of the dewar so that, in effect, the areas outlined by the individual turns of wire in the coil

could be matched. This adjustment is called "field balancing." Our first such instrument (Brenner et al., 1975) employed an rf-SQUID which permitted us to detect fields that were as weak as one billionth the strength of the earth's steady field. Ultimately the rf-SQUID was replaced by an even more sensitive dc-SQUID, so that the limiting factor at low frequencies was no longer SQUID sensitivity but the residual ambient magnetic noise.

The Need for Multi-Channel Instruments

At one time it was widely believed that the next most important advance in neuromagnetic instrumentation would be the introduction of refrigerators capable of keeping superconducting instruments at liquid helium temperatures by appropriate use of helium gas (Cohen, 1983). This would obviate the need for large dewars filled with liquid helium, which require refilling on a regular basis. However, without denying the advantages of refrigerators (in fact we are currently involved in a successful effort to develop one), it was our view the the single most important "next step" in instrumentation would be the introduction of multi-channel instruments to measure the field simultaneously at a number of positions. The higher priority given to multi-channel instruments stemmed from our learning that it is possible to determine the location of active groups of neurons in the brain by mapping the way in which the extracranial magnetic field varies in amplitude as a function of position over the scalp (Brenner et al., 1978). This would make it possible to create a new kind of image, a "neuromagnetic image," for which we propose the acronym NMI. This is a functional image, to contrast it with the structural images provided by CT scan and by magnetic resonance imaging. As we shall emphasize here, the generation of the NMI requires the use of multi-channel instruments, so we set out to develop a prototype device to determine its feasibility. Toward this end, we collaborated with Biomagnetic Technologies Inc. (BTi) of San Diego, California, in developing a five-channel instrument (Williamson et al., 1985). We were not alone in taking this approach, as colleagues at the Low Temperature Laboratory of the Helsinki University of

Technology anticipated us by constructing and installing a four-channel SQUID magnetometer for use in a magnetically shielded environment (Ilmoniemi et al., 1984), and our colleagues in Rome (Romani & Leoni, 1985) were working along similar lines.

As already intimated, the reason for developing multi-channel magnetometers is that they make it possible to conveniently and economically determine the location of the source of the field inside the head. Thus, for example, an equivalent current dipole source of the observed field can be determined by mapping the radial component of the field across the surface of the head. The measurements of the field at many different positions allow one to generate a contour map representing isofield contours. An example of such a contour plot is shown in Figure 2. This figure is based upon data obtained in an experiment in which the subject was presented with auditory stimuli consisting of clicks repeated at a rate of 32 Hz, and the steady state response at this frequency was measured (Romani et al., 1982a). It will

be noted that the pattern is dipolar, i.e., displaying two field extrema of opposite polarity.

Although responses of this type from the primary sensory areas tend to be quite stable over time for any given subject, one cannot be sure of the stability of responses that are more readily affected by levels of arousal or by shifts in the deployment of attention. To study these "event-related fields" it is necessary to avoid the assumption of stationarity. The only simple way in which to do this is to measure the field at several places outside the head at the same time. Replications of measurements at or near some of these places while measuring the field at more distant places enable one to determine if the source of the observed field is indeed the same from one trial to the next. This is particularly important when studying cogntive processes like attention, since the state of attention may fluctuate from one time to another.

Experimental economy is another reason justifying multi-channel instruments. The creation of several contour maps which show field distributions over the head when different stimuli are used can require many long hours of experimentation. If the field could be measured at only one place at a time, the dewar and perhaps the head of the subject would have to be repositioned from one trial to the next. Moreover, it is vital to know the spatial position at which the field is measured with a high degree of precision. Otherwise it would be impossible to make accurate contour maps for the purpose of identifying the position and orientation of the source within the head. We will not discuss the latter problem here except to say that new methods have already been developed for the automatic recording of the head's position and orientation relative to the detection coils within the dewar, and these new methods are currently being tested. However, we shall discuss the development of multiple channel instruments and their use at NYU.

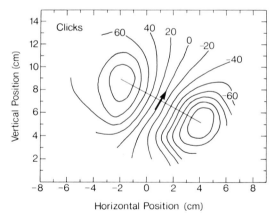

Figure 2. Constant field contours across the right hemisphere for the neuromagnetic response to auditory clicks presented at 32 Hz. Values indicate the strength of the field perpendicular to the scalp in femtotesla, with positive values for outward direction. The orientation of the underlying equivalent current dipole source is indicated by the arrow, whose center indicates the dipole's lateral position. The origin of the coordinate system is the ear canal, with the horizontal axis directed toward the corner of the eye (at position +9) and vertical position measured perpendicular to this axis.

Five- and Seven-Channel Systems

Figure 3 shows the dewar containing the 5-sensor probe together with the SCANNER device used to hold it. Figure 4 is a schematic of the cryogenic instruments contained within

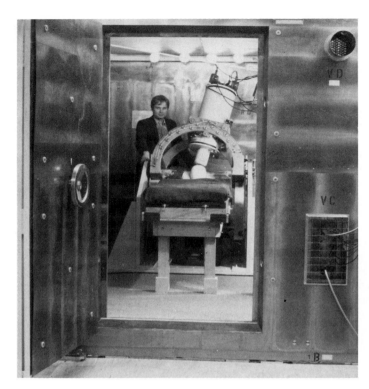

Figure 3. Cylindrical dewar containing a 5-sensor probe at the Neuromagnetism Laboratory of the Departments of Physics and Psychology at NYU. The dewar is supported by a fiberglass carriage that is moved by a scanning device (SCANNER) from one position to another across the head for accurate placement.

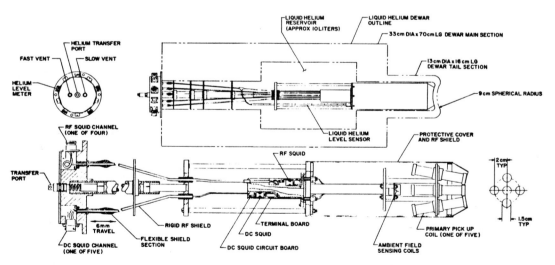

Figure 4. Diagram of the dewar (upper right) and 5-sensor probe (bottom) for neuromagnetic studies, shown on their sides. The cross section for the top mounting flange of the probe is at the upper left and for the array of detection coils at the lower right. Courtesy of Biomagnetic Technologies Inc.

the dewar. The individual coils of the five second-order gradiometers are 1.5 cm in diameter with the end sets separated from the middle set by 4 cm (the "baseline" of the gradiometer). The bottommost coils ("pick-up coils") of the gradiometers have a center-to-center separation of 2 cm from each other, with the axes of the outer four coils tipped by $10°$ from the dewar axis so that each coil points to a common position 9 cm below the bottom of the dewar. While we relied upon the mechanical positioning of superconducting tabs to obtain field balance in our single-sensor system, as did Romani and Leoni (1985) for a 4-sensor system, we adopted a totally new procedure in this system. Instead we incorporated three rf-SQUID magnetometers for monitoring the field in three orthogonal directions just above the detection coils and a simple first-order gradiometer for monitoring the field gradient along the axis of the dewar. The outputs of these ancillary devices are given empirically determined weights, and then subtracted from the outputs of each of the five signal channels. This "electronic" field balancing yields results comparable to those obtained with the mechanical field balancing for the single-channel instrument. The noise level above about 4 Hz in each channel, after subtracting the weighted outputs of the references, is about 20 femtotesla (fT) per root Hz of bandwidth. However, at lower frequencies the noise amplitude increases at a rate that is slightly faster than the inverse of the frequency. This effect of ambient magnetic noise is pervasive, and it seriously restricts our ability to measure very slowly changing fields. Excess noise at power line frequencies is largely removed by comb filters.

Our experience with this system convinced us that it is indeed possible to place a large number of channels in close proximity to each other within a single dewar, i.e., the "cross talk" between channels was less than 1%. Since we were also thinking in terms of clinical applications, it became increasingly obvious that it will ultimately be necessary to monitor the field over the entire scalp at once. Although many technical problems remain, we consider it feasible to construct a system composed of about 100 channels within a single dewar. This is a long-term development project, so in order to make it possible to conduct studies using a relatively large number of channels, we, together with Dr. Rodolfo Llinas and Dr. Charles Nicholson, collaborated with BTi in the design and installation of two 7-sensor probes that could be used concurrently to provide 14 channels of information for analysis of field patterns. Our goal is to use this twin dewar system (GEMINI) in clinical cases to permit the early evaluation of the promise of neuromagnetic recordings for medicine in areas other than epilepsy. Figure 5 illustrates the arrangement in Bellevue Hospital of the NYU Medical Center, where an overhead gantry supports two carriages from which the dewars of GEMINI are suspended. The detection coils in each probe have the same dimensions and arrangement as for the 5-sensor probe described earlier, except that there are six outer coils instead of four. Control of the SQUID electronics settings, electronic gains, and cut-off frequencies for high- and low-pass filters is by computer.

Another feature of GEMINI is a change in one of the reference detection coils used for electronic balancing. Studies with the 5-sensor probe showed that the residual noise after carrying out field balancing with the field references did not appreciably correlate with the reference signal from the first-order gradiometer. In other words, the detection coils were sufficiently well balanced with respect to a uniform field gradient so that there was no advantage in providing for electronic balancing as well. The residual low-frequency noise from ambient field fluctuations must be due to higher-order gradients of the field. Therefore, in place of a first-order gradiometer the GEMINI probes each have a second-order gradiometer as a reference to supplement the three orthogonal field references. Initial tests indicate that after electronically balancing for field the residual noise in certain situations does indeed correlate with the second-order gradient reference, and by subtracting the latter after proper attenuation the noise level below approximately 2 Hz can be reduced by about a factor of 2.

After extensive tests of the performance of the GEMINI system we found that even with electronic balancing for field and its second-order gradient the low-frequency noise level

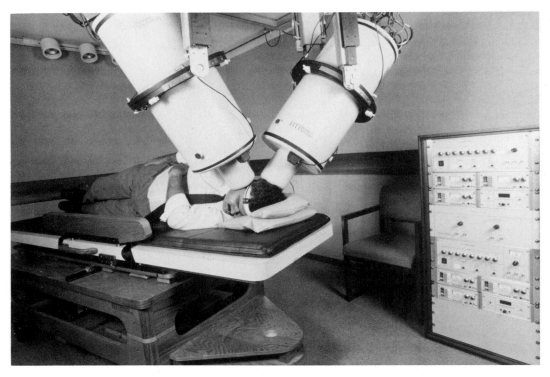

Figure 5. Arrangement of two 7-sensor probes supported by an overhead gantry at the Center for Neuromagnetism of the NYU Medical Center. Courtesy of Biomagnetic Technologies Inc.

may not be acceptable for all state-of-the-art neuromagnetic measurements. In particular, it is not possible to study slowly varying phenomena related to cognitive processes because of the high level of residual low-frequency noise, even after optimum system balancing. Such phenomena can best be studied in a magnetically shielded environment.

Magnetic Shielding

SQUID systems using a second-order gradiometer for the detection coil are capable of a wide range of useful measurements in an unshielded setting, including laboratories and clinics. However, ambient noise increases dramatically at low frequencies in noisy locations, and there may be additional noise at discrete frequencies from nearby machinery. High levels of radio frequency noise may also interfere with the operation of the SQUID. A room constructed with magnetic and radio-frequency shielding is one effective way to

minimize these problems. The first rooms built for biomagnetic applications had four or more widely-spaced, concentric shells of high-permeability material (e.g., Mager, 1982) and are very effective. However, this requires a large room for installation, and the space inside is small, having a characteristic dimension of 2 m. Newer magnetically shielded rooms (MSRs) have fewer shells, provide more working space, and yield acceptable shielding for most purposes (Kelhä et al., 1982; Buchanan et al., 1987). Figure 5 shows the GEMINI system installed in such a room.

The two MSRs at NYU were prefabricated by Vacuumschmeltze GmbH of West Germany The interior of the room has floor dimensions of 3 m × 4 m and a height of 2.4 m. As such it is comparable to, or exceeds in size, conventional rf-shielded rooms and Faraday shields commonly used in EEG research.

The MSR consists of an inner shield of mumetal mounted on 8-mm thick aluminum plate that serves as an eddy-current magnetic and radio-frequency shield. It has a conventional stretch-wall covering over interior and exterior for protection and attractive appearance. The inner wall montage is supported on the outside by a stiff aluminum framework of 15 cm thickness, and the outer surface of the framework is covered by a second mu-metal shield and stretch-wall partitions. A single door, balanced on heavy-duty ball bearings, provides magnetic continuity for the two layers of magnetic shielding. The door is secured by a wheel-type of locking mechanism that can be opened from either the inside or outside.

The strength of the MSR frame is sufficient to support a 300 kg weight attached to the center of the ceiling which causes a sag of less than 0.3 mm. This makes it possible for the ceiling to support a pair of aluminum rails used to suspend a gantry for supporting the 5-sensor system. Furthermore, the stiff framework in the wall will support the gantries for a pair of CryoSQUID sensors, which are based on a refrigerator that continually recycles helium to maintain the SQUIDs at the temperature of liquid helium (Buchanan et al., 1987). These sensors are about to be delivered to NYU. With this arrangement a total of 7 sensors can be positioned independently over three different areas of the subject's head.

MSR Performance

After a 60-Hz shaking field is applied, the steady earth's field is attenuated by a factor of 1000. Shielding is less effective for very low-frequency fields as is usual with such materials, being only about 30 dB. The effect of eddy-current shielding becomes apparent above about 1 Hz, and the attenuation rises to a value of about 10,000 at 100 Hz with a tendency toward saturation at higher frequencies. The shielding is not quite as effective as for MSRs having many more separated layers of magnetic shielding, but the present room is considerably less expensive and has greater interior space. Furthermore, when second-order gradiometers are used as detection coils in the room, the noise spectrum is similar to that of the more expensive MSRs. For further details the reader is referred to Buchanan et al. (1987).

Analysis

Source Localization

The overriding advantage of magnetic measurements is the possibility of determining more accurately the location within the brain of confined regions of activity, when the activity can be modeled as a *current dipole*, i.e., a short element of current. Accurate localization is central to the process of constructing functional maps of the brain. One example is the discovery of a tonotopic organization across the auditory cortex of human subjects (Figure 6).

If the source is a current dipole, there will be one region of the scalp where the field emerges, and another region where it reenters the head. There is one location within each of these two regions where the field is stronger than at other locations. These strongest emerging and reentering fields are referred to as "field extrema." Where the source is close to a flat portion of the skull it can be approximated by a flat surface covering a semi-infinite, uniform conducting region (the *half-space model*). When this model is applicable, then the source would lie midway between the field extrema and at a depth that is equal to the distance between the extrema divided by $\sqrt{2} = 1.42$. Similarly, for a current dipole in a sphere (which may be fitted to the local curvature of a portion of the skull), the depth of the source can be deduced from the ratio of the distance between the extrema to the radius of the sphere (Williamson & Kaufman, 1981). Such simple recipes, which are useful for making first estimates, can be refined by more accurate numerical models describing the head.

There are cases where the field patterns from two or even three simultaneously active sources have been analyzed to reveal the positions of underlying activity; but in general the problem of dealing with multiple sources is still in its infancy. Nevertheless, Hari et al. (1987) recently reported that it is theoretically possible to resolve current dipoles separated by as little as 1 mm when they are within about 3 cm of the scalp, with some loss of precision as the dipoles move more deeply into the brain. Despite this promising result, more theoretical and experimental work is needed to deal with the more interesting problems of the time sequence of multiply active areas in the brain. It should be kept in mind that there is no unique solution for determining the configuration of electrical sources that can be deduced from electrical potential measurements, or magnetic field measurements, or a combination of the two. Furthermore, it is theoretically possible for electrically and magnetically "silent" sources to exist, in the sense that there are source configurations that produce no skin potential distribution or external fields.

Implications for Multi-Channel Systems

While work is progressing along several different lines toward the goal of resolving and locating sources of neuromagnetic fields, in this section we shall focus on the implications of using multiple sensors for source localization. Our motivation for employing 14 sensors is perhaps best explained by considering the precision with which field measurements can locate the simplest neural source: a confined region of activity that can be modeled by an equivalent current dipole. Such a dipole is characterized by 5 parameters: the strength Q of its moment tangential to the scalp (the normal component is magnetically silent); transverse position x and y in the tangent plane; depth D beneath the scalp; and orientation PSI in the tangent plane. Therefore, in principle, a 5-sensor probe is sufficient to determine the parameters with simultaneous measurements at a single, appropriate position. Computations for the case where the probe is centered on one of the two field extrema show that while this is indeed true, the presence of a typical level of magnetic noise introduces considerable uncertainty in the values of these parameters (Costa Ribeira et al., 1988). Table 1 compares the uncertainties associated with single sensor systems with 7-sensor as well as a pair of 7-sensor systems. For a 10% noise level the uncertainties in strength and depth exceed 30% for both 5- and 7-sensor probes, although the latter provides a significant advantage in determining the lateral position and orientation. By comparison the 14-sensor system provides a marked advantage in the precision of all parameters, with less than 16% uncertainty in strength and depth, 2 mm uncertainty in lateral coordinates, and 3° in orientation. We hasten to add that these computations are for a favorable situation where the dipole is relatively shallow, i.e., when its depth is comparable to the distance separating the detection coils within a given probe. For deeper sources the uncertainties will be greater. Furthermore, this illustration is based on a simplified spherical model of the cranium where the electrical conductivity is assumed to depend on radial but not angular position (the external magnetic field pattern then being independent of the exact functional description). Nevertheless, the results shown in Table 1 clearly display the relative advantage of using a large array of sensors.

Table 1. Uncertainties in best-fitting current dipole parameters for various levels of noise, expressed as a percentage of the dipole field sensed at a field extremum. The dipole is located at a depth of 2 cm in a spherical head of 9-cm radius. For the 5- and 7-sensor systems, the probe was centered on one of the field extrema; the 14-sensor system consists of two 7-sensor probes which were centered on the two extrema.

Probe	Noise (%)	Q/Q (%)	D/D (%)	x (mm)	z (mm)	PSI (deg)
5-sensor	5	21	16	4.6	13.6	40
	10	42	31	6.7	20.0	64
7-sensor	5	20	15	1.2	4.0	12
	10	44	31	2.6	8.1	14
14-sensor	5	8	6	0.4	1.0	3
	10	16	11	0.8	1.9	6

Examples from Sensory-Evoked Fields

One of the principal advantages of neuromagnetic methods is the possibility of locating sources of neural activity by a relatively simple procedure (Williamson & Kaufman, 1981; Romani et al., 1982c). The procedure does not require knowledge of the exact shape of the head, but merely the sphere that best fits the relevant region of the head. Recently it was argued that the sphere fitting the inner surface of the skull nearest the source is most appropriate (Hari & Illmoniemi, 1986). In any event, if the source is sufficiently confined to allow it to be reasonably well modeled as an equivalent current dipole in a spherical head, the resulting pattern across the scalp of the radial component of the field is always composed of one region of outward directed field and another of inward field. This universal duality is due to the fact that only the tangential component of the dipole contributes to the field outside the head—the radial component is magnetically "silent." Magnetic field lines form closed loops around the dipole, and the extrema indicate where the loops are most dense where they emerge from and enter the scalp. As already indicated, to determine the lateral position and depth of the current dipole, it is only necessary to locate the positions of the maximum outward and inward radial field. Once the three dimensional position of the dipole is determined, that information, together with knowledge of the strength of the field, allows one to compute the strength of the dipole (the current dipole moment). Thus, it is now possible to determine the strength of the underlying neural activity as opposed to the amplitude of an epiphenomenon such as scalp potential or external field strength. The latter are imperfect indicators of what is actually going on in the brain, but the strength of the underlying neural activity is indicative of actual brain function, and therefore will play a central role in NMI.

The first evidence that neural sources may be located by the positions of the field extrema was presented by Brenner et al. (1978) in a study of the somatically evoked field. This work led to obvious refinements in the determination of the location, orientation and strength of a current dipole by employing a least-squares fit of the data over and near the field extrema. Okada et al. (1984) used such methods to show that it is possible to identify from field patterns the cortical representations of the digits of the hand along the Rolandic fissure. Depth determinations placed the individual source locations between 6 and 22 mm beneath the inner surface of the skull, which is an anatomically reasonable depth for sources within the fissure.

To exploit this ability to locate sources of fields, Romani et al. (1982a) and Romani et al. (1982b) studied the steady-state response to a tone whose amplitude was sinusoidally modulated at a rate of 32/s. Mapping the field patterns for tones of different frequencies

showed that the depth of the source increased monotonically with frequency, with the cumulative distance across the auditory cortex within the Sylvian fissure from one source to the next varying as the logarithm of the frequency. This demonstrated the existence of a tone map across the auditory cortex which extends over a distance of about 2 cm for the range 100—5000 Hz. Thus, using a simple sphere model we were able to demonstrate the tonotopic organization of a portion of the human auditory cortex (Figure 6).

The potential evoked by a long tone burst differs from steady-state responses such as those occurring when tones are modulated at some high frequency, e.g., 32 Hz. The evoked electrical response to a tone burst typically contains four major components, i.e., P1 (latency of about 45 ms), N1 (90 ms), P2 (160 ms) and a steady potential (SP). In their study of the N1-P2 complex, Vaughan and Ritter (1970) observed a reversal of scalp potential polarity along a line corresponding to the approximate location of the Sylvian fissure, which is consistent with the hypothesis that the source or sources of this complex lie in the auditory cortex, oriented normal to the fissure. This interpretation is widely accepted despite some earlier controversy. However, Wood and Wolpaw (1980) also showed that the morphology of the waveform varies with position over the scalp. The N1 component has a longer latency over temporal areas than in the frontal areas or near the vertex. The distribution of potential for N1 also appears to differ in detail from that associated with P2, as previously reported by Simson, Vaughan and Ritter (1976). Thus, the N1-P2 complex must be modeled by more than one equivalent current dipole. This is supported by the finding of McCallum and Curry (1979; 1980) that there are three successive peaks in the N1 time-frame in measurements made on the surface of the cortex. It is possible to associate each peak with a different source.

These findings are nicely complemented by auditory evoked field studies. First, however, we should mention the convention of affixing an "m" after the symbol for an evoked potential component to indicate that we are discussing a neuromagnetic correlate of that component. Thus, "N1m" is the neuromagnetic

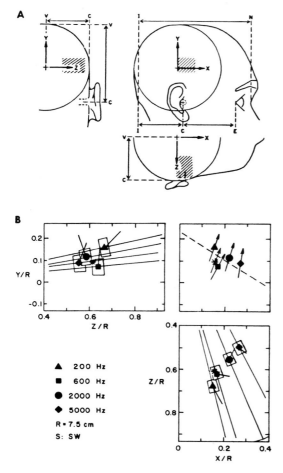

Figure 6. Tonotopic organization of activity across auditory cortex represented by locations of the equivalent current dipole sources, for steady state responses to amplitude modulated tones of the indicated frequencies. The star indicates the position of the response to click stimuli presented at 32/s, whose power spectrum peaks at 900 Hz. Shaded areas in A indicate the locations of the enlarged lower panels in B. The orientation of each dipole is indicated by a line, and the uncertainty in position by a box. Long straight lines correspond to radii of the sphere used to model the head, which is shown schematically in A. The dashed line is the independently estimated position of the Sylvian fissure.

made over the temporal area by Reite et al. (1978) for click stimuli, but Farrell et al. (1980) were the first to note an anterior-posterior polarity reversal for P1m, which implied that the position of its source was in or near the primary auditory cortex. Elberling et al. (1980) studied responses to tone bursts of long duration and found a polarity reversal for N1m suggesting that its source lay in the same general area. Hari et al. (1980) also reported a reversal of polarity of N1m and P2m, as well as the steady field (SF), where the positions of the extrema were consistent with dipole sources in or near primary auditory cortex with moments oriented perpendicular to the lateral sulcus. Thus, all of these major components of the transient auditory response, viz. P1m, N1m, P2m and SF, seem to originate in the vicinity of the auditory cortex. It is to be noted that unlike scalp potentials, there is no evidence of latency shifts with positions from which these components are recored and, unlike direct recordings from the surface of the cortex, no evidence for several peaks within the time frame of N1.

As intimated above, electrical potential data suggest that N1 may well reflect the activity of more than one source. This is further substantiated by Hari et al. (1982) who found that the amplitudes of N1m and the vertex-recorded N1 increased with interstimulus interval (ISI), but not at the same rates. The amplitude of N1m saturated at substantially shorter ISIs than did that of N1, thus suggesting that more than one source from different regions of the brain contribute to the electrical N1. Since N1m is primarily sensitive to sources that are tangential to the scalp while the electrical N1 is sensitive to both tangential and to radial sources, it is possible that the radial sources contribute to the differences between the two measures. Moreover, sources at distant cerebral positions may well contribute to electrical potential differences, while this is far less likely to happen in magnetic recordings (Kaufman & Williamson, 1982).

Assuming that the evoked field does not reflect the activity of all of the same sources that contribute to the evoked potential, it is of some interest to note that the sources of N1m and of P2m are not in precisely the same place on the auditory cortex as is the region that re-

counterpart to the potential referred to as "N1," and the "m" emphasizes that the magnetic and electric components may not in general be attributable to identical sources.

The first observations of the auditory evoked field components P1m and N1m were

sponds to steady-state stimulation (Pelizzone et al., 1984). Also, Pelizzone, Williamson and Kaufman (1985) found that the sources of P2m in two subjects were as much as 1 cm anterior to the source of N1m along the projection of the lateral sulcus onto the head. The source of P2m in these subjects could not be resolved from that of the steady-state response, but they are functionally different: P2m seems to be "indifferent" to the tonal properties of the acoustic stimulus, while there is a tonal dependency of the steady state response. Furthermore, although the source of the steady-state response differs in spatial location from that of the N1m response, both sources are tonotopically organized (Pantew et al., 1988). This is consistent with results of animal experiments showing that there are multiple auditory areas (Woolsey, 1981).

It is important to emphasize that at least two regions of auditory cortex respond differentially to tones that vary only in frequency, whereas one or more other regions are essentially indifferent to the simple spectral composition of the stimuli and obviously have different functions. We shall now see that activity of one of the tonotopically organized portions of the auditory cortex is modulated by selective attention where the selection is based on pitch. Thus, groups of neurons tuned to different frequencies respond differently, depending upon whether or not attention is being paid to specific tonal frequencies.

Attention and the Event-Related Field

Background

Some of the most important event-related potential (ERP) research deals with the effect of selective attention on the auditory response. This topic was originally explored using behavioral methods, such as the shadowing of a message delivered to one ear in the context of a dichotic listening experiment (cf. Cherry, 1953; Moray, 1959; Treisman, 1960). This type of research led to the formulation of several competing "filter" theories. One of the controversies in this area concerns the location in

the chain of sensory processing of selective attention so that it becomes possible to disregard one message while shadowing a concurrent message. It has been found that attention may be deployed to one of the two ears, or even to one position in auditory space rather than another position. Moreover, physical features alone, such as the pitch of a voice, may, if sufficiently distinctive, allow attention to that voice while disregarding another voice. To make matters even more complicated, the semantic content of the message may be used to guide attention. Clearly, multiple capacities must be involved in selective attention.

The finding by Treisman and Geffen (1967) that a message is analyzed in some degree up to the level of its semantic content even though the subject is not aware of attending to it suggests a high level of processing prior to perception. However, Deutsch and Deutsch (1963) suggested that the filter might well be located between conscious perception and the motor activity to which perceptions can lead. This idea has an intuitive appeal, since it too is consistent with the fact that messages are processed to a high level. However, both views may be right. The ability of subjects to adopt different strategies, e.g., stimulus set vs. response set, implies that the filtering process, and the stage at which it occurs, may well be partially determined by the situations of the subjects and the strategies they adopt. ERP and the complementary event-related field (ERF) techniques may be helpful in determining the level at which the filtering process occurs in the context of a particular task.

Hillyard et al. (1973) failed to demonstrate any effect of selective attention on the auditory brainstem evoked response. This would seem to rule out a role for peripheral gating, as suggested by Hernandez-Peon et al. (1956). Hillyard et al. (1973) employed a dichotic listening procedure quite similar to that used by Treisman (1960) and found that attending to a train of stimuli resulted in an enhanced negativity in the time frame of the N1 component as compared to the corresponding component related to the stimuli that were being ignored. Many earlier studies, beginning with that of Spong et al. (1965), demonstrated similar effects when subjects selectively attended to either a visual or an auditory stimulus. However, many of these studies were considered to be flawed because stimuli were presented periodically, thus allowing subjects to anticipate their occurrence. According to Naatanen (1967) and Karlin (1970) this procedure does not discriminate between fluctuations in general arousal (a general anticipatory effect) and may be fundamentally different from an effect of selective attention (a modality specific effect). It is not entirely clear that general anticipatory effects are unrelated to selective attention. Thus, for example, Neisser (1967) and Hochberg (1970) specifically reject a simple filter theory and suggest that attention entails the ongoing matching of the events being monitored with an internal model of the set of events (a "schema"). Such matching entails anticipation. Nevertheless, Hillyard et al. (1973) avoided effects of anticipation as well as other potential pitfalls and showed that midlatency components are differentially affected by selective attention during a dichotic listening task.

It is worth drawing attention to two features of the experiment by Hillyard and his coworkers. First, the period between stimuli varied from an interval of 100 ms to one of 800 ms. On the average, these are short periods of time as compared with many experiments of this type. This makes the task relatively difficult, as does the fact that the difference in pitch between target and non-target stimuli in one ear was very small. This level of task difficulty seems more likely to engage selective attention than would slowly delivered and easy-to-detect stimuli. These considerations were also factors in the design of our experiments. Secondly, the stimuli that were ignored and to which attention was paid differed from each other both in pitch and in apparent location.

Schwent et al. (1976) went on to determine whether the attended and ignored signals had to be differentiated from each other by both pitch and perceived location. Thus, they compared responses obtained when the stimuli to the two ears were of the same pitch, but differed in perceived location. For tone bursts of lowest and highest pitch the effect was about the same whether or not the two stimuli were perceived as being at the same location or at different locations. In general, they found that

the effect can occur with equal strength even when the two trains of stimuli differ along only one dimension, e.g., pitch or perceived location, provided that the difference within that dimension is sufficiently salient.

Selective attention to visual stimuli often gives a different pattern of results. As pointed out by Hillyard et al. (1985), N1 is enhanced with attention to a chain of events occurring in a specific spatial location. Stimuli at other locations result in relatively weaker N1 components. However, this effect appears only after the first event in the train of visual events, a point to which we shall return later. When visual stimuli are selected on the basis of color, orientation, size or brightness, the P1-N1-P2-N2 pattern differs remarkably from that produced by stimuli selected on the basis of spatial location. These authors consider their results as strong evidence for early selection, since there should be no difference in the ERPs if the selection were post-perceptual. The conclusions of Hillyard et al. (1985) are somewhat more complicated than as described here, but we shall use this simplified version as a starting point for describing our own work.

Methods

In this section we describe the methods used in experiments involving selective auditory attention and selective visual attention. Our goal is to exploit the method of neuromagnetism to determine if activity of regions of the primary sensory areas of the brain is modulated by selective attention. Thus, we want to test the hypothesis that selective attention entails some filtering process along the sensory pathways. Alternatively, selective attention may entail a general (non-specific) process, which would be reflected by modulation of activity that is not restricted to specific sensory areas.

Auditory Experiment

All our experiments described in this paper made use of the 5-channel neuromagnetometer described above. This particular experiment (Curtis et al., 1987) required that the field be measured at many points over and near the temporal regions of both sides of the head, so that we could obtain sufficient information to permit location of sources in or near the auditory cortex. This means that the field was sampled from 30 different positions on each side of the head by placing the probe sequentially at six locations. Subsequently these data were used to construct maps of isofield contours, and the underlying sources were then fit by equivalent current dipoles. Three subjects were studied in detail, and one additional subject was studied only partially.

A dichotic listening paradigm was employed in which tone bursts were delivered at a rate of 3/s to one ear and at a rate of 3.5/s to the other ear. Since neither the fundamental frequencies nor their first 5 higher harmonics coincided, it was possible to simultaneously average the band-limited responses and then obtain the separate response at 3 Hz together with its first 5 higher harmonics and at 3.5 Hz together with its first 5 harmonics. The 3/s stimulus train was composed of 50-ms tone bursts that alternated between the frequencies of 1500 Hz and of 1550 Hz. The two tones were perceptibly different in pitch. The 1500-Hz and 1550-Hz bursts were presented in random order, but the randomly chosen pattern was repeated after 40—50 bursts (a pseudorandom sequence). Similarly, the 3.5/s bursts were also composed of tones of different frequencies. These were 3000 and 3050 Hz. The length of the random string was different from that of the tones of lower pitch, and the ordering of these two tone bursts was independent of the order of the 3/s tone bursts.

This arrangement made it possible for the subject to attend to one of the trains of tone bursts while ignoring the other. In fact, the task of the subject was to determine the number of tone bursts that occurred before the pseudorandom pattern repeated itself. Subjectively this seems to capture attention about as well as the usual shadowing task does. In fact, subjects were unable to describe the concurrently given pattern that they were trying to ignore.

With the 5-sensor probe placed over a given position on one side of the head, the subject listened to the 3/s train presented to the contralateral ear and 3.5/s train to the ipsilateral ear. He was instructed to determine the length of the pattern of one train while ignoring the other train. In this main experiment the entire procedure was repeated with the subject paying attention to the tone bursts recurring at the other repetition rate. Hence, we were able to compare responses to tones presented to one ear when they were attended to and when they were ignored, but when they had the same repetition rate and the same spectral composition. The probe was then moved across the head to another position, and similar measurements of the field were made. This was continued until at least six different positions on one side of the head were covered.

The pair of stimuli used in this experiment differed in pitch and also in perceived location. Several control experiments were run to determine whether these or other physical aspects of the stimuli could affect our results. In one control experiment we presented both signals over two loudspeakers placed close to each other so that the position cue would be eliminated. In another control experiment we deliberately attenuated the loudness of one signal by 20 dB. The subject attended to this signal while ignoring the other louder signal. Then the subject attended to the louder signal and ignored the attenuated signal.

Since we were using rapid stimulus repetition rates that verged onto the steady state domain, we also conducted a control experiment in which the interstimulus interval was randomized between 1000 and 1500 ms to determine if our 50-ms duration tone bursts would produce the classic waveform of the transient evoked potential. Subjects listened to these tone bursts passively, since they received no instructions other than to listen. Isofield contour maps were made and dipole fits completed to determine whether the position of the source of the classic N1m component was discriminable from the peak observed at about 100 ms after stimulation by the same tone bursts presented with a repetition rate of 3/s.

Vision Experiment

As this particular experiment is still underway, the results are incomplete. Even so, they are sufficiently interesting to warrant presentation here. We are conducting this experiment in collaboration with Bruce Luber. The purpose of the experiment is to determine whether the activity of visual cortex is differentially affected by selective attention to events in visual space. Since our concern here is with the visual cortex, mapping of the field external to the head was done in the occipital and parietal regions. The subject lay prone on a bed and looked through an aperture down into a mirror which reflected the image on the screen of a display oscilloscope to his eyes. This made it possible to move the neuromagnetic probe around the occipital and parietal regions of the head while the subject fixated a mark on the screen.

The stimuli were two bar gratings placed one above the other on one side of a screen of uniform luminance. Each grating pattern subtended 3° horizontally and 2° vertically, with a 0.5° strip of uniform luminance separating them. The fixation point was at the center of the screen, on the midline of the strip and 0.5° to the side of the nearest edges of the gratings. The mean luminance of the grating matched the background luminance of the screen. The gratings were generated using an Inisfree Picasso Image Generator driven by a PDP 11/34 computer. One of the gratings had a spatial frequency which was alternated between 1.25 c/° and 2.50 c/°. The other grating had a spatial frequency which alternated between 3.5 and 7.0 c/°. The two spatial frequencies in one of the gratings were presented in random order at a presentation rate of 3/s. At the same time the other two spatial frequencies in the second quadrant of the display were presented in random order at a rate of 2.75/s. Each grating in the former sequence was presented for 200 ms, and those in the latter sequence for 250 ms.

Thus far the basic procedure is analogous to that used in the auditory experiment. None of the first 10 harmonics of 3/s and 2.75/s coincide, so the averaging computer can accept the band-limited signal and selectively analyze responses at these two repetition rates. However, following the suggestion of Dr. Risto Ilmoniemi, we modified the procedure slightly. Rather than employ a pseudo-random sequence where the length of the pattern prior to its repetition had to be detected, the

pattern in one quadrant had one of two possible spatial frequencies which were always selected at random. However, the trial simply stopped after a randomly selected interval of time which could range from 4 to 40 s. The subject never knew whether a trial would be long or short. His only instruction was that he had to keep track of one of the two stimuli so that when the train stopped he could tell the experimenter the spatial frequencies of the four or five patterns immediately preceding cessation of the trial. The average responses to the attended and ignored patterns were accumulated and then averaged together subsequently. This was to assure that at least 600 events entered a particular average.

This procedure has some advantages over the one we had used previously. The most obvious of these is that the strategy used by the subject in performing the task does not change so markedly as it might when performing the original auditory task. The subject must keep track of the stimulus to give an accurate answer to the question concerning the preceding four or five stimuli in a given quadrant. In fact, we have data from one male subject who was unable to perform the task, and his responses failed to show differentiation related to the instruction to attend to one stimulus and ignore the other.

Results

Auditory Experiment

Typical auditory responses from the vicinity of one extremum on the scalp are shown in Figure 7. The five vertically separated traces in each column correspond to the outputs of the five sensors of the neuromagnetometer. In this paradigm the N1m and P2m components have somewhat longer latencies than for the classic transient response, being about 110 ms and 250 ms, respectively. The most important aspect of these traces is that their amplitudes depend upon whether or not the subject is attending to a particular stimulus train. For example, the traces evoked by stimuli having a 3/s repetition rate are greater in amplitude than are the corresponding traces obtained at the same positions but where the subject was ignoring the same stimulus train.

3/sec Presentation 3.5/sec Presentation

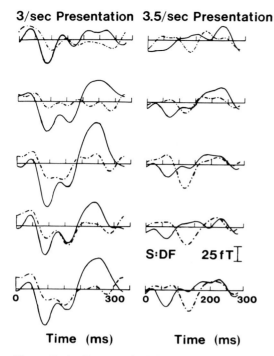

Time (ms)   **Time (ms)**

Figure 7. Auditory evoked fields obtained with a 5-sensor probe placed over the anterior extremum of the left hemisphere of subject DF, averaged at 3/s (left column) and 3.5/s (right column). Solid lines are responses when the subject attends to the 3/s train, and dashed lines are for the 3.5/s train. Each trace corresponds to 500 repetitions for the 3/Hz train and includes the fundamental and 4 harmonics.

As a first step in the evaluation of these data, we performed an ANOVA using data from one probe position over each field extremum of each hemisphere for each subject. Thus there were a total of 20 measurement positions per subject. We examined the effects of instruction (to attend or to ignore), the repetition rate of the stimuli, the "components" of the response (two peaks that correspond to N1m and P2m), the 5 channels used to detect the fields, the hemisphere over which the measures were taken, and whether the channel is positioned over the anterior or posterior field extremum. Other than amplitude differences across channels, attributed to the spatial variation of the field pattern, the only significant main effect was instructions. For instructions F was significant with p = .028. It may be of

some interest that we found no consistent hemispheric differences. Nor did we find any significant difference between the mean amplitudes of N1m and P2m.

Plots of isofield contours indicated that the N1m and P2m sources were located at close proximity to each other in or near the auditory cortex. Since Pelizzone et al. (1985) showed that these two components are related to sources that are about 1 cm apart, we may also assume that the N1m and P2m components of this study are also related to different sources.

To be sure that the N1m component examined here is the same as that found in the classic transient response, we conducted a control experiment as described in the Methods section. Isofield contour plots based on this study are quite precise, since the amplitudes of the responses are much larger than the background noise. We could not establish any significant difference in the locations of N1m generated in the transient response and the nominal N1m of the quasi steady-state response of this experiment.

When one of the stimuli was reduced in intensity by 20 dB it had no effect on the relative amplitude difference related to attention. Causing both stimuli to be heard over loudspeakers aimed at one ear, which severely reduced the effect of the spatial location cue but did not affect the difference in the pitch dimension between the two trains of stimuli, did not affect the results in any significant manner.

Dipole fits demonstrated that the current dipole moment of the source of N1m during attention for the subject characterized in Figure 6 is about 12 nA-m. By contrast, assuming that the depth of the source is the same, when comparable stimuli are ignored the current dipole moment is about 6 nA-m, or about 50% less. The depths of the sources of N1m and P2m were about 3 cm beneath the scalp. However, the certainty of this estimation is far less for the ignore condition because the weaker signal reduced the signal-to-noise ratio.

Vision Experiment

The results of the vision experiment are incomplete. Thus far we have completed full sets of measurements on only two subjects.

However, qualitatively the two sets of data are alike, and because the findings reveal a significant feature of these subjects' attentional effect, we report the results here. Also, we had one subject who showed no effect of instructions to attend, but he did not provide any behavioral evidence that he was able to perform the task.

Figure 8 is an isofield contour plot for the 150-ms component of the response that was in step with the attended 3.5/7.5 c/° stimulus presented at a rate of 3/s. Figure 8A displays the response for attended stimuli in the upper right quadrant of the visual field. The classic description of the cortical representation of the visual field, the cruciform model, indicates that if fixation was as instructed the stimulus had its first cortical effect in the floor of the calcarine fissure and adjacent wall of the longitudinal fissure of the left hemisphere. Indeed, the current dipole that best explains the pattern in the upper panels of Figure 8 is tipped slightly toward the upper right, which is consistent with this region of cortical excitation if the balance of intracellular current flows toward the surface of the cortex.

Figure 8C depicts responses for attended stimuli in the lower right visual field. The corresponding current dipole is more horizontal, indicating a different distribution of cortical activity than for stimuli in the upper right visual field. However, we would expect from the cruciform model that the dipole would be oriented toward the lower right, indicating excitation across the ceiling of the carcarine fissure and adjacent, longitudinal fissure. The data do not support this picture.

When the same stimuli are ignored (Figures 8B, 8D) there is a significant reduction in dipole source strengths for gratings presented in both the upper and lower right visual field. This establishes the principle that activity can be affected by attention in the corresponding different regions of visual cortex. There is no significant change in source position or orientation. Similar results are seen in the responses to stimuli presented at 2.75/s.

The 85-ms component, as well, displays marked attentional effects. While the corresponding sources evoked by upper right and lower right presentations in general behave quite similarly to those for the 150-ms compo-

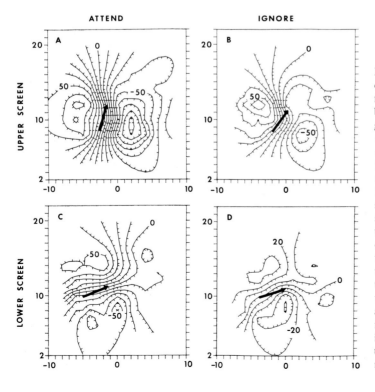

Figure 8. Magnetic field patterns over the occipital area of a subject for the 150 ms component evoked by visual presentation at 3/s of gratings randomly selected to have spatial frequencies of 3.5 or 7.0 c/°. The stimuli were presented in the upper right visual field (A, B) and lower right visual field (C, D). Responses to attended stimuli are shown in A and C and to ignored stimuli in B and D. Arrows show the positions of equivalent current dipole sources as determined by the positive and negative field extrema. Horizontal distances across the scalp from the midline and vertical distances from the inion are indicated in centimeters. Isofield contours are given at 10 fT intervals, which is comparable to the noise level in the measurements.

nent, there are also some differences. These will be the subject of a future publication.

The foregoing results are suggestive of the power of NMI. It is conventional to measure eye movements during an ERP experiment by means of the electrooculogram. At best, this has an accuracy of $0.5°$. Near the fovea an eye movement of nearly this magnitude results in a rather large change in the center of gravity of the portion of striate cortex affected by the visual stimulus. In fact, it is possible to conclude that the changes in the contour maps (and, ipso facto, those in any neuromagnetic image based on such maps) are more accurate indicators of average eye position during a set of experimental trials than is the EOG.

Conclusions

It is clear from the foregoing neuromagnetic evidence that activity in auditory and visual areas of sensory cortex is affected by attention. This is consistent with the notion that selective attention takes place at or prior to the level of conscious perception. We find no evidence for a non-specific control of attention localized elsewhere in the brain, although this cannot be ruled out.

As was pointed out earlier, evidence exists that the first responses to sequences of stimuli do not show the same effects of attentional modulation as do later responses. It should be borne in mind that all of the responses we describe are average responses based upon hundreds of individual responses. As yet we cannot rule out the possibility that activity related to early stimuli is not modulated by attention, but it is only later, after subsequent stages of neural processing have had time to become effective, that the activity of these earlier stages becomes modified by feedback from the subsequent stages. One of the more tantalizing aspects of our more recent results is that when attention is paid to a region in visual space, this is reflected in differential activity of the retinotopically organized portions of the visual cortex.

In view of these findings using a multi-channel instrument, it is clear that further developments of larger arrays of sensors will make neuromagnetic measurements more efficient for conducting studies of higher-order processing by the brain. Fewer trials are required, and the corresponding shorter time required for data acquision translates into better control of the subject's attention, as well as more stable responses. Furthermore, the prospects for an imaging system based upon neuromagnetism are quite promising. The integration of NMI with MRI and CT images can well reveal the functioning of the brain that is related to normal cognitive processes, and, most tantalizing, to abnormal cognitive processes as well.

References

Brenner D, Williamson SJ, Kaufman L, (1975) Visually evoked magnetic fields of the human brain. *Science, 190,* 480−482.

Brenner D, Lipton J, Kaufman L, Williamson SJ (1978) Somatically evoked magnetic fields of the human brain. *Science, 199,* 81.

Buchanan DS, Paulson D, Williamson SJ (1987, in press) In Fast RW (Ed.) *Advances in cryogenic engineering.* Plenum Press, New York.

Cherry C (1953) On the recognition of speech with one, and with two, ears. *J Acoustic Soc Amer, 25,* 975−979.

Cohen D (1972) Magnetoencephalography: Detection of the brain's electrical activity with a superconducting magnetometer. *Science, 175,* 664−666.

Cohen D (1983) Introduction. In Williamson SJ, Romani GL, Kaufman L, Modena I (Eds.) *Biomagnetism: An interdisciplinary approach.* Plenum Press, New York, 5−16.

Costa Ribeira P, Williamson SJ, Kaufman L (1988, submitted) *Method for calibrating a SQUID magnetometer array for locating neural sources in the human brain with minimal data.*

Curtis S, Kaufman L, Williamson SJ (in prep.) *The modulation of activity of the auditory cortex by selective attention.*

Deutsch JA, Deutsch D (1963) Attention: Some theoretical considerations. *Psychol Rev, 70,* 80−90.

Elberling C, Bak C, Kofoed B, Lebech J, Saermark K (1980) Magnetic auditory responses from the human brain. A preliminary report. *Scand Audiol, 9,* 185−190.

Farrell DE, Tripp JH, Norgren R, Teyler TJ (1980) A study of the auditory evoked magnetic field of the human brain. *Electroenceph clin Neurophysiol, 49,* 31−37.

Hari R, Ilmoniemi RJ (1986) Cerebral magnetic fields. *Crit Rev Biomed Eng, 14,* 93−126.

Hari R, Aittoniemi K, Jarvinen ML, Katila T, Varpula T (1980) Auditory evoked transient and sustained magnetic fields of the human brain. *Exp Brain Res, 40,* 237—240.

Hari R, Kaila K, Katila T, Tuomisto T, Varpula T (1982) Interstimulus interval dependence of the auditory vertex response and its magnetic counterpart: Implications for their neural generation. *Electroenceph clin Neurophysiol, 54,* 461—569.

Hari R, Joutsiniemi S-L, Sarvas J (1987, in press) Spatial resolution of neuromagnetic records: Theoretical calculations in a spherical model. *Electroenceph clin Neurophysiol.*

Hernandez-Peon R, Scherrer H, Jouvet M (1956) Modification of electrical activity in the cochlear nucleus during attention in unanaesthetized cats. *Science, 123,* 331—332.

Hillyard SA, Hink RF, Schwent VL, Picton TW (1973) Electrical signs of selective attention in the human brain. *Science, 182,* 177—180.

Hillyard SA, Munte TF, Neville HJ (1985) Visual-spatial attention, orienting, and brain physiology. In Posner MI, Marin OS (Eds.) *Mechanisms of attention: Attention and performance XI.* Erlbaum, Hillsdale, NJ, 63—84.

Hochberg JE (1970) Attention, organization and consciousness. In Mostofsky DI (Ed.) *Attention: Contemporary theory and analysis.* Appleton-Century-Crofts, New York, 99—124.

Ilmoniemi RJ, Hamalainen M, Knuutila J (1985) The forward and inverse problems in the spherical model. In Weinberg H, Stroink G, Katila T (Eds.) *Biomagnetism: Applications and Theory.* Pergamon, New York, 278—282.

Ilmoniemi RJ, Hari R, Reinikainen K (1984) A four-channel SQUID magnetometer for brain research. *Electroenceph clin Neurophysiol, 58,* 467—473.

Karlin L (1970) Cognition, preparation, and sensory-evoked potentials. *Psychological Bulletin, 73,* 122—136.

Kaufman L, Williamson SJ (1982) Magnetic location of cortical activity. *Ann NY Acad Sci, 388,* 197—213.

Kaufman L, Williamson SJ (1986) The neuromagnetic field. In Cracco RQ, Bodis-Wollner I (Eds.) *Evoked potentials, 3,* 85-98.

Kelhä VO, Pukki JM, Peltonen RS, Penttinen AJ, Ilmoniemi RJ, Heino JJ (1982) Design, construction, and performance of a large-volume magnetic shield. *IEEE Trans Magn, 18,* 260—270.

Mager A (1982) Magnetisch abgeschirmte Kabine zur Aufnahme kleinster magnetischer und elektrischer Biosignale. *Naturwiss, 69,* 383—388.

McCallum WC, Curry SH (1979) Hemisphere differences in event related potentials and CNVs associated with monaural stimuli and lateralized

motor responses. In Lehmann D, Callaway E (Eds.) *Human evoked potentials: Applications and problems.* Plenum Press, New York, 235—250.

McCallum WC, Curry SH (1980) The form and distribution of auditory evoked potentials and CNVs when stimuli and responses are lateralized. In Kornhuber HH, Deecke L (Eds.) *Motivation, motor and sensory processes of the brain: Electrical potentials, behaviour and clinical use. Progress in brain research Vol. 54.* Elsevier, Amsterdam, 767—775.

Moray N (1959) Attention in dichotic listening: Affective cues and the influence of instruction. *Quart J Exp Psychol, 11,* 56—60.

Naatanen R (1967) Selective attention and evoked potentials. *Annales Academiae Scientiarum Fennicae B., 151,* 1—226.

Neisser U (1967) *Cognitive psychology.* Appleton-Century-Crofts, New York.

Nunez P (1981) A study of the origins of the time dependencies of the scalp EEG: I—Theoretical basis. *IEEE Trans Biomed Eng 28,* 271—280; II—Experimental support of theory. *IEEE Trans Biomed Eng, 28,* 281—288.

Okada Y, Tanenbaum R, Kaufman L, Williamson SJ (1984) Somatotopic organization of the human somatosensory cortex revealed by neuromagnetic techniques. *Exp Brain Res, 56,* 197—205.

Pantew C, Hoke M, Lehnertz K, Lütkenhöher B, Anogianakis G, Wittkowski W (1988, in press) Tonotopic organization of the human auditory cortex revealed by transient auditory evoked magentic field. *Electroenceph clin Neurophysiol.*

Pelizzone M, Williamson SJ, Kaufman L, Schafer KL (1984) Different sources of transient and steady state responses in human auditory cortex revealed by neuromagnetic fields. *New York Acad Sci, 435,* 570—571.

Pelizzone M, Williamson SJ, Kaufman L (1985) Evidence for multiple areas in the human auditory cortex. In Weinberg H, Stroink G, Katila T (Eds.) *Biomagnetism: Applications and theory.* Pergamon, New York, 326—330.

Reite M, Edrich J, Zimmerman JT, Zimmerman JE (1978) Human magnetic auditory evoked fields. *Electroenceph clin Neurophysiol, 45,* 114—117.

Romani GL, Leoni R (1985) Multichannel instrumentation for biomagnetism. In Hahlbohm HD, Lubbig H (Eds.) *SQUID '85: Superconducting quantum interference devices.* Walter de Gruyter, Berlin, 919.

Romani GL, Narici L (1986) Principles and clinical validity of the biomagnetic method. *Med Progr through Technol, 11,* 123—159.

Romani GL, Williamson SJ, Kaufman L (1982a) Tonotopic organization of the human auditory cortex. *Science, 216,* 1339—1340.

Romani GL, Williamson SJ, Kaufman L (1982b) Characterization of the human auditory cortex by the neuromagnetic method. *Exp Brain Res, 47,* 381—393.

Romani GL, Williamson SJ, Kaufman L (1982c) Biomagnetic Instrumentation. *Rev Sci Instrum, 53,* 1815—1845.

Schwent VL, Snyder E, Hillyard SA (1976) Auditory evoked potentials during multichannel selective listening: Role of pitch and localization cues. *J Exp Psych: Human Percep and Perform, 2,* 313—325.

Simson R, Vaughan HG Jr, Ritter W (1976) The scalp topography of potentials associated with missing visual or auditory stimuli. *Electroenceph clin Neurophysiol, 40,* 33—42.

Spong P, Haider M, Lindsley DB (1965) Selective attentiveness and cortical evoked responses to visual and auditory stimuli. *Science, 148,* 395—397.

Treisman A (1960) Contextual cues in selective listening. *Quart J Exp Psychol, 12,* 242—248.

Treisman A, Geffen G (1967) Selective attention—perception or response? *Quart J Exp Psychol, 20,* 139—150.

Vaughan HG Jr, Ritter W (1970) The sources of auditory evoked responses recorded from the human brain. *Electroenceph clin Neurophysiol, 28,* 360—367.

Williamson SJ, Kaufman L (1981) Magnetic fields of the cerebral cortex. In Erne SN, Hahlbohm HD, Lubbig H (Eds.) *Biomagnetism.* Walter de Gruyter, Berlin, 353—402.

Williamson SJ, Kaufman L (1987) Analysis of neuromagnetic signals. In Gevins AS, Remond A (Eds.) *Methods of analysis of brain electrical and magnetic signals* (Handbook of electroencephalography and clinical neurophysiology, Vol. 1). Elsevier, Amsterdam, 405—448.

Williamson SJ, Romani GL, Kaufman L, Modena I (1983) *Biomagnetism: An interdisciplinary approach.* Plenum Press, New York.

Williamson SJ, Pelizzone M, Okada Y, Kaufman L, Crum DB, Marsden JR (1985) Five channel SQUID installation for unshielded neuromagnetic measurements. In Weinberg H, Stroink G, Katila T (Eds.) *Biomagnetism: Applications and theory.* Pergamon, New York, 46—51.

Wolpaw JR, Wood CC (1980) Scalpdistribution of human auditory evoked potentials: I. Evaluation of reference electrode sites. *Electroenceph clin Neurophysiol, 54,* 15—24.

Wood CC, Wolpaw JR (1980) Scalp distribution of human auditory evoked potentials: II. Evidence for multiple sources and involvement of auditory cortex. *Electroenceph clin Neurophysiol, 54,* 25—38.

Woolsey CN (1981) *Cortical sensory organization, Vol. 3: Mutiple auditory areas.* Humana Press, Clifton, NJ.

The Influence of Various Head Models on EEGs and MEGs

J. W. H. Meijs*, B. J. ten Voorde*,
M. J. Peters*, C. J. Stok**,
F. H. Lopes da Silva***

The construction from magnetic resonance images of a realistically formed four-compartment model of the head is described. From this model four less realistic head models are constructed for which the numerical effort necessary to compute the EEG or the MEG is less. The influence of using the four restricted head models for computing the magnetic fields is studied for sources described by current dipoles, which are located throughout the occipital region of the head. Simulations show that the influence on the EEG and MEG distributions due to the use of the different head models varies for different locations of the dipole within the head. This influence on the MEG is given quantitatively.

The interpretation of the electroencephalogram (EEG) and the magnetoencephalogram (MEG) in terms of the underlying brain activity raises some major problems. These problems are related to experimental variables, such as the noise level or the configuration of the measuring device, but also to more fundamental features like the models of the source and the head. In order to be able to localize sources of functional brain activity mathematical models of both the source and the volume conductor are necessary. These models should reflect the physical reality adequately, meaning that the models should be as simple as possible while also fitting the experimental data. For some models there exist analytical expressions which allow the computation of the electrical potential and the magnetic field with little numerical effort. The single current dipole within the four concentric spheres are

such models. The latter restricted models are commonly used, but whether they adequately simulate the physical reality is a matter of discussion.

In order to determine the adequacy of different restricted head models we have constructed a realistically shaped four compartment model of the head and computed the MEGs using this model and other, more restricted, head models.

Both EEG and MEG are caused by the same electrical processes within the brain. Whether the EEG and MEG give complementary information on the sources of brain activity has often been discussed (Plonsey, 1972; Cuffin & Cohen, 1979; Plonsey, 1982). An important argument in this discussion is the frequently stated opinion that the magnetic field is far less affected by the shape of the head than the EEG is. In a study of visually evoked responses, in which the EEG and the MEG were recorded under the same experimental conditions, it was found that the equiv-

* Twente University, PO Box 217, 7500 AE Enschede, The Netherlands
** P. T. T. Telematics Laboratory, PO Box 570, Groningen, The Netherlands
*** Biological Centre, University of Amsterdam, Kruislaan 320, Amsterdam, The Netherlands
We would like to thank Philips Medical Systems (the Netherlands) and the University Hospital Leiden for the use of the Philips Magnetic Resonance scanner.

alent sources, estimated on the basis of the measured EEGs or MEGs of a subject, did not always coincide (Stok, 1986). The observed discrepancies might be due to the influence of the restricted modelling of the shape of the subject's head. In this paper the dependency of EEGs and MEGs on various models of the head is simulated for sources in the visual cortex area.

Methods

Model of Brain Activity

The activity of the neurons in the cortex is the origin of the EEG and MEG, which can be measured at the scalp, remote from the microscopic sources. These signals can be recorded if the active neurons are regularly distributed in space and firing sufficiently synchronized. This is the case in the cortex, where the neurons are aligned in palisades. The active cortical areas can be described mathematically by a current multipole expansion (Romani, this volume). For each measured field distribution, the minimal number of multipole terms has to be determined that will give an adequate approximation of the measured electric and magnetic field distributions. Whether such a multipole model of the source can be matched by the physiology of the source will be discussed here.

The events taking place at the microscopic level are considered first. When the neurons are activated in an approximately synchronous way, postsynaptic potentials will be generated in a more or less restricted layer along their soma-dendritic membranes. In this way intra- and extracellular currents will flow between the active and the passive patches of the membrane. In those cases where the dendrites have relatively short electrotonic lengths and the active synaptic patches of membrane occupy a small part of the soma-dendritic membrane, fields due to the total neuronal activity can be considered to contain a current quadrupolar term (Mitzdorf, 1985; Lopes da Silva & van Rotterdam, 1982). However, in most cases the active synaptic patches of membrane have a rather extensive electronic length and since the dendrites are arranged

asymetrically, the total current configuration may be reduced to that generated by single current dipoles. Therefore we may assume that, in general, the microscopic sources of neuronal activity may be considered as a set of current dipoles distributed in palisade. In this way a dipole layer is formed, which from a large distance can be considered as a single current dipole.

At the macroscopic level we consider that at a certain moment in time several areas of the cortex are active that may contribute to the fields recorded at points of observation located relatively far away. These different areas are assumed to form the "functional macroscopic source." In some cases such a source may be accounted for by the "two-dipole model" (Maier et al., 1987) in which two spatially separated single current dipoles describe the functional source(s) more adequately. However, since the field resulting from two spatially separated current dipoles does not differ much from a pure dipolar field in many cases (Cuffin, 1985; Meijs et al., 1988), we assume that such a two-dipole model is not a more appropriate source model than the single current dipole one. Disk-like layers covered with a homogeneous dipole distribution also do not give rise to EEGs that deviate much from the pure dipolar field (Munck et al., submitted).

If the active cortex area is folded, the quadrupolar term, or even higher order terms in the multipole expansion, might become apparent and should be included in the source description. Although the two-dipole model can also contribute to quadrupolar terms within the EEG or MEG patterns, the multipole expansion is a preferable source model for describing the active brain region.

Models of the Head

The geometrical model of the head should describe the physiological reality of the volume conductor as accurately as possible. Each tissue within the head takes a volume which has a complex shape and the conductivity of a tissue is usually anisotropic and not homogeneous. In the case of complex models of the head, the numerical computations necessary to solve the forward problem become very elaborate or even unsolvable. Computers and appropriate computational methods can, however, handle rather complex head models.

The Realistic Head Model

Our most complex model consists of four realistically shaped compartments representing the scalp, the skull, the Cerebro Spinal Fluid (CSF) and the brain. The compartments are considered to be homogeneous and isotropic. This head model was constructed using Magnetic Resonance Images (MRI). In order to do so, 22 transversal cross-sectional images of the head of a person were made ranging from the top of the head to 30 mm under the chin. The slice thickness represented in each MRI map is 10 mm (Figure 1).

The proton spin density (H-density), which is different in different tissues, is registered in an MRI map. Therefore it is possible to distinguish a tissue from its surroundings when the H-densities of the tissues are converted into gradations of greyness in an MRI map. However, the actual range of the H-values of the soft tissues within the head is restricted with the effect that the tissue boundaries cannot be sharply recognized. To enhance the tissue contrast within the images the original H-value distributions have to be rescaled. A particular tissue within the head can be enhanced using an appropriate grey-value rescaling of that tissue. An adequate transformation of the H-values to grey values within the MRI maps is found in the "smoothed band-pass grey transformation" (Figure 2).

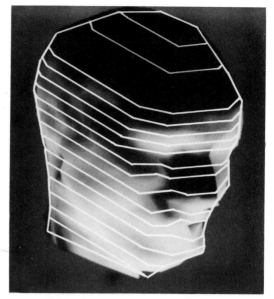

Figure 1. Representation of the head of our subject. Transversal slices through the head are indicated by the horizontal lines. These slices coincide with the Magnetic Resonance scans through the subject's head.

Using this transformation, the scalp, the skull and the brain tissues were enhanced. Examples of some transformed MRI maps are given in Figure 3 (a) through (f). Each figure shows three different representations of the same slice which are more discriminative with respect to a certain tissue: the first one shows the scalp, the second one the skull and the last one the brain tissue in detail.

Using these reconstructed images, the boundaries of the tissues were traced with the

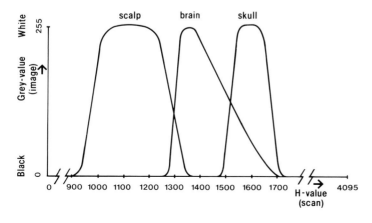

Figure 2. The grey value transformation schemes used to reconstruct the MRI maps. The H-values, representing the proton spin density of the tissues, are given along the horizontal axis. The gradations of greyness within the reconstructed images are given vertically. The three curves indicate the transformations used to elicit the scalp, the brain tissue and the skull.

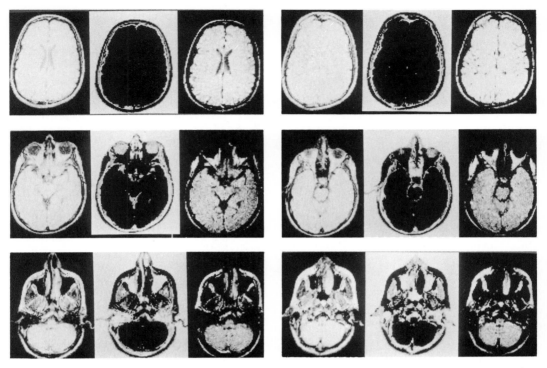

Figure 3. Six reconstructed cross-sections of the head. In each set of three images of the same cross-section of the scalp, the skull or the brain tissue is enhanced.

so-called "eight neighbourhood tracing method" (Rosenfeld & Kak, 1982). This method provides picture elements of 1×1 mm located on the boundaries of the tissues chosen within the image. The relative position of the slices within the head is well defined since the subject did not move during the MRI scan. By assigning CSF to the space between the inner side of the skull and the outer boundary of the brain tissue, four realistically shaped compartments were composed.

The large number of point-locations obtained using this procedure defines the boundaries of the scalp, the skull, the CSF and the brain tissue within the head. Very fine triangular grids can be composed from these data (Figure 4), and although these pictures are aesthetically attractive, from a numerical point of view such fine grids are not desirable since they will result in time-consuming computations (Meijs et al., 1987 b).

The large number of points had to be reduced to attain an appropriate triangular paneling of the tissue boundaries. These trian-

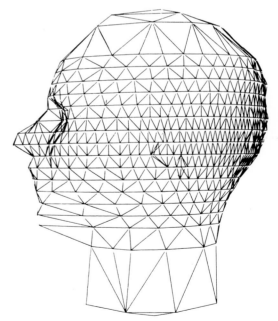

Figure 4. A representation of the scalp of our realistically shaped head model consisting of 1800 triangles.

gular representations of the compartment boundaries are given in Figure 5, where the scalp, the skull, the CSF and the brain compartments are drawn as viewed from the left and back of the head.

Other Head Models

In a first-order approximation, the skull can be considered as an electrical insulator. In this approximation, no current will flow in the two outer compartments. Consequently, the two outer compartments will not contribute to the observed magnetic field (Hämäläinen & Sarvas, 1987). Based on this assumption, two other head models are deduced from the same MRI maps: (i) a model which consists of only the CSF and the brain tissue. Taking into account that the conductivities of the brain tissue and the CSF do not differ very much, the latter model is simplified by assigning the conductivity of the brain tissue to the CSF compartment resulting in (ii) a model which consists of brain tissue only. An advantage of

using these simplified head models is that the time necessary to compute the EEG and the MEG is far less than in the case where four compartments are taken into account.

Two further models are considered: (iii) the "four eccentric spheres model" (Meijs & Peters, 1987), obtained by fitting a sphere to each compartment boundary individually (Figure 5); and (iv) the classic "four concentric spheres model," which is obtained by fitting the outer sphere to the surface of the scalp. The radii of the four concentric shells are based on the MRI maps. Table 1 shows the sphere parameters as determined for these two spherical models.

Sources

Above we have argued that in most cases the source model can be considered as a single current dipole although sometimes higher order terms of the multipole expansion have to be included to obtain a more adequate representation of the source. The influence of

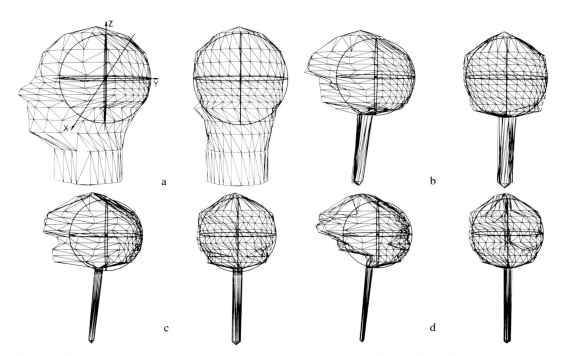

Figure 5. Triangular representation of the four compartment boundaries of the realistically shaped model of the head. The discrete boundaries of the scalp (a), the skull (b), the CSF (c) and the brain tissue (d) are represented. The side and back view are given for each compartment. In these figures the spheres, fitting the compartments best at the back of the head, are drawn as well.

Table 1. Sphere parameters of the concentric and eccentric sphere models. The locations of the centres of the eccentric spheres are given by (x_m, y_m, z_m) and the radii of these spheres are given by R. The center of the concentric spheres is (0,0,0), the radii are given by R_c.

Tissue	x_m	y_m	z_m	R	R_c
	(mm)	(mm)	(mm)	(mm)	(mm)
Scalp	0.0	0.0	0.0	75.0	75.0
Skull	0.0	7.3	6.0	64.5	71.0
CSF	0.4	6.0	7.2	60.0	65.0
Brain	1.1	7.9	8.2	56.2	63.0

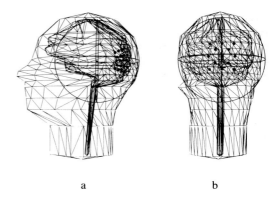

a   b

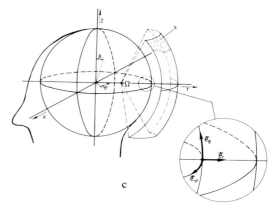

c

Figure 6. Side view (a) and back view (b) of the triangulated brain tissue as positioned within the scalp compartment. The sphere fitting the scalp best is represented as well. The dots represent the projections of the source locations within the brain compartment. In Fig. 6 (c) the coordinate systems used are presented. The solid angle (Ω) subtended by the recording sphere's segment (S) with respect to the source, is a constant for all source locations.

using the simplified head models on the EEG or MEG is determined using a single current dipole as the model of the source. The location of this dipole is varied systematically throughout the occipital section of the head. The dipoles are located along lines which intersect at the centre of the sphere fitting the scalp best (Figure 6). Sources lying outside the brain, for example those in a fissure, are omitted. The source depths (i. e., the depth relative to the sphere fitting the scalp) are confined to 20.0, 25.4, 31.4 and 38.3 mm, respectively. All dipoles are orientated in the azimuthal ($\vec{e}_\varphi$-) direction.

The Boundary Element Method

The boundary element method which is used to compute both the EEG and MEG is based on the numerical solution of the integral equations derived by Barnard et al. (1967) and Geselowitz (1970). These equations show that the contributions of the volume currents in a piecewise homogeneous volume conductor can be considered to be equivalent to the influence of secondary sources which lie at the interfaces between regions of different conductivities. The orientation of these secondary sources is normal to the interfaces and their strengths are proportional to the potential on and to the conductivity differences of the two tissues at both sides of the interfaces considered. The electrical potential due to the secondary sources is added to the electrical potential caused by the primary source (i. e., the single current dipole) in order to obtain the total observed electrical potential. Analo-

gously, the total observed magnetic field is composed of the field caused by the primary source and the field due to the secondary sources. The conductivities of the tissues are adopted from the literature (Geddes & Baker, 1967) and have values of 0.33, 0.0042, 1.00 and 0.33 S/m for the scalp, skull, CSF, and brain tissue, respectively.

Conditions to be met by the triangles describing the various interfaces between the tissues are imposed by the boundary element method (Lynn & Timlake, 1968 a). If the spatial gradient of the potential on a triangle is large, the area of the triangle has to be reduced since the potential distribution on each triangle is assumed to be a constant within the boundary element method. In the present study each realistically shaped compartment boundary is described by about 600 triangles. The areas of the triangles in the occipital part of the head (in the source area) are smaller than the ones in the front.

Recording Procedure

The component of the magnetic field studied is the normal component on a sphere which is concentric with the sphere fitting the scalp best. The radius of this "scalp sphere" is 75 mm and that of the recording sphere 100 mm. As a consequence, the contribution of the volume currents, and hence of the secondary sources at the compartment boundaries, to this magnetic field component is zero if the concentric spheres model is used (Grynszpan & Geselowitz, 1973). Although this contribution is non-zero if the realistically shaped head model is used, it is found to be small in comparison to the other field components (Meijs et al., 1987a). In addition, the normal component of the magnetic field on a spherical recording surface can be measured with high accuracy. In our laboratory a cryostat-holder was constructed in which the normal orientation of the cryostat with respect to the recording sphere is controlled by means of a "parallelogram construction" (Figure 7a). The head has to be so positioned within this device that the centre of the recording sphere coincides with the midpoint of the sphere fitting the scalp best. The mean value of the inaccuracy in the positioning of the angular coordinates of the cryostat, using this device, is 0.2 degrees. The error vectors which represent the inaccuracy within the positioning of the cryostat are indicated in Figure 7b.

The segment of the recording sphere is chosen such that the extremes of the field patterns are incorporated into the map. To be able to compare the values of the RDM (see below) for sources with different source depths, the solid angle (Ω) of the recording segment with respect to the source location is constant for all sources (Figure 6; Meijs et al.,

1988). There are 196 measuring points in the recording sphere.

Inverse Computations

The inverse problem is the estimation of the single current dipole parameters of the source from a field distribution outside the head. To solve this inverse problem, a model of the head is required. In the present study we used for the inverse computations the previously mentioned concentric spheres model. The algorithm used to estimate the parameters of the Equivalent Current Dipole (ECD), minimizes the difference between the measured and the estimated distributions in the least-square-error sense i.e., the sum of the quadratic differences. The search method which is used to estimate the parameters of the ECD is the Marquardt algorithm (Marquardt, 1963). This method was shown to be successful in ECD source estimations (Kavanagh et al., 1978; Stok, 1987).

Measures

A measure of fit is necessary to quantify the influence of different head models on the computed magnetic field. Two measures are used in this study. The first one will be denoted by the Relative Difference Measure (RDM) (Meijs et al., 1988) which is defined as:

$$RDM = \left[\frac{\int\limits_{S} (F_r - F)^2 \, dS}{\int\limits_{S} F_r^2 \, dS} \right]^{\frac{1}{2}} \qquad (1)$$

where,

F_r is the reference field computed using some reference model of the head.

F is the field computed for the same source as used for F_r but using one of the other head models.

S is the segment of the recording surface considered.

The other measure, the so-called Dipolar Difference Measure (DDM), is based on the fact that the computed distributions are all derived from single current dipoles. The

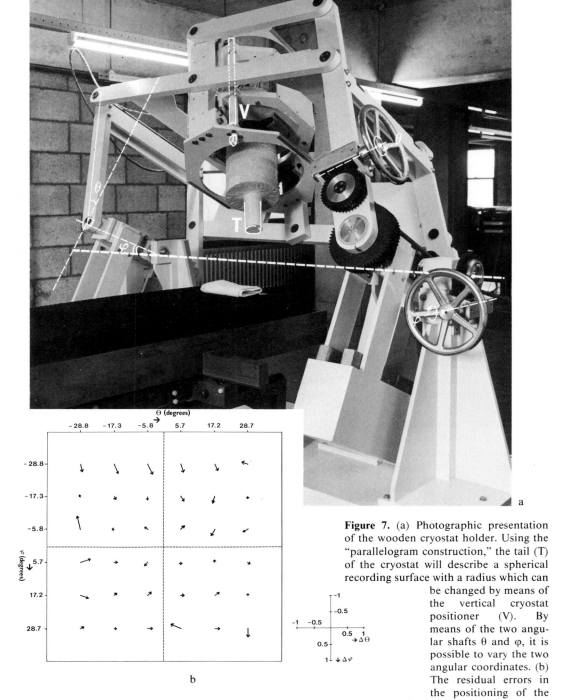

Figure 7. (a) Photographic presentation of the wooden cryostat holder. Using the "parallelogram construction," the tail (T) of the cryostat will describe a spherical recording surface with a radius which can be changed by means of the vertical cryostat positioner (V). By means of the two angular shafts θ and φ, it is possible to vary the two angular coordinates. (b) The residual errors in the positioning of the two angular coordinates are indicated in a grid in the recording sphere covering an area of approximately 60 × 60 degrees. The arrows reflect the inaccuracy in the angular positioning of the grid points.

DDM couples forward and inverse calculations and is defined as:

$$\overrightarrow{DDM}_x = (DDM_r, DDM_\theta, DDM_\varphi) = \vec{X}_r - \vec{X} \quad (2)$$

$$DDM_\alpha = \arccos (\vec{p}_r \cdot \vec{p}) / (p_r \cdot p)) \quad (3)$$

where,

$\vec{X}_r - \vec{X}$ represents the distance between the location of the ECD estimated from a field distribution based on the reference model (indicated by $\vec{X}_r$) and the ECD estimated from a field distribution based on one of the other models ($\vec{X}$).

$\vec{p}_r$ represents the equivalent current dipole moment based on the reference model.

$\vec{p}$ represents the equivalent current dipole moment based on another head model.

To eliminate the coupling between the source depth of the ECD and the estimated source strength and therefore the DDM_α, the dipole moments in (3) are normalized. A visual explanation of the methods used to quantify the differences due to the use of several models of the head is given in Figure 8.

Accuracy and Estimation of Errors

In order to estimate the accuracy of the numerical procedures, the field distribution generated by a single current dipole within the model consisting of four concentric, triangulated spheres is computed. Each sphere is panelled with 320 triangles (Meijs et al., 1987 b). The reference field distribution for the same source within the same concentric spheres model is computed by means of an analytic expression. This reference distribu-

tion is exactly known, which implies that the RDM value obtained by comparing these two distributions is due to the numerical errors in the boundary element method. Because there are no analytical expressions for determining the accuracy using the other head models, we assume that the numerical accuracy for the other models is of the same order of magnitude (Lynn & Timlake, 1968 b).

In order to estimate the accuracy of the numerical procedures by means of the DDM, the field distribution generated by a dipole within the triangulated four concentric spheres model is computed using the forward procedure. From this distribution an ECD is computed. The inverse computations are based on the analytic expression for the four concentric spheres model. The difference in location and direction between the initial dipole and this ECD is caused by both the algorithm used for the inverse procedure and the boundary element method. We again assume that the estimation of the accuracy as based on this concentric spheres model is of the same order for the other head models.

Results

Table 2 shows the mean values and the standard deviations of the RDM and DDM values obtained for the various models of the head. The reference field is based on the realistically shaped four compartment model of the head since this model imitates the physical reality as closely as possible. Therefore, we assume that the reference field distribution is the best approximation of the measured isomagnetic field maps. The values are averaged for all sources studied.

For all models considered, the mean error in the ECD location, reflected by the magnitude of the DDM_x, is about 4 mm. The vari-

Measure	Concentric spheres	Eccentric spheres	Brain and CSF	Brain	Numerical test
RDM	0.14 ± 0.05	0.13 ± 0.05	0.15 ± 0.10	0.16 ± 0.08	0.01
DDM_x (mm)	4.5 ± 3.5	3.8 ± 2.6	3.7 ± 2.1	4.0 ± 2.0	0.1
DDM_α (o)	3.2 ± 1.5	3.2 ± 1.4	3.3 ± 1.8	3.7 ± 1.7	0.1

Table 2. Mean values and standard deviations of the RDM, the DDM_x and the DDM_α, using several head models. The averages presented here include all sources studied. The mean values of the accuracy are given in the last column.

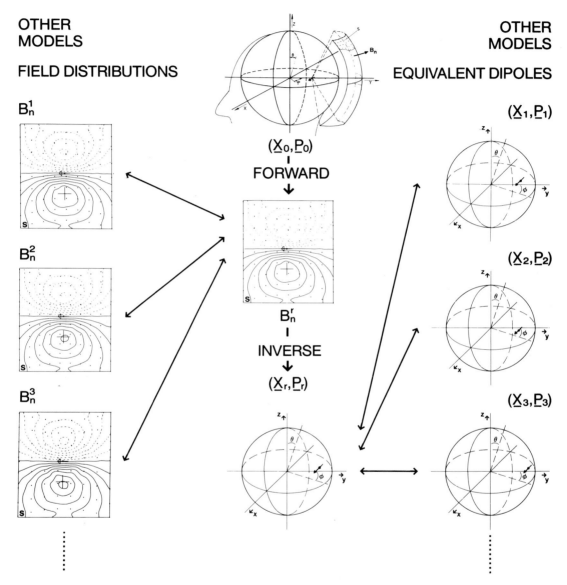

Figure 8. Schematic presentation of the methods used to quantify the influence of using different head models to compute the MEG. The initial current dipole $\vec{P}_0$, located in $\vec{X}_0$, is used to compute the MEGs using several head models. The fields are presented in the left column. The reference field is computed using the most realistically formed four compartment model of the head (presented in the middle column). The RDM is used to quantify the differences between the reference field and the fields presented in the left column. An ECD can be estimated from this reference field. This ECD, indicated by $(\vec{X}_r, \vec{P}_r)$, acts as the reference ECD. Fitting ECDs to the field distributions represented in the left column results in the set of ECDs which are presented in the right column. These ECDs are compared with the reference ECD by means of the DDM.

ation in the direction of the ECDs is small, the mean values of the DDM_α are smaller than 4 degrees. Since the influence of the four concentric spheres model on the chosen magnetic field component is zero, the values in the first column of Table 2 represent the contribution of the volume currents to the magnetic field in the realistically shaped four compartment model of the head which acts as the reference. In the last column of Table 2 the accuracy, averaged over all sources, is given. The accuracy of the numerical procedures quantified by the RDM is one order of magnitude smaller than the RDM values due to the use of the differing head models. This implies that the accuracy of the boundary element method is sufficient to analyse the influence of the various head models. The same can be said for the DDM.

A horizontal "equatorial" plane passing through the centre of the sphere fitting the scalp best, divides the sources into three groups (Figure 9): (a) the upper sources, (b) the equatorial sources and (c) the lower sources. Table 3 shows that for the two spherical models the source estimation is more adequate for the lower sources but less so for the upper ones. For the other realistically shaped head models the estimation is better for the upper sources but worse for the lower sources. The distance between the ECD location based on the reference model and that based on another head model, given by the DDM_x value, is for the substantial values of the DDM_x mostly due to a difference in the source depth, denoted by DDM_r (Table 3). The difference in the locations of the ECDs in the tangential direction is about 2 mm. Table 3 also shows that the depth of the lower sources is overestimated for all models. For the spherical models the depth is underestimated for the upper sources.

Table 4 shows that the values of the error measures averaged for one source depth increase with the source depth. This is found for all models considered in this study.

Discussion

The influence of using the realistically shaped four compartment model of the head for computing the MEG instead of other, more re-

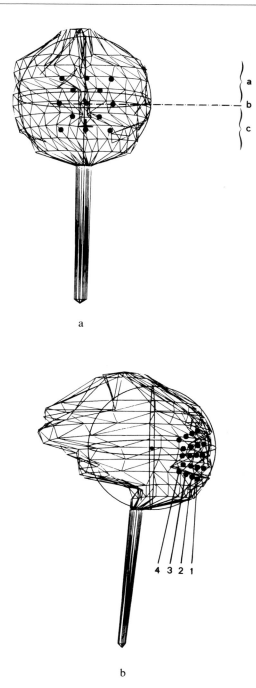

Figure 9. Source subdivisions, in the back view of the head (a), the "equatorial" plane through the midpoint of the scalp sphere is given. This divides the source into the three subsets of sources (a through c). In the side view (b), the sources having the same source depths are indicated (1 through 4).

Measure		Concentric spheres		Eccentric spheres		Brain and CSF		Brain
DDM$_x$	(a)		8.4		6.4		1.6	2.3
	(b)	4.5	2.0	3.8	2.0	3.7	2.6	4.0 3.2
	(c)		2.3		2.4		6.6	6.3
DDM$_r$	(a)		−8.1		−6.1		0.5	0.1
	(b)	−3.0	−1.0	−1.7	0.4	2.5	1.8	2.4 2.0
	(c)		0.7		1.2		5.1	4.8

Table 3. Mean values of the DDM$_x$ and DDM$_r$ for subsets of sources within the brain compartment. Mean value for each subset of sources (a through c) is given to the right of "all-over" averages. The radial component, DDM$_r$, is given in the lower part.

depth (mm)	Measure	Concentric spheres	Eccentric spheres	Brain and CSF	Brain
20.0		0.12±0.03	0.11±0.03	0.12±0.08	0.13±0.06
25.4	RDM	0.15±0.08	0.14±0.08	0.13±0.09	0.15±0.08
31.4		0.13±0.05	0.12±0.04	0.14±0.10	0.15±0.08
38.3		0.15±0.04	0.13±0.03	0.20±0.12	0.20±0.10
20.0		2.3±1.4	1.8±0.8	1.7±1.0	1.8±0.8
25.4	DDM$_x$	3.7±2.8	3.0±2.1	2.4±1.9	2.6±1.4
31.4	(mm)	4.4±3.5	3.7±2.5	3.6±3.1	4.0±2.4
38.3		6.9±6.2	6.0±4.8	6.6±3.4	7.1±3.2
20.0		2.2±1.6	2.3±1.5	2.7±1.7	2.8±1.6
25.4	DDM$_\alpha$	2.5±1.4	2.5±1.3	2.8±1.6	3.1±1.5
31.4	(o)	3.1±1.6	3.1±1.5	3.3±2.0	3.7±1.8
38.3		3.2±1.3	3.3±1.2	3.2±1.9	3.5±1.8

Table 4. Mean values and standard deviations of RDM, DDM$_x$ and DDM$_\alpha$ as a function of the depth of the source.

stricted, head models increases with source depth. This can be explained by the fact that the source term, which is the same for all head models, will be much smaller for deeper sources whereas the volume term, which depends on the specific head model, will decrease relatively less since the secondary sources are located on the compartment boundaries close to the recording sphere. The contribution of the volume term to the MEG compared with that of the source term will therefore increase. Another factor which can account for this phenomenon is that the inverse algorithm which is used for the source estimation is less accurate for deeper sources.

The fact that the source estimation for the spherical models is more adequate for the lower sources may be explained by the fact that the fit of the spheres for points on the various interfaces between regions with different conductivities was better for points under the plane mentioned. For the realistically shaped head models with a restricted number of com-partments, the source estimation was better for the upper sources but it was worse for the lower ones. This may be explained by the fact that there was no conducting neck present in these two models.

The potential distribution on the scalp (the EEG) has to be computed to obtain the magnetic field (Meijs et al., 1987 b). The accuracy interval for the potential distribution reflected in the RDM and DDM are obtained in a similar way as described for the magnetic field (see above, "Accuracy and Estimation of Errors"). For the electrical potential the numerical errors were in the same order of magnitude as the effects due to the use of different head models. This implies that for the potential distribution the accuracy has to be improved, for instance, by using more triangles in the source region. This strategy has been followed to compute the EEGs accurately using the triangulated four eccentric spheres model of the head (Meijs & Peters, 1987). It was found that the influence of the eccentricity of the spheres on the EEG was significant, but not on the MEG. Examples demonstrating these differing influences are given in Figures 10 and 11. The values of the RDMs are in the order of 0.5 for the potential distributions and 0.05 for the magnetic field distributions.

The results presented in this paper are valid for sources located at the back of the head. This area is particularly interesting since visually evoked responses have been investigated in more detail (Kouijzer et al., 1985; Stok et al., submitted). The sources due to these stimuli are located in the occipital region of the head. The head models would have to be adapted for other source locations and the results would probably be different for other sites within the head. For example, the eye sockets and the internal ear may play an important role for sources located in the frontal or temporal regions of the brain.

We have used both the RDM and the DDM as quantitative measures to evaluate the field differences. We found that both measures have supplementary advantages. In order to compute the value of the RDM, only the field distributions in the recording plane have to be known and no inverse techniques are necessary. Field differences due to different causes can be easily compared by means

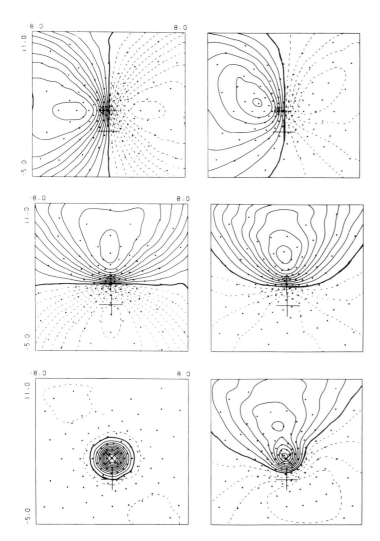

Figure 10. Potential distributions at the outer sphere, representing the scalp. The projected grid points are indicated by the small dots. The projection is such that the distances in the x- and z-directions are conserved. The cross represents the inion and the arrow the projected dipole. The dimensions of the maps, in cm, are indicated in the first map of the series. The interval between successive contours is 0.06 mV. The maps in the first column represent the potential computed for the model consisting of four concentric spheres and those in the second column the potential for the model consisting of the four eccentric spheres. In the first row the dipole is pointing in the x-direction, in the second in the z-direction, and in the third row in the y-direction.

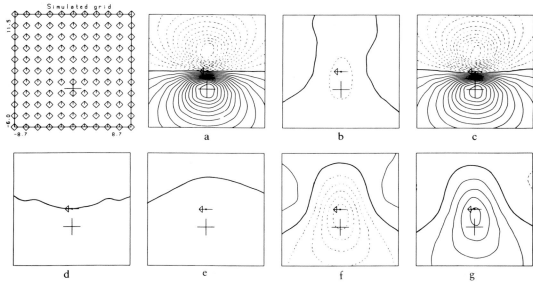

Figure 11. Isocontour maps of the magnetic field component normal to the recording sphere. The depth of the source below the recording sphere is 32 mm. The interval between successive contours is 10 fT. Solid lines indicate that the field leaves the head, dotted lines indicate that the field enters the head. The sequence of maps given is: (a) the magnetic field using the concentric spheres model of the head, (b) the contribution of the volume currents in the four eccentric spheres model to Bn and (c) the recorded magnetic field using the eccentric spheres model. Maps (d) through (g) show the separate contributions of the scalp (d), the skull (e), the CSF (f) and the brain tissue (g). The volume term (b) is equal to the sum of these four contributions. Other symbols used are the same as in Figure 10. The field distribution represented in (a) is equal to the field distribution due to the source only, since the contribution to the magnetic field due to the volume currents is zero for the concentric spheres model.

of the values of the RDM. Obviously, this measure implies a large data reduction, yet it is a useful measure for comparing dipolar field distributions. For example, in the case of two parallel dipoles separated by a distance of 30 mm, the RDM due to the use of these two dipoles instead of one current dipole in the middle will be in the order of 0.1. The same RDM value will be caused by adding Gaussian noise to the field having zero mean and a standard deviation of 5% of the extremes of the dipolar pattern (Meijs et al., 1988). A large data reduction, however, also results in a loss of information. This loss of information is less for the DDM, in which the rotation, translation or a relative displacement of the extremes is reflected in both the position and direction of the ECDs. This measure is interesting since it defines the inaccuracy in the estimated ECD location and direction (in mm and degrees) when the estimation of the ECD is based on a restricted head model such as the

four concentric sphere model. By combining the RDM and the DDM in the analysis of the EEG and MEG patterns, their complementary qualities are used.

Conclusions

The common statement that the magnetic field can pass through the skull is, of course, true but the skull is an obstacle for the volume currents. Therefore, the contribution of the volume currents to the MEG depends on the model of the head used. We have shown in this study that the influence of the realistically shaped head on the MEG can be considerable. The Equivalent Current Dipoles (ECDs), based on the four concentric spheres model of the head are found to be displaced up to 16 mm with respect to the ECDs based on the realistically formed head model. The direction of the ECDs is not influenced by use of the different head models and is retained within 4 degrees. We have found that the influence of the head models on the MEG strongly depends on the location of the source within that head model. For superficial sources this influence is small: displacements of the ECDs are less than 3 mm, but the influence increases with source depth. The two spherical models studied are adequate for sources in the "neck area": the two other realistically shaped but yet restricted head models perform well for sources in the "top area" of the head. For MEG studies, the concentric spheres model is an adequate head model for cortical sources.

References

Barnard ACL, Duck JM, Lynn MS, Timlake WP (1967) The application of electromagnetic theory to electrocardiology II. *Biophys J, 7*, 463–491.

Cuffin BN (1985) A comparison of moving dipole inverse solutions using EEG's and MEG's. *IEEE Trans Biomed Engng, 32*, 905–910.

Cuffin BN, Cohen D (1979) Comparison of the magnetoencephalogram and the electroencephalogram. *Electroenceph clin Neurophysiol, 47*, 132–146.

Geddes LA, Baker LE (1967) The specific resistance of biological material: A compendium of data for the biomedical engineer and physiologist. *Med and Biol Engng, 5*, 271–293.

Geselowitz DB (1970) On the magnetic field outside an inhomogeneous volume conductor by internal sources. *IEEE Trans on Magn, 6*, 346–347.

Grynszpan F, Geselowitz DB (1973) Model studies of the magnetocardiogram. *Biophys J, 13*, 911–925.

Hämäläinen MS, Sarvas J (1987) Feasibility of the homogeneous head model in the interpretation of neuromagnetic fields. *Phys Med Biol, 32*, 91–97.

Kavanagh RN, Darcey TM, Lehmann D, Fender DH (1978) Evaluation of methods for three-dimensional localization of electrical sources in the human brain. *IEEE Trans Biomed Engng, 25*, 421–429.

Kouijzer WJJ, Stok CJ, Reits D, Dunajski Z, Lopes da Silva FH, Peters MJ (1985) Neuromagnetic fields evoked by a pattern on-offset stimulus. *IEEE Trans Biomed Engng, 32*, 455–458.

Lopes da Silva FH, Rotterdam van A (1982) Biophysical aspects of EEG and MEG generation. In Niedermeyer E, Lopes da Silva FH (Eds.) *Electroencephalography.* Urban & Schwarzenberg, Baltimore, 15–26.

Lynn MS, Timlake WP (1968 a) The use of multiple deflations in the numerical solution of singular systems of equations with applications to potential theory. *Siam J Numer Anal, 5*, 303–322.

Lynn MS, Timlake WP (1968 b) On the numerical solution of the singular integral equations of potential theory. *Numer Math, 11*, 77–98.

Maier J, Dagnelie G, Spekreijse H, Dijk van BW (1987) Principal components analysis for source localization of VEPs in man. *Vis Res, 27*, 165–177.

Marquardt DW (1963) An algorithm for least-squares estimation of non-linear parameters. *J Soc Indust Appl Math, 11*, 431–441.

Meijs JWH, Peters MJ (1987) The EEG and MEG, using a model of eccentric spheres to describe the head. *IEEE Trans Biomed Engng, 34*, 913–920.

Meijs JWH, Bosch FGC, Peters MJ, Lopes da Silva FH (1987a) On the magnetic field distribution generated by a dipolar current source situated in a realistically shaped compartment model of the head. *Electroenceph clin Neurophysiol, 66*, 286–298.

Meijs JWH, Peters MJ, Oosterom van A, Boom HBK (1987 b) The application of the Richardson extrapolation in simulation studies of EEGs. *Med and Biol Engng and Comp, 25*, 222–226.

Meijs JWH, Peters MJ, Boom HBK, Lopes da Silva FH (1988, in press) The relative influence of model assumptions and measurement procedures in the analysis of the MEG. *Med and Biol Engng and Comp.*

Mitzdorf U (1985) Current source-density method and application in cat cerebral cortex: Investigation of evoked potentials and EEG phenomena. *Physiol Rev, 65*, 37–100.

Munck de JC, Dijk van BW, Spekreijse H (submitted) An analytic method to determine the effect of source modeling errors on the apparent location and direction of biological sources. *J Appl Phys.*

Plonsey R (1972) Capability and limitations of electrocardiography and magnetocardiography. *IEEE Trans Biomed Engng, 19*, 239–244.

Plonsey R (1982) The nature of sources of bioelectric and biomagnetic fields. *Biophys J, 39*, 309–312.

Rosenfeld A, Kak AC (1982) *Digital picture processing* (2nd edn.). Academic Press, New York.

Stok CJ (1986) *The inverse problem in EEG and MEG with application to the visual evoked responses.* Thesis, Twente University, The Netherlands.

Stok CJ (1987) EEG/MEG single dipole source estimation. *IEEE Trans Biomed Engng, 34*, 289–296.

Stok CJ, Lopes da Silva FH, Spekreijse H, Peters MJ, Boom HBK (submitted) A comparative EEG/MEG equivalent dipole study of the pattern on-set response. *Electoenceph clin Neurophysiol.*

Functional Localization
by Topographic Magnetic Brain Mapping

G. L. Romani

Neuromagnetic investigations performed during the last few years have repeatedly shown an impressive capability to perform a three-dimensional source localization on the basis of the measured spatial distribution of magnetic fields over the scalp. The development of multi-channel systems, although still only in a partially satisfying configuration with just a few adjacent magnetic sensors, has given further impulse to the field and is providing a large amount of novel results, particularly interesting for the understanding of brain functioning. In the present paper, after a brief description of the state of the art of instrumentation and modeling, including related problems and perspectives, the most recent results obtained using the multi-channel system operating at the IESS since 1984 will be reviewed. In particular a topographic mapping of somatosensory evoked fields will be shown, with particular emphasis on the possibility of performing source localization and following the location of the equivalent generator(s) corresponding to both subcortical and cortical components in the evoked magnetic response to median nerve stimulation.

The application of the biomagnetic method to the investigation of cerebral functioning is providing larger and larger amounts of important results and, consequently, is raising increasing interest among scientists and clinicians. As is well known (Williamson & Kaufman, 1981a; Romani et al., 1982; Romani & Narici, 1986), the study of magnetic fields associated with bioelectric currents flowing in neural tissue represents—under specific experimental conditions—a unique tool for gathering information directly from intracellular activity, with only a minor contribution from volume currents. Consequently, starting from a measurement of the magnetic field distribu-

tion over the scalp, as produced by a particular normal or abnormal cerebral function, it is possible to solve the inverse problem and achieve a three-dimensional localization of an equivalent generator responsible for that function, provided a suitable model source has been identified. As was pointed out on several occasions (Williamson & Kaufman, 1981b; Romani & Leoni, 1985; Romani & Narici, 1986), this avenue could lead to a unique means for functional imaging of fast occurring events in the brain, like, for instance, information processing or the onset and propagation of epileptic seizures.

To fully achieve this goal, however, two major problems are still to be solved: the first is strictly related to technological progress, the second to appropriate development of the theoretical approach and of adequate analytical tools. Indeed, the present state of the art of instrumentation, although improving rapidly, is only partially satisfying: magnetic signals can be measured simultaneously only at a few sites on the scalp. This hardly permits detecting the overall field distribution usually associated with a cerebral response. In order to

Istituto di Elettronica dello Stato Solido — CNR, Via Cineto Romano 42, 00156 Roma, Italy.
The author is indebted to Drs. M. Cilli, M. Peresson, V. Pizzella and G. Torrioli for the help provided during daily collaboration. In particular he wants to thank Drs. S. N. Ernè and L. Narici, and Profs. I. Modena, G. B. Ricci and P. Rossini for the many fruitful discussions. Special thanks are due to Prof. R. M. Chapman for a critical revision of the manuscript and to Prof. A. Paoletti for continuous encouragement.

cover more of the field distribution, the measurement must be repeated several times, with the inevitable consequence of some variability in the response itself, the degree of which is difficult to quantify. Additionally, the choice of the optimal sensor configuration is still to be definitively identified. On the other hand, the solution of the inverse problem—not unique by definition—is based on the choice of an appropriate model source to account for the measured field distribution: traditionally, a current dipole in a homogeneously conducting sphere has been used so far with relatively satisfying results. Nevertheless, in many cases this simple source model is not adequate and more sophisticated models and/or source configurations must be used. Consequently the localization algorithms become more and more complicated and time consuming, with a subsequent need for more powerful computers.

Both problems—which will be briefly described in the following sections—will certainly be solved in the near future, and the experimentalists should not be discouraged by these difficulties: rather, they should be stimulated by the impressive quality of the results which have been, and are being, collected in the study of brain physiology and pathology, only a minimal part of which will be presented in the present article.

Instrumentation

As we said, the present generation of multichannel systems represents only a first step toward the development of a neuromagnetometer appropriate to the task of achieving real-time functional localization. It is therefore preferable to briefly describe the possible configurations for this "final" system, rather than dwell on what is available now.

Topographic brain mapping is achieved by simply measuring the magnetic field at a certain number of positions over the subject's head. This measurement, which as yet is not simultaneous but in fact requires several successive replications, will be performed in a single shot in the near future, and each measuring site will most probably correspond to a specific position on a "measuring grid."

Romani and Leoni (1985) have shown that grid spacing (D) and grid size (W) are two fundamental parameters in successful investigation of a specific cerebral source. Figure 1 a schematically illustrates these parameters, D and W. As far as a single current dipole source is concerned (see below), D establishes the depth of the shallowest localizable source, and W, that of the deepest. In other words, as immediately inferable from basic concepts of spatial sampling, D represents the sampling rate and sets the value of the Nyquist frequency, $F_n = (2D)^{-1}$. On the other hand, W affects the low spatial frequency range. W is obviously limited by the physical dimensions of the dewar containing the system. On the basis of the present state of the art in dewar manufacturing, it is likely that a "large" system will be contained in a dewar with a cylindric tail and a concave bottom surface, following a spherical surface with a radius of perhaps 12 cm. According to a "maximum packing" criterion, the sensor displacement in the tail would not follow the grid illustrated in Figure 1 a, but rather the configuration shown in Figure 1 b. In this case the sensors would be located on concentric circles at sites spaced D apart, and D would also be the radial increment for different circles. This criterion would establish some "magic numbers" for the total number of sensors: 7, 19, 37, etc. Another, more important consequence would be the establishment of particular symmetry condi-

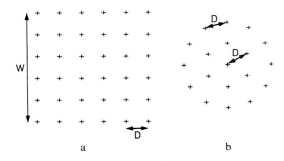

Figure 1. (a) Traditional shape of a measuring grid for neuromagnetic measurements. The total width is W and the spacing between adjacent sites is D. (b) Measuring grid according to the maximum packing criterion (for 19 sensors) described in the text. D is both the radial increment and the spacing between adjacent sites.

tions in the spatial Fourier transform along concentric circles which could be of remarkable importance in the localization procedure.

A second point is the choice of the sensor geometry. So far only "wound-wire" detection coils have been used in neuromagnetic systems. Depending on the amount of ambient noise or, rather, on the degree of shielding, magnetometers, first-order, second-order, and even third-order gradiometers have been used to pick up cerebral fields (Romani & Narici, 1986). With rare exceptions (Cohen, 1979), all the gradiometric configurations were based on a "vertical" geometry (see Figure 2), where the fundamental parameter becomes the "baseline" b, i.e., the distance between the planes of different sub-coils of the gradiometer. The rapid development of microfabrication techniques and of a new generation of highly sensitive DC SQUIDs, has given impulse to the study of alternative geometries which, in a planar configuration, could combine spatial discrimination and integration with the SQUID itself (Figure 2). Even if, so far, the experimental approach has been developed only to a limited extent (Carelli & Foglietti, 1983; Ketchen M, personal communication), many simulation studies have been carried out by several groups (Ernè & Romani, 1985; Tesche, 1985; Carelli & Leoni, 1986; Bain et al., 1987; Romani, 1987) on the performances of planar gradiometers (see Figure 2b). Although this is not the proper place to discuss the topic in detail, it

should be borne in mind that the major advantages of microfabricated devices include a high discriminating power against unwanted fields, no need for superconducting contacts between the SQUID and the loops, and the lack of a superconducting flux transformer, as the loops themselves are directly inserted in the SQUID (Ernè & Romani, 1985). This last property well repays the disadvantage of having a short baseline. On the other hand, we should point out a lack of symmetry for rotation of the source with respect to the gradiometer; this significantly complicates the measured pattern. Figure 3 shows an example of the pattern produced by the same model source, a current dipole in a homogeneously conducting sphere, as detected by an array of 36 vertical second-order gradiometers and by an array of 36 planar "quadratic" gradiometers. Figure 3b—d illustrate pattern modifications versus source orientation.

There is another important aspect related to the choice of sensor configuration. Bruno et al. (1986) showed that a gradiometric geometry can be regarded as a spatial filter tending to enhance higher spatial frequencies. Planar devices feature similar but even more pronounced property (Ernè & Romani, 1985; Tesche, 1985). Consequently these configurations are somewhat less suitable for investigating deep sources, whereas they can always be recommended when the pattern features a large content of high spatial frequencies. Ernè and Romani (1985) showed that planar gradi-

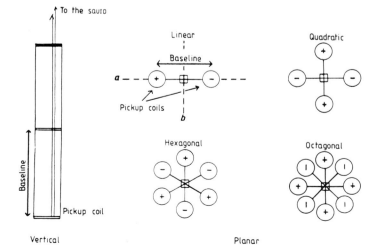

Figure 2. Schematic drawing of a "vertical" second-order gradiometer and of the four simplest geometries for planar gradiometers. The square in the center of each planar device schematically represents the DC SQUID.

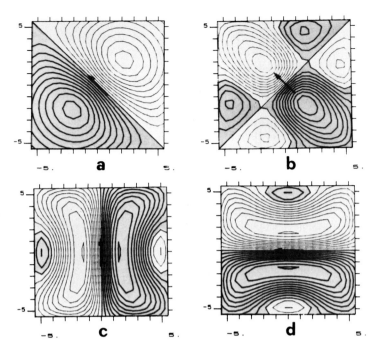

Figure 3. (a) Simulated iso-field contour map illustrating the field distribution from a current dipole (arrow, 5 cm depth) as detected by an array of 36 vertical gradiometers (1 cm pickup coil diameter, 5 cm baseline). (b) The same simulation performed for an array of 36 planar quadratic gradiometers (0.5 cm pickup coil diameter, 1.5 cm baseline). The dependence of pattern shape on source orientation is shown in (c) and (d). It is worth remarking the different field polarity in (c) and (d).

ometers are in fact particularly useful in identifying complex source configurations; here they have an unrivaled advantage over vertical gradiometric geometries.

Modeling and Source Localization

It has been shown repeatedly that the most convenient approach to the solution of the inverse problem by magnetic measurements consists of (a) the choice of a simple model, (b) calculating from it the magnetic field distribution, and (c) comparing the calculated distribution to the experimentally measured one (Williamson & Kaufman, 1981b; Romani et al., 1982; Romani & Leoni, 1985). This source should be simple enough to be mathematically tractable but sufficiently realistic from a physiological point of view. Considering the basic process underlying the propagation of activation along the neural system, namely the action potential, the current dipole model has been repeatedly proposed and adopted (Grynzpan & Geselowitz, 1973; Williamson & Kaufman, 1981b). Figure 4a schematically illustrates the ionic current flows

inside and outside a neutral branch and Figure 4b the source used to model this activity. A theoretical analysis (see for instance Williamson & Kaufman, 1987) of the properties of this source shows that, as long as the source is immersed in a homogeneously conducting medium, the magnetic field at a point P is independent of volume currents, i.e., extracellular currents. This property, which immediately points out one of the advantages of the magnetic approach, is maintained also in the presence of a spherical boundary to the medium, provided that only the component of the magnetic field normal to the sphere is measured. The theoretical pattern displayed by this component onto the sphere surface is symmetric, shows two regions of maximum field with opposite polarity (see Figure 5), and maintains this symmetry for rotation of the current dipole from a tangential direction to a radial one. Radial current flows do not produce any external field as do dipoles in the center of the sphere. This drawback, however, can prove to be a significant advantage, in that it "cancels" part of the effects of cerebral activity and most likely makes things easier to interpret.

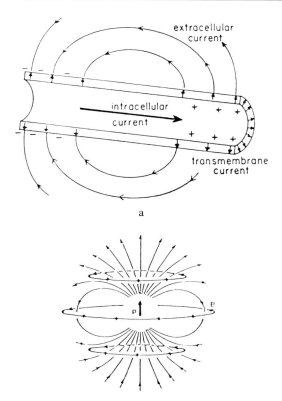

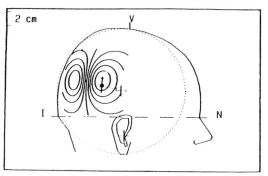

Figure 5. Spatial distribution of the normal component of the magnetic field from a current dipole over the surface of a spherical medium with homogeneous conductivity. The smallest loops identify regions of maximum field with opposite polarity.

Figure 4. (a) Schematic representation of a dendritic trunk, illustrating the different current flows occurring at a cellular level (courtesy of S. J. Williamson). (b) The current dipole model source is immersed in an infinite medium with homogeneous conductivity: the thin lines represent the "volume" currents, i.e., the current lines closing the loop created by the "primary" current (thick arrow). The transverse circles are the magnetic field lines.

It should be clear that the magnetic measurement provides a tool to directly investigate primary sources of cerebral activity, with no contribution in the ideal case, and only a minor "spoiling" in the real one, due to volume currents and the intervening tissue. A localization algorithm (Romani & Leoni, 1985) can be used to compare the theoretical and experimental field distributions—typically based on a least squares fit—and source localization can be achieved. Simple statistical procedures can be adopted to get the level of significance of the fit and the 95% confidence interval.

There are, however, some considerations which must be pointed out. First, to fully evaluate whether the localization is correct, we should be at least aware of, or better yet calculate, the effect of volume curents on the measured field distribution in the "real" case, when an actual head is measured and not a sphere. Several authors have estimated this contribution to be on the order of a few percent of the total field (Barth et al., 1986; Ricci et al., 1987). This problem is of remarkable importance now, but will be even more important for "large" multi-channel systems, where a wide portion of the head will be simultaneously measured and significant discrepancies will occur for the distances between the head surface and the dewar.

Second, it has been stressed on several occasions (see, for instance, Romani, 1984) that fortunately most of the primary areas are located inside fissures, and consequently current flows associated with cortical activity at a pyramidal cell level feature a preferential direction tangential to the surface. This certainly is one of the reasons why the most impressive and accurate results have been obtained in the study of evoked fields from primary areas. Nevertheless, it is relatively infrequent to have current flows concentrated in a tiny volume, or to activate a single "source" at a time. The brain is a much more complex machine, and the configuration of the sources underlying a specific cerebral activity is generally complex. This statement holds even more strictly if the investigation is shifted to paroxysmal activity, as in epilepsy, where larger areas of the cortex may be involved. Additionally, it is commonly agreed that evoked fields and potentials from the scalp, as far as "near fields" are concerned, originate mainly from post-synaptic activity, whereas "far fields"—generated in sub-cortical structures as well as within the peripheral nervous system—are likely to be related to propagating action potentials (Rossini, personal communication). It is usually assumed that a single dipole holds also for post-synaptic activity. Experimentally it has been shown in a number of presentations that the post-synaptic activity elicited by electrical stimulation in a patch of cortex can be represented as a dipole layer oriented perpendicularly to the cortical surface (Landau, 1967; Creutzfeldt et al., 1969; Freeman, 1975; Nunez, 1981; Lopes da Silva & van Rotterdam, 1987; Mitzdorf, 1985). The same holds also for the cortical alpha rhythm (Lopes da Silva & van Rotterdam, 1987; Mitzdorf, 1985).

On the basis of these considerations it is clear that the simple single-dipole-source is often not appropriate to the task and that either more dipoles or more sophisticated sources should be used. Ernè and co-workers (1987) have recently performed a detailed analysis of the properties of a quadrupolar source, which represents a higher term in the multipole expansion of the magnetic field. Put simply, a multipole analysis, even if truncated at the quadrupolar term, might be regarded as adding a correction term to the traditional dipole analysis, which may account for a relatively widespread current distribution. On the other hand, we should consider that a quadrupole is a tensorial quantity, the five components of which may be considered as combinations of two current dipoles with antiparallel orientation and separated by an infinitesimal gradient in each of three orthogonal directions. According to this definition, Q_{xy} for example represents two antiparallel dipoles oriented along the X axis and separated by a small gradient dy in the Y direction, and so on. Figure 6 shows the five components of a current quadrupole. It is worth stressing that the last two components, Q_{xz}

and Q_{yz}, must be considered as pseudo-dipolar in that they are indistinguishable from a real dipolar source. From this point of view, it is clear that current flows like those schematically depicted in Figure 6 are not completely unrealistic from a physiological perspective, and that the use of a quadrupolar term may improve the localization accuracy or even permit localization when the simple dipole is not effective, as shown in the next section.

Functional Localization for Somatosensory Evoked Fields

As mentioned in the introduction, a few multichannel instruments are currently in operation all over the world. All these systems consist of a few adjacent magnetic sensors and, consequently, adequate field mapping can be achieved only by a sequence of successive measurements—with all the limitations and drawbacks pointed out in the previous section. Nevertheless, the quality of results so far obtained is definitely impressive and promises further and more significant achievements. In this section we will briefly describe some of the results obtained since 1984 in the study of somatosensory evoked fields using the four-channel instrumentation operating at the Istituto di Elettronica dello Stato Solido—CNR in Rome. This system consists of four second-order vertical gradiometers, with a long baseline (b = 7 cm), designed to be particularly suitable for deep source investigation. It should be noted that the same system has been and is being used for several other studies, including auditory and visual evoked fields (Narici et al., 1987a; Narici et al., 1987b), spontaneous activity and clinical study of patients affected by focal and photosensitive epilepsy (Ricci et al., 1987).

Figure 7 shows an example of evoked responses from a normal subject in response to electrical stimulation of the median nerve at the wrist. Details of the experimental paradigm are reported elsewhere (Rossini et al., 1987; Rossini et al., submitted), and are typical for this kind of measurements. The recording bandwidth was 1–1000 Hz, which is somewhat novel for magnetic measurement. Two

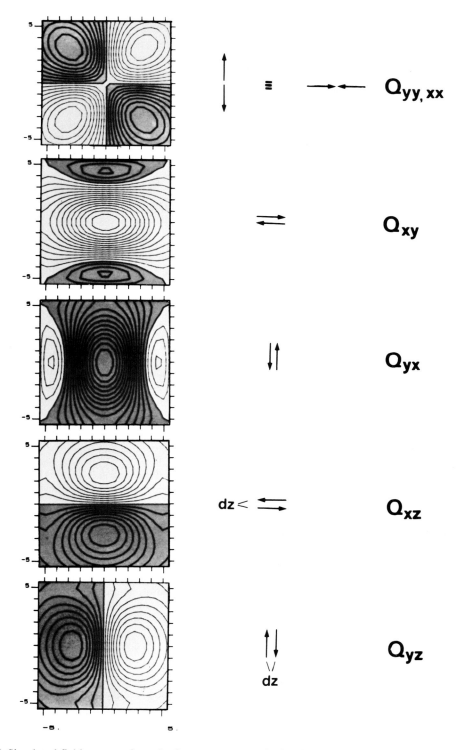

Figure 6. Simulated field patterns from the five components (depicted on the right) of a current quadrupole (5 cm depth) as detected by an array of 36 vertical gradiometers (see captions Figure 3).

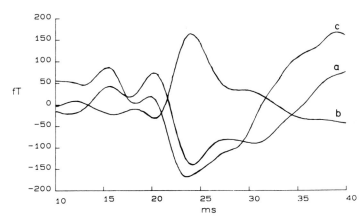

Figure 7. Evoked magnetic and electric response (subj. FZ) under median nerve electric stimulation at the wrist. (a) and (b) were recorded at the scalp sites of maximum field with opposite polarity for the 20 ms component. (c) is the evoked potential measured simultaneously with (a).

magnetic traces (a, b) and one electric (c) are shown in the figure. The first two correspond to the positions of maximum field with opposite polarity (for the N20 component) whereas c) was recorded simultaneously with a) from the derivation C_x-left ear lobe, where C_x was located midway between C_4 and P_4. The electric signal simultaneous with b) is not shown as it is identical to c). The traces show several components, some of which feature the same latency in the EFs and in the EP, whereas others do not. In particular, the first component clearly appreciable in the EFs had a peak latency of about 15 ms, the same as that for the corresponding component in the EP. It should be remarked that the polarity of this early component reverses in the two EFs, although its amplitude appears significantly reduced in b). The following components undergo a mirror-reflection behavior in the EFs, but are not always in phase with the corresponding EP. This immediately addresses the problem of interpreting the cortical activity produced by median nerve stimulation as due to a single generator, located in the posterior bank of the Rolandic fissure, or to multiple generators in both the somatosensory and motor cortex. This is not the place to discuss this long-standing question in detail. The interested reader is directed to more specific references (Wood et al., 1985; Rossini et al., 1987; Rossini et al., submitted). We want to stress here only what is evident from magnetic data.

For our purposes it is preferable to „trans-form" the information contained in the temporal traces of the EFs into isofield maps, illustrating the spatial distribution of the magnetic field over the scalp at successive latencies from the stimulus. This is shown in the color maps of Figure 8. They permit following the scalp distribution of the field in steps of 1 ms. The reference frame has its origin at the crossing of the nasion-inion horizontal line, i.e. Frankfort line, with the ear-to-ear line through the vertex. The vertical lines are all perpendicular to the Frankfort line and to the vertical line joining nasion to inion. The spatial units are in cm and the step between adjacent isofield contours is 5 fT. The field distribution undergoes several polarity reversals in the time window illustrated by the maps. A clearcut dipolar feature appears evident in, and constitutes a stable pattern across, many of the maps. Consequently we are allowed to apply the source localization procedure whenever possible. Figure 9 illustrates the result of this procedure obtained for the 15, 20 and 24 ms components. The localized equivalent dipoles are positioned inside the actual profiles of the subject's head and are included in their respective 95% confidence intervals. The position of the equivalent source for the early component with 15 ms latency is relatively deep (about 5 cm), suggesting a sub-cortical location of the active area. The other two sources are shallower, about 2 cm and 3.5 cm respectively, thus suggesting a cortical location. For the moment, no further consideration is made of the significant forward dis-

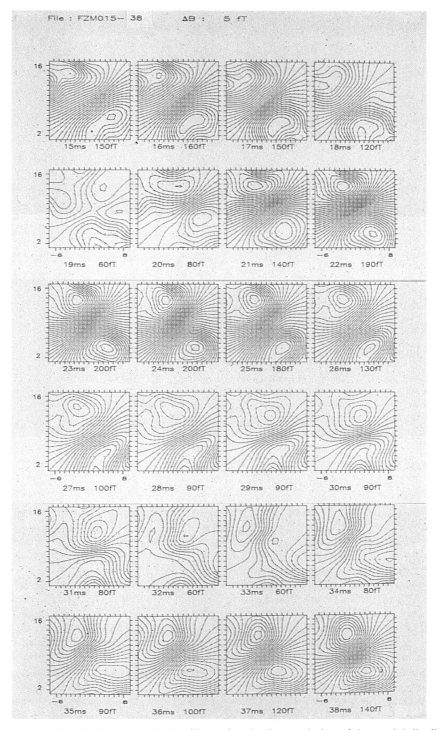

Figure 8. Sequence of iso-field maps (subj. FZ) illustrating the time evolution of the spatial distribution of the magnetic field in the latency range 15–38 ms. The step between adjacent iso-field lines is 5 femtoTesla. The reference frame is described in the text.

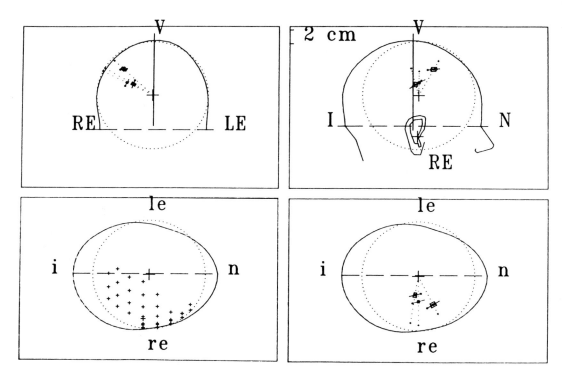

Figure 9. Three-dimensional localization (sub. FZ) carried out from the maps of the previous figure with latencies 15 (middle size box), 20 (large size box) and 24 ms (small size box), respectively. The localization is shown in the actual profiles of the subject's head. Crosses in the lower left panel represent the positions of the experimental points over the scalp.

placement of the source of the 20 ms component, suggestive of possible involvement of the motor cortex. The equivalent source for the 24 ms component could well be located at the bottom of the Rolandic fissure. A similar localization procedure performed on the last map of the series shown in Figure 8, gives a localization radially consistent with that of the 24 ms component, but at a shallower depth (2.7 cm). This is in agreement with previous findings (Narici et al., 1987 a) that demonstrated for the 40 ms component a dependence of depth of source location on stimulus repetition rate.

Before concluding, it should be stressed that although dipolar characteristics are common in most of the magnetic field maps recorded under electric stimulation of the median nerve, it is not infrequent to detect more complicated field patterns, particularly in the "transition" between one stable dipolar distribution and another. Figure 10 shows the isofield maps obtained with a quite similar procedure on a different subject. Again, three equivalent sources can easily be localized for components with 18, 23, and 26 ms latencies. Again their location is first quite deep (5 cm), then shallow (1.8 cm) and then in a place which could well be at the bottom of the Rolandic fissure (3.8 cm). Nevertheless, the map at 24 ms latency has a particular feature which merits discussion in some detail. This map probably represents a situation in which the immediately preceding activity is not completely finished, whereas the immediately following one is still growing. Such a condition cannot be represented by a single source, and in fact the map shows a much more complicated pattern. It is, however, possible to use a multipole expansion analysis—even if trun-

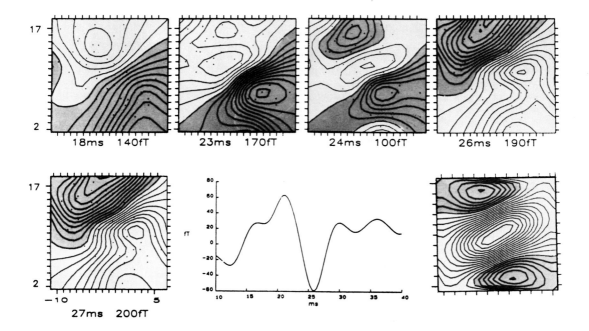

Figure 10. Sequence of iso-field contour maps, measured from subj. RT, illustrating the temporal evolution of the field distribution under median nerve stimulation, in correspondence to the latencies indicated below each map. The step between adjacent iso-field lines is 5fT. The insert shows the evoked field as measured at position (−5,13) of the recording grid. The unlabeled map shows the simulated iso-field map from two equally intense components Q_{xx} and Q_{xy} of a current quadrupole at 5 cm depth. This map should be compared qualitatively with the experimental map with 24 ms latency.

cated at the quadrupolar term. The theoretical field distribution obtained by a simple combination of Q_{xx} and Q_{xy} at a depth of 1.5 cm and with the same intensity is shown at the bottom right of Figure 10. It permits a qualitative comparison of the two maps. The agreement— even if only qualitative at this stage—is surprisingly good and holds promise of fruitful use for a multipole analysis.

Conclusions

Space limitations prevented providing more than just a hint of what is going on in the field. Instrumentation is improving rapidly with several "few-channel" systems in use all over the world, and many projects on "class 100" multi-channel systems in progress. The technology is already adequate for the task, even if additional advantages can come from the adoption of novel geometries for the detection coils, i.e., planar gradiometers. At the same time, the localization procedures, presently based on the simple single-dipole model, should be improved and include more sophisticated modeling, like for instance multipole analysis. In fact, although the dipolar source works quite well in specific cases, it fails when more sources are simultaneously present or widespread activity occurs. In this case we have seen that the inclusion of a quadrupolar term may surprisingly improve the quality of the results. Nevertheless, while awaiting the "ultimate" system, important findings may be collected both in basic research on brain function and on the clinical side, and bring us closer to the goal of "real-time" functional localization.

References

Bain RJP, Jones AE, Donaldson GB (1987) Design of high-order superconducting planar gradiometers with shaped asymmetric near-source response. *Proc Appl Sup Conf Baltimore, USA.*

Barth DS, Sutherling W, Broffman J, Beatty J (1986) Magnetic localization of a dipolar current source implanted in a sphere and a human cranium. *Electroenceph clin Neurophysiol, 63,* 260—273.

Bruno AC, Costa Ribeiro P, von der Weid JP (1986) Discrete spatial filtering with SQUID gradiometers in biomagnetism. *J Appl Phys, 59,* 2584—2589.

Carelli P, Foglietti V (1983) A second-derivative gradiometer integrated with a dc superconducting interferometer. *J Appl Phys, 54,* 6065—6067.

Carelli P, Leoni R (1986) Localization of biological sources with arrays of superconducting gradiometers. *J Appl Phys, 59,* 645—650.

Cohen D (1979) Magnetic measurement and display of current generators in the brain. Part I: The 2-D detector. *Proc V Inter Conf Med Phys, Jerusalem, Israel,* 15—19.

Creutzfeldt OD, Rosina A, Ito M, Probst W (1969) Visual evoked response of single cells and of the EEG in primary visual area of the cat. *J Neurophysiol, 32,* 127—139.

Ernè SN, Romani GL (1985) Performances of higher order planar gradiometers for biomagnetic source localization. In Hahlbohm HD, Lubbig H (Eds.) *SQUID85: Superconducting quantum interference devices and their applications.* Walter de Gruyter, Berlin-New York, 951—961.

Ernè SN, Trahms L, Trontelj Z (1987, in press) Current mulitpoles as sources of biomagnetic and bioelectric data. *Proc 6th Inter Conf on Biomagnetism, Tokyo, Japan.*

Freeman WJ (1975) *Mass action of the nervous system.* Academic Press, New York.

Grynzpan F, Geselowitz DB (1973) Model studies of the magnetocardiogram. *Biophys J, 13,* 911-925.

Landau WM (1967) Evoked potentials. In Quarton GC, Melnechnk T, Schmidt FO (Eds.) *The neurosciences – A study program.* Rockefeller University Press, New York.

Lopes da Silva FH, van Rotterdam A (1987) Biophysical aspects of EEG and MEG generation. In Niedermayer R, Lopes da Silva FH (Eds.) *Electoencephalography.* Urban and Schwarzenberg, Baltimore, 29—41.

Lopes da Silva FH, Storm van Leeuwen W (1978) The cortical alpha rhythm in dog. The depth and surface profile of phase. In Brazier MA, Petsche H (Eds.) *Architectonics of cerebral cortex.* Raven Press, New York, 319—333.

Mitzdorf U (1985) Current source-density method and application in cat cerebral cortex: Investigation of evoked potentials and EEG phenomena. *Physiol Rev, 65,* 37—100.

Narici L, Romani GL, Salustri C, Pizzella V, Torrioli G, Modena I (1987a) Neuromagnetic characterization of the cortical response to median nerve stimulation in the steady state paradigm. *Int J Neuroscience, 32,* 837—843.

Narici L, Romani GL, Salustri C, Pizzella V, Modena I, Papanicolaou (1987b) Neuromagnetic evidence of synchronized spontaneous activity in the brain following repetitive sensory stimulation. *Int J Neuroscience, 32,* 831—836.

Nunez PL (1981) *Electric fields of the brain: The neurophysics of EEG.* Oxford University Press, New York.

Ricci GB, Romani GL, Salustri C, Pizzella V, Torrioli G, Buonomo S, Peresson M, Modena I (1987) Study of focal epilepsy by multichannel neuromagnetic measurements. *Electroenceph clin Neurophysiol, 66,* 358—368.

Romani GL (1984) Biomagnetism: An application of SQUID sensors to medicine and physiology. *Physica, 126B,* 70—81.

Romani GL (1987) The inverse problem in MEG studies: An instrumental and analytical perspective. *Phys Med Biol, 1,* 23—31.

Romani GL, Leoni R (1985) Localization of cerebral sources with neuromagnetic measurements. In Weinberg H, Stroink G, Katila T (Eds.) *Biomagnetism: Applications and theory.* Pergamon Press, New York-Toronto, 205—220.

Romani GL, Narici L (1986) Principles and clinical validity of the biomagnetic method. *Med Progr through Technol, 11,* 123—159.

Romani GL, Williamson SJ, Kaufman L (1982) Biomagnetic instrumentation. *Rev Sci Instrum, 53,* 1815—1845.

Rossini P, Cilli M, Narici L, Peresson M, Pizzella V, Romani GL, Salustri C, Traversa R, Di Luzio S (1987, in press) Short-latency somatosensory evoked activity to median nerve stimulation: Differences in electric and magnetic scalp recordings. *Proc 6th Intern Conf on Biomagnetism, Tokyo, Japan.*

Rossini P, Narici L, Romani GL, Traversa R, Cecchi L, Cilli M, Urbano A (submitted) Short-latency somatosensory evoked responses in healthy humans: electric and magnetic recordings. *Ex Brain Res.*

Tesche C (1985) Design of compensated planar input coils for biomagnetic measurements. In Hahlbohm HD, Lubbig H (Eds.) *SQUID85: Superconducting quantum interference devices and their applications.* Walter de Gruyter, Berlin-New York, 933—937.

Williamson SJ, Kaufman L (1981a) Biomagnetism. *J Magn Mat, 22,* 129—201.

Williamson SJ, Kaufman L (1981 b) Magnetic fields of the cerebral cortex. In Ernè SN, Hahlbohm HD, Lubbig H (Eds.) *Biomagnetism.* Walter de Gruyter, Berlin-New York, 353–402.

Williamson SJ, Kaufman L (1987) Analysis of neuromagnetic signals. In Gevins A, Remond A (Eds.) *Methods of analysis of brain electric and magnetic signals* (Handbook of Electroencephalography and Clinical Neurophysiology, Vol 1). Elsevier, Amsterdam, 405–448.

Wood CC, Cohen D, Cuffin BN, Yarita M, Allison T (1985) Electrical sources in human somatosensory cortex: Identification by combined magnetic and potential recording. *Science, 227,* 1051–1053.

Evoked Magnetic Fields
in the Study of Somatosensory Cortical Areas

J. Huttunen

This paper describes examples of topographical distribution of somatosensory evoked magnetic fields (SEFs) in healthy subjects. The data were obtained with 1st order SQUID gradiometers, with either 3 or 7 channels for simultaneous recording. After stimulation of an upper limb nerve, the SEF consists of a small N20m deflection, followed by more prominent peaks with opposite polarity at 40 ms and 80 ms, and a late wave between 100 ms and 200 ms. The topographical field patterns of these deflections may be interpreted in terms of single equivalent current dipoles, lying close to each other within or near the primary hand projection cortex. Similarly, after lower limb stimulation, the SEF complex measured on top of the head reflects a sequential activation of several current sources, which lie near the foot primary projection area. Apart from these primary sensorimotor areas, SEFs may be recorded at the lateral aspects of the head. These bilateral responses may be explained by equivalent current dipoles at the second somatosensory cortex (SII). A novel somatosensory offset response from the primary sensorimotor cortex is additionally described. It is concluded that MEG recordings provide a useful aid in the attempt to identify the neural generators of somatosensory evoked responses.

In order to study processing of sensory information in the human cerebral cortex by means of non-invasive electro- or magnetoencephalographic recordings (EEG and MEG, respectively), it is necessary to attempt to identify the neural sources of various evoked response deflections. Using electrical recordings, this question has been approached in three ways: intracranial potential recordings, correlation of scalp potential changes with cerebral pathology, and recording topographical distribution of scalp potentials. Although these methods have provided valuable information about evoked response generators, they all have some limitations. For example, intracranial recordings are restricted to those justified on clinical grounds and brain lesions are often widespread and poorly delineated. Interpretation of scalp topography is hampered by the multitude of possible current sources for a given scalp distribution. Accordingly, the events underlying, for example, somatosensory evoked potentials (SEPs) after the earliest cortical deflections are still poorly understood.

Topographical mapping of evoked magnetic fields gives information complementary to EEG about cortical activation patterns after sensory input, and may help to identify current sources of evoked responses (for reviews on MEG, see Hari & Ilmoniemi, 1986; Williamson & Kaufman, 1987). In the case of spherical symmetry, modelling of the neutral sources is expected to be simpler for evoked magnetic fields than evoked potentials, because in MEG the possible generators are restricted to tangential current sources. In EEG both radial and tangential current sources, alone or in combination, must be con-

Low Temperature Laboratory, Helsinki University of Technology, 02150 Espoo, Finland.
The author wishes to thank all members of the neuromagnetism group of the Low Temperature Laboratory of Helsinki University of Technology for encouragement and collaboration. These studies were financially supported by the Academy of Finland and the Sigrid Juselius Foundation.

sidered as possible generators. In addition, MEG is more selectively sensitive to superficial, i.e. mainly cortical, current sources than EEG.

Although the selectivity of MEG to tangential sources holds only for spherical symmetry, recent modelling studies indicate that, locally, the spherical model is a good approximation of the human head. For example, in the case of realistic head geometry, radial current sources do not seem to contribute much to the radial component of the magnetic field over posterior temporal and occipital areas (Hämäläinen & Sarvas, 1987).

Further differences between MEG and EEG include the fact that the magnetic field extrema on the head produced by a given current dipole source are nearer to each other than the extrema of the corresponding EEG distribution. This results from the transparency of biological tissues to magnetic signals and contrasts the distorting effect especially of the skull on volume conducted potentials. Because of this difference, essential features of the MEG pattern of a given source are confined to a smaller area than those of the corresponding EEG pattern, and hence the magnetic signals are less likely to be contaminated by simultaneous activity elsewhere in the brain. Finally, MEG, unlike EEG, is not a referential recording. This difference is relevant for topographic studies, because using an "active" reference may cause misleading interpretations on visual inspection of a potential map. Similar ambiguities do not exist for magnetic field maps.

Taking into account that cortical current flow mainly occurs perpendicular to the surface of the cortex, it follows from the preceding discussion that MEG is a useful tool in studying fissural cortical areas. These include parts of the primary sensorimotor cortex (SMI) in the walls of the central sulcus and the entire second somatosensory cortex (SII) within the upper wall of the lateral sulcus. This paper gives examples of activation of these areas following stimulation of peripheral nerves as studied by recording somatosensory evoked magnetic fields (SEFs) in healthy human subjects. Previously, SEF studies have been reviewed by Hari and Kaukoranta (1985).

Activation of the Primary Sensorimotor Cortex

Hand Projection Area

Figure 1 shows averaged SEFs measured at different locations over the right hemisphere after electrical stimulation of the left median nerve. These responses represent preliminary data recorded with a novel, low-noise (5–6 fT/Hz) 1st-order gradiometer (Knuutila et al., 1987). The SEF consists of several peaks, all of which reverse polarity between medial and lateral recording locations over SMI. Within 100 ms after the stimulus, three peaks may be invariably identified, although some of the subjects show more complex waveforms.

The first deflection starts at 16 ms and peaks at 20 ms. By analogy to the SEPs, it is called N20m, where m stands for magnetic. At the recording locations of Figure 1, no activity can be discerned before 16 ms. The peak latency of N20m is the same at all measurement locations. This is at variance with SEPs, which may show different peak latencies at different recording sites, indicating overlapping activation of tangential (N20) and radial current sources (P22 or P25). The magnetic field distribution is simpler, because of lack deflections corresponding to the P22 and P25 potentials.

The next deflection peaks at 30–45 ms in different subjects and is opposite in polarity to N20. We have called this peak P40m. It is followed by another peak in the same direction, designated as P80m. Figure 2, illustrating a response with a longer time window, shows that a slow deflection appears between 100 and 200 ms in the same direction as N20m. Sometimes this may last beyond 200 ms, or it may be followed by yet another slow deflection. The maximum amplitude of N20m and of the slow deflection after 100 ms is usually 100–300 fT, whereas P40m and P80m may exceed 1000 fT with an interstimulus interval of 1 s. No magnetic responses have been observed arising at SMI cortex ipsilateral to the stimulated side (Hari et al. 1984).

Figure 2 illustrates examples of topographic isocontour maps, based on measurements at 84 locations over the right SMI, at different latencies after stimulation of the left median

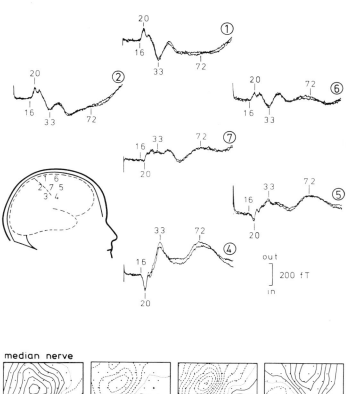

Figure 1. SEFs recorded over the right hemisphere with a 7-channel 1-st order dc-SQUID gradiometer (baseline 60 mm, pickup coil diameter 20 mm); data from channel 3 are not shown because of malfunction during this measurement. The approximate recording locations are shown on the schematic head. Each trace is an average of 1000 responses, Recording bandwidth is 0.5—2000 Hz. Two averaged responses from successive measurements are superimposed.

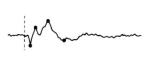

Figure 2. Isofield contour maps at the peak latencies of N20m, P40m, P80m and a late deflection at 170 ms, produced by left median nerve stimulation in one subject. The field maps were calculated with a weighted least-squares approximation; all amplitudes were measured with respect to a prestimulus baseline. Solid lines indicate flux out of the head and dotted lines flux into the head. Difference between isocontour lines is 60 fT. The dots on the hexagonal lattice show the gradiometer pickup coil locations and the insert illustrates the measurement area on the scalp. Arrows indicate sites and orientations of the equivalent current dipoles. Open circles mark the location of C4. Goodness of fit is denoted by g.

nerve. The field pattern appears dipolar at the peak latencies of all four main deflections of the response. For N20m, the field emerges from the head at locations near the midline and enters it at lateral locations. The distance between field extrema is 6—7 cm. Similar field maps for N20m have been reported by other authors (Hari et al., 1984; Wood et al., 1985; Kaukoranta et al., 1986a; Rossini et al., 1987). The equivalent current dipole, found by a least-squares fit in a spherical head model, is located beneath the zero isofield line midway between the field extremes, and the depth estimates vary between 2 cm and 4 cm. This loca-

tion is 12—14 cm above the ear canal and corresponds well with the site of the SMI hand area contralateral to the stimulated wrist. The probable site of origin for N20m, which represents the first cortical activation, is Brodmann's area 3b at the posterior wall of the central sulcus. Pointing anteriorly, the equivalent current dipole is consistent with current flow toward cortical surface at area 3b, being consistent with excitation of pyramidal neurones near cell somata at cortical layers IIIb and IV. Such a pattern of excitation is thought to be the first cortical event after sensory stimulation (Creutzfeldt, 1983).

The field pattern of P40m also appears dipolar, but now the field emerges from the head at lateral locations and enters it medially. While the exact generator of P40m in terms of cytoarchitectonic areas may not be identified from the field maps, some conclusions are possible based on comparison with the field pattern of N20m. The equivalent current dipole for P40m points posteriorly and is located near but slightly more medial to the N20m dipole. Therefore the neural populations underlying N20m and P40m cannot be identical. We have consistently observed this tendency of P40m dipoles to be located more medially than the N20m for both median and ulnar nerve stimulation (Huttunen et al., 1987a). Therefore, because it has been reported that the precentral motor hand area is more medially located than the corresponding postcentral sensory hand area (Woolsey et al., 1979; Celesia, 1979), one possibility is that P40m arises at the motor cortex within the anterior wall of the central sulcus. However, it is possible that after the initial cortical activation the SEF reflects summated activity of multiple generators. For example, postexcitatory inhibitory potentials in the same cells that underlie N20m may also contribute to generation of P40m. We have not observed systematic anteroposterior differences between N20m and P40m dipole locations; this may be due to the fact that the localizing error is greater in the direction of the dipole than perpendicular to it. More extensive studies, possibly correlating the SEF with pre- and postcentral cortical lesions, are therefore needed to fully establish to what extent a precentral generator may be assigned to P40m.

The field pattern of P80m is also dipolar and similar to the pattern of P40m, but the location of the equivalent current dipole differs significantly from that of N20m and P40m. A comparison of field patterns in response to ulnar and median nerve stimulation (Huttunen et al., 1987a) revealed that the N20m and P40m dipoles were more medially located for ulnar nerve than for median nerve stimulation. This difference is attributable to the somatotopical organization of SMI where the thumb is the most laterally represented of the fingers. On the other hand, P80m dipoles were very close to each other, disclosing no mediolateral differences for ulnar and median nerve stimulation. Therefore, P80m appears to represent more widespread activity than the earlier deflections, perhaps including parietal association areas, where somatotopic organization becomes less accurate (Hyvärinen & Poranen, 1978; Iwamura et al. 1983). However, postexcitatory inhibition at area 3b may also contribute to P80m, which, then, may reflect activity of several distinct sources. This interpretation agrees with the conclusion of Arezzo et al. (1981), based on epi- and transcortical recordings in monkeys, that with increasing latency wider areas within SMI and adjacent association areas are responsible for the generation of the somatosensory potential.

The slow SEF deflection between 100 and 200 ms demonstrates a remarkable difference between SEFs and SEPs. During this magnetic deflection, the field emerges from the head near the midline and enters it at lateral locations. The pattern again resembles one produced by a current dipole, which lies near those for the earlier deflections, suggesting that the underlying activity occurs near SMI. By contrast, the scalp SEP is dominated after 100 ms by the widespread vertex potential whose generators are unknown and which masks simultaneous activity at SMI (Goff et al., 1980). An equivalent of the vertex potential is not seen in the SEFs, which demonstrate activation of sources near SMI up to 200 ms after stimulation; therefore, recording of magnetic fields appears to be more suitable than recording of scalp potentials in the study of long-latency events in SMI.

Because the dipole locations significantly differ from each other at the peak latencies of the four main deflections, the SEF complex as a whole reveals a sequential activation of multiple current sources within or near SMI up to 200 ms after stimulation. We have assessed goodness of fit of the dipole model with the measured field patterns by calculating the amount of variance in the measured patterns that can be accounted for by the dipole model. In the example of Figure 2, the fit of the dipole model with the data 88—92% for N20m, P40m and P80m, but only 73% for the late deflection peaking at 170 ms. Figure 3 shows goodness-of-fit values at different latencies for the median nerve SEF. Least-

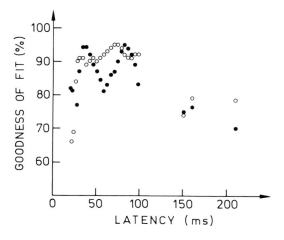

Figure 3. Goodness-of-fit values of the dipole model with the measured field patterns at different latencies after median nerve stimulation in one subject.

After 100 ms the single dipole model does not explain the magnetic fields maps as well as before 100 ms; at present, it is not clear whether this is due to the relatively small amplitude of the long-latency deflection or to the complex nature of the source itself.

It should be emphasized that even good agreement of the data with the dipole model does not mean that the real current source is a pointlike current dipole. For example, modelling experiments have shown that, in the presence of experimental noise, field patterns produced by current dipole layers extending over several centimetres are indistinguishable from ideally dipolar patterns (Okada, 1985; Hari et al., 1988). Therefore, the location of an equivalent current dipole is considered to represent the center of mass of underlying activity. Changes of dipole locations with time, then, may be interpreted as changes in net neural activity.

Foot Projection Area

The lower limb SEF from the SMI foot area, illustrated in Figure 4, starts with a P40m deflection, whose field pattern may be accounted for by a parasagittally located equivalent current dipole pointing toward the opposite hemisphere and posteriorly (Huttunen et al., 1987b). P40m corresponds to the N20m of the upper limb SEF and represents the first cortical activation. The field pattern is again compatible with excitation within the middle cortical layers in the primary sensory projection area. The scalp distribution of the corresponding evoked potential, P40, likewise resembles one produced by a similar equivalent current dipole (Desmedt & Bourquet,

squares dipole fittings were performed every 4 ms from 20 to 100 ms and every 10 ms thereafter. It is seen that much of the variance in the measured pattern may be explained by a single current dipole throughout the period from 20 to 100 ms. This indicates that during the first 100 ms after stimulation, tangential current sources are constantly activated at SMI. Because these tangential sources must influence the scalp topograhpy of SEPs as well, the magnetic data might be used to extract the contribution of radial sources from the potential maps. This could be done by calculating the electric potential distribution caused by tangential sources detected with MEG mappings and subtracting potential maps obtained in this way from potential maps actually measured.

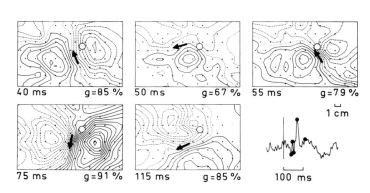

40 ms   g=85 %   50 ms   g=67 %   55 ms   g=79 %

1 cm

75 ms   g=91 %   115 ms   g=85 %   100 ms

Figure 4. Magnetic responses to stimulation of left posterior tibial nerve at the ankle, measured 2 cm anterior to the vertex (marked with the open circle), and corresponding isocontour field maps at the peak latencies of the response. Isofield separation is 50 fT. Other details as in Figure 2.

1985; Kakigi & Jones, 1986). However, the peak latencies of the P40 potential differ at the positive and negative maxima of the scalp distribution (Desmedt & Bourquet, 1985), indicating that a simple dipolar source does not fully explain the EEG pattern. Therefore, in the case of lower limb stimulation as well, the MEG pattern appears to be simpler to interpret. The equivalent current dipole for P40m, being almost perpendicular to the sagittal plane, explains the "paradoxical lateralization" of the corresponding evoked potential, namely that the positive potential maximum of P40 is measured over the hemisphere ipsilateral to stimulation (Lüders et al., 1987).

After P40m and before 100 ms, there are several peaks, whose configuration varies considerably from one subject to another. During these deflections the field patterns are not always dipolar. When they are, the source location is consistent with the site of the primary foot projection area but differs from the location of the P40m dipole. The non-dipolar nature of some of the field patterns is in contrast to upper limb SEFs, which are well accounted for by single equivalent current dipoles up to 100 ms after stimulation. This disparity may be due to anatomical differences between the hand and foot projection areas: the foot is represented both at the walls of the central and sagittal sulci which are almost perpendicular to each other, but at the hand area the sulci lie more in parallel to each other. The deflections after P40m of the lower limb SEF exemplify the need for more complex source models than the single dipole model.

In any event, the field patterns of the deflections following P40m differed considerably from those for P40m, indicating sequential activation of several generators at or near the primary foot projection area. In this respect, the results parallel the results of upper limb SEF studies.

Offset Response from the Primary Hand Projection Area

Figure 5 shows examples of responses from the right SMI when the thenar eminence was stimulated with electric pulse trains of 3 seconds' duration (Huttunen & Hari, 1987). In the trace showing any individual response, a prominent onset deflection is seen to occur after the first stimulus, followed by a steady-state response following the 10-Hz stimulation, and a large-amplitude, reproducible offset response peaking at 200 ms after the last stimulus in train. The offset response could be elicited at stimulation frequencies from 10 to 240 Hz, causing tetanization of thenar muscles without systematic changes in peak latency; it did not however occur with 5-Hz stimulation, which produced separate muscle twitches. Median nerve stimulation at the wrist also elicited onset-, offset- and steady-state responses, but stimulation of the cutaneous branches at the thumb only evoked a steady-state response. No off-response was observed at stimulation intensities below motor threshold.

The topographic field patterns of both on- and off-responses were dipolar and in agreement with neural currents at or near SMI. In

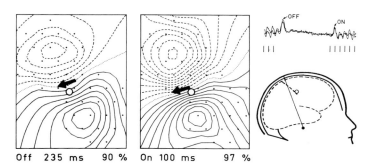

Figure 5. Responses to off- and onsets of 10-Hz stimulus trains delivered to the thenar eminence, and isocontour field maps at the peak latencies of the on- and off-responses. The responses are centered on the pause (1.1 s) between trains, so that the vertical lines on the left indicate the last stimuli and the lines on the right the first stimuli of the trains. The curves are filtered from 0.5 to 45 Hz. N = 200. Isofield contour separation is 50 fT. Other details as in Figure 2.

Off   235 ms   90 %   On 100 ms   97 %

two subjects with extensive field mappings, the dipole locations of on- and off-responses differed from each other by about 1 cm, indicating separate current sources.

This type of off-response has not been reported previously from SMI. It differs from the amply documented electrical auditory and visual off-responses by having a much longer latency than the corresponding onset response. Although our field mappings show an origin at SMI, the generation mechanism of the off-response may, of course, not be deduced from the mappings. However, because a tetanization of thenar muscles was necessary for its occurrence, the off-response might be related to the function of muscle spindle afferents. Studies correlating the offset response with pathology of afferent pathways might help to elucidate which ascending tracts participate in mediating this response.

Activation of the Second Somatosensory Cortex

Apart from locations near SMI, SEFs may be recorded at lateral aspects of the head (Hari et al., 1983; Kaukoranta et al., 1986 b). Figure 6 shows that a prominent response to stimulation of both ipsi- and contralateral peroneal nerves at the ankle is obtained about 6 cm above the ear canal. The peak latency of the response is about 100 ms and no activity can be discerned before 60 ms. The field pattern is dipolar, with equivalent current dipoles

located 1—2 cm above the T3/T4 points of the international 10—20 system, at a depth of 25—30 mm from scalp surface. This site corresponds well with the approximate location of SII in the upper wall of the lateral sulcus, in the region where the central and lateral sulci come close to each other.

Evidence for the existence of a human SII relies on cortical stimulation studies (Penfield & Jasper, 1954) and epicortical recording of evoked potentials (Lüders et al., 1985). With both methods, activity arising at SII has been found only in a minoritiy of brains studied. This may be due to the poorly accessible site of SII in the sulcal wall. The first deflection recorded from the exposed human SII cortex in response to median nerve stimulation peaked at 20—30 ms, only a few milliseconds after the first response at SMI (Lüders et al., 1985). Kaukoranta et al. (1986 b) did not observe comparable short-latency responses from SII. This disparity may be due to the different properties of MEG and EEG: the short-latency potentials recorded by Lüders and coworkers did not reverse polarity over the lateral sulcus and may hence have reflected activity at the convexial cortex rather than at the depth of the sulcal wall. On the other hand, it is possible that small early deflections have not been discerned in the SEFs because of noise.

Since both SMI and SII may be simultaneously activated by afferent input from peripheral nerves, it is of interest to look at the EEG and MEG distributions produced by

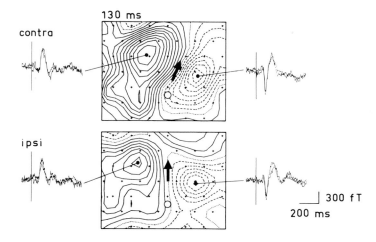

Figure 6. Responses from the lateral aspects of the head to stimulation of ipsi- and contralateral peroneal nerves at the ankle and corresponding isofield contour maps at the peak latencies of the main deflection. Bandwidth is 0.05—100 Hz. N = 150—200. T3 location is marked by a circle. Isofied contour separation is 30 fT. Other details as in Figure 2.

such co-activation. Figure 7 shows a computer simulation, which mimics the situation 100 ms after stimulation of a left limb nerve. Due to the considerable overlapping of the EEG patterns produced by the individual dipoles, the potential distribution is not suggestive of the sources causing it on either hemisphere. It rather resembles a potential distribution produced by a radial source near the SMI hand area. This may be one of the reasons why, in the scalp SEP, no components have been assigned with certainty to activation of SII. On the other hand, the magnetic field patterns are clearly separable and immediately suggest dipolar sources at correct locations. This is due to the smaller spatial extent of the magnetic field patterns and the fact that the dipoles are more favourably oriented for MEG. The simulation shows that studying the human SMI and SII separately is more feasible with evoked magnetic fields than with electric potentials.

ELECTRIC POTENTIAL   MAGNETIC FIELD

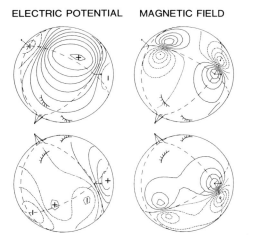

THREE-DIPOLE MODEL

Figure 7. A computer simulation of the electrical potential and magnetic field distributions 100 ms after stimulation of the left peroneal nerve. The arrows represent current dipoles at the right primary foot projection area and at both second somatosensory cortices. The simulation is done in a spherical volume conductor (radius 106 mm) with four layers of concentric inhomogeneities, corresponding to the brain, liquor space, skull and scalp; the corresponding conductivities are 0.33 S/m, 1.4 S/m, 0.006 S/m and 0.28 S/m. The dipole moments are 6 nAm, except for the ipsilateral dipole at SII for which it is 4 nAm. Separation between isofield lines is 100 fT and between isopotential lines 0.2 μV.

Conclusion

Much of evoked potential research still suffers from lack of exact knowledge of neural generators of the various potential deflections. Studies on SEFs have so far shown that MEG may be useful in generator identification, mainly because source modelling is simpler for magnetic fields than for volume conducted scalp potentials. So far, the SEF studies clearly have shown that areas at or near the site of primary sensory projection of afferent impulses are activated up to 200 ms after stimulation; MEG is therefore especially well suited for studying events at the primary projection cortex after sensory stimulation. Another major application of MEG lies in the apparently unique possibility to study SII, whose functional role is still poorly understood in man.

However, it should be noted that the exact generators, in terms of activated cytoarchitectonic areas, are still unknown for most SEF deflections from SMI. For example, reliable separation of pre- and postcentral activities has not yet been possible. It is hoped that this goal will be reached with mappings using the novel, sensitive multichannel gradiometers. Valuable information in this regard might be obtained by correlating SEFs with circumscribed lesions of pre- and postcentral cortex.

References

Arezzo JC, Vaughan HG, Legatt AD (1981) Topography and intracranial sources of somatosensory evoked potentials in the monkey. II. Cortical components. *Electroenceph clin Neurophysiol, 51,* 1—18.

Celesia GG (1979) Somatosensory evoked potentials recorded directly from human thalamus and SM I cortical area. *Arch Neurol, 36,* 399—405.

Creutzfeldt OD (1983) *Cortex cerebri.* Springer-Verlag, Berlin.

Desmedt JE, Bourquet M (1985) Color imaging of parietal and frontal somatosensory potential fields evoked by stimulation of median and posterior tibial nerve in man. *Electroenceph clin Neuropsyhsiol, 62,* 1—17.

Goff WR, Williamson PD, VanGlider JC, Allison T, Fisher TC (1980) Neural origins of long latency evoked potentials recorded from the depth and from cortical surface of the brain in man. In Desmedt JE (Ed.) *Clinical uses of cerebral, brainstem and spinal somatosensory evoked potentials. Progress in clinical neurophysiology, Vol. 7.* Karger, Basel, 125–145.

Hämäläinen M, Sarvas J (1987) Feasibility of the homogeneous head model in the interpretation of neuromagnetic fields. *Phys Med Biol, 32,* 91–97.

Hari R, Ilmoniemi R (1986) Cerebral magnetic fields. *CRC Crit Rev Biomed Engin, 14,* 93–126.

Hari R, Kaukoranta E (1985) Neuromagnetic studies of the somatosensory system: Principles and examples. *Progr Neurobiol, 24,* 233–256.

Hari R, Hämäläinen M, Kaukoranta E, Reinikainen K, Teszner D (1983) Neuromagnetic responses from the second somatosensory cortex in man. *Acta Neurol Scand, 68,* 207–212.

Hari R, Reinikainen K, Kaukoranta E, Hämäläinen M, Ilmoniemi R, Penttinen A, Salminen J, Teszner D (1984) Somatosensory evoked cerebral magnetic fields from SI and SII in man. *Electroenceph clin Neurophysiol, 57,* 254–263.

Hari R, Joutsiniemi S-L, Sarvas J (1988, in press) Spatial resolution of neuromagnetic recordings: theoretical calculations in a spherical model. *Electroenceph clin Neurophysiol.*

Huttunen J, Hari R (1987) Long-latency off-responses from the human sensorimotor cortex to tetanizing stimulation of thenar muscles. *Neurosci Lett, 74,* 63–68.

Huttunen J, Hari R, Leinonen L (1987a) Cerebral magnetic fields to stimulation of ulnar and median nerves. *Electroenceph clin Neurophysiol, 66,* 391–400.

Huttunen J, Kaukoranta E, Hari R (1987b) Cerebral magnetic responses to stimulation of tibial and sural nerves. *J Neurol Sci, 79,* 43–54.

Hyvärinen J, Poranen A (1978) Receptive field integration and submodality convergence in the hand area of the post-central gyrus of the alert monkey. *J Physiol, 283,* 539–556.

Iwamura Y, Tanaka M, Sakamoto M, Hikosaka O (1983) Converging patterns of finger representation and complex response properties of neurons in area 1 of the first somatosensory cortex of the conscious monkey. *Exp Brain Res, 51,* 327–337.

Kakigi R, Jones SL (1986) Influence of concurrent tactile stimulation on somatosensory evoked potentials following posterior tibial nerve stimulation in man. *Electroenceph clin Neurophysiol, 65,* 118–129.

Kaukoranta E, Hämäläinen M, Sarvas J, Hari R (1986a) Mixed and sensory nerve stimulations activate different cytoarchitectonic areas in the human somatosensory cortex. *Exp Brain Res, 63,* 60–66.

Kaukoranta E, Hari R, Hämäläinen M, Huttunen J (1986b) Cerebral magnetic fields evoked by peroneal nerve stimulation. *Somatosens Res, 3,* 309–321.

Knuutila J, Ahlfors S, Ahonen A, Hällström J, Kajola M, Lounasmaa OV, Vilkman V, Tesche C (1987) *A large-area low-noise sevenchannel DC SQUID magnetometer for brain research.* (Report of Helsinki University of Technology, TKK-F-A 613.)

Lüders H, Lesser RP, Dinner DS, Hahn JF, Salanga V, Morris HH (1985) The second sensory area in humans: Evoked potential and electrical stimulation studies. *Ann Neurol, 17,* 177–184.

Lüders H, Lesser RP, Dinner DS, Hahn J, Morris H, Wyllie E, Resor S (1987) The source of "paradoxical lateralization" of cortical evoked potentials to posterior tibial nerve stimulation. *Neurology, 37,* 82–88.

Okada YC (1985) Discrimination of localized and distributed current dipole sources and localized single and multiple sources. In Weinberg H, Stroink G, Katila T (Eds.) *Biomagnetism: Applications and theory.* Pergamon Press, New York, 266–272.

Penfield W, Jasper H (1954) *Epilepsy and functional anatomy of the human brain.* Little, Brown and Company, Boston.

Rossini PM, Caramia M, Romani GL, Salustri C, Pizzella V, Narici L, Modena I (1987) Scalp topography of electrical and magnetic somatosensory evoked signals: preliminary findings in healthy humans. In *Abstracts of the 3rd International Evoked Potentials Symposium,* Berlin.

Williamson SJ, Kaufman L (1987) Analysis of neuromagnetic signals. In Gevins A, Remond A (Eds.) *Methods of analysis of brain electrical and magnetic signals* (Handbook of Electroencephalography and Clinical Neurophysiology, Vol. 1). Elsevier, Amsterdam, 405–448.

Wood CC, Cohen D, Cuffin BN, Yarita M, Allison T (1985) Electrical sources in the human somatosensory cortex: identification by combined magnetic and potential field recordings. *Science, 227,* 1051–1053.

Woolsey CN, Erickson TC, Warren EG (1979) Localization in somatic sensory and motor areas of human cerebral cortex as determined by direct recording of evoked potentials and electric stimulation. *J Neurosurg, 51,* 476–506.

Source Localization of Human Brain Potentials Estimated by the Dipole-Tracing Method

S. Homma, Y. Nakajima, S. Watanabe*, H. Kamoshita, Y. Kawashima

Somatosensory evoked potentials (SEPs) elicited by electrical stimulation of the median nerve were simultaneously recorded in humans using twenty-one surface electrodes positioned on the scalp. Source generators of P14, N18, P22 and P40 were estimated by the dipole-tracing method. These generators were located in the brainstem, thalamus, and cortex, respectively. Double shock stimulation at an interval of less than 30 ms failed to elicit a discriminative sense of two stimuli. The component at 40 ms elicited by the second stimulus of the double shock did not show positivity. In this case, the location and vector direction of the equivalent dipole of P40 were different from those of P40 elicited by single shock. By subtracting SEPs elicited by single shock from those elicited by double shock, the equivalent dipole of the potential corresponding to P40 and generated by the second stimulus was calculated. The resulting dipole was located in the same region, but the vector was in the inverse direction of that of the dipole elicited by the single shock. It seems that the generation of this inverse potential in the cortex is closely related to loss of discriminative sense of the double shock.

We have developed a computer-aided method, designated the dipole-tracing (DT) method, to estimate the location of source generators of brain activity as an equivalent current dipole. The detailed mathematical expressions have been previously described (He et al. 1987; Homma et al., 1987). According to this method, the potential distribution, Φ_{obs}, is recorded in humans using twenty-one surface electrodes placed on the scalp. A separate potential distribution induced by a current dipole within a head model is calculated as φ_{cal}. The location and vector moment of the current dipole are iteratively changed within the head model until the squared difference between Φ_{obs} and Φ_{cal} is at a minimum. The location and vector moment of the dipole at this minimum is estimated as those of the source generator of brain activity.

Somatosensory evoked potentials (SEPs) elicited by electrical stimulation of the median nerve at the wrist were recorded using 21 surface electrodes attached to the scalp according to the international 10-20 method. In the present study, the source generators of several peaks such as P14, N18, P22 and P40 were estimated by this DT method.

Watanabe et al. (1985) preliminarily reported that when a double electrical shock is applied to the median nerve at stimulus intervals less than 30 ms, the subjects were not able to identify the successive double stimuli, and that the component at 40 ms elicited by the second stimulus did not show a clear positivity in this stimulus condition. It was found in the present study that the location and vector direction of the equivalent dipole of P40 elicited by the second stimulus are different from those of P40 elicited by single shock stimulation. This difference seems to be due to generation of another current dipole elicited by this stimulation condition. In the present study, this second dipole was estimated by subtracting SEPs elicited by single shocks from those of double shocks. This method was designated as the subtraction DT method.

Three-dimensional coordinates of 21 surface electrodes were measured by a special device, in which the x-y plane coincided with orbitomeatal lines and Cz was set as (O,O,z).

Department of Physiology, School of Medicine, Chiba University, Chiba 280, Japan.
* Chiba College of Health Science, Chiba 260, Japan.

For calculation of the potential distribution of Φ_{cal}, it was assumed that the head is embedded in an infinite and homogeneous medium. The accuracy of the DT method was expressed in terms of dipolarity (percentage) derived from normalized residue (the minimum squared difference between Φ_{obs} and Φ_{cal}). Thus a low dipolarity percentage means that the residue is large, and that the electrical phenomenon cannot be correctly expressed by a single equivalent dipole. The influence of diffuse electrical sources or more than two dipoles is a plausible reason of low dipolarity. In contrast, high dipolarity means that the electrical sources can be estimated as a single equivalent dipole and are restricted to a small region. In the present study, equivalent dipoles with greater than 90% dipolarity were adopted for further analysis.

Equivalent Dipoles of SEP

SEPs elicited by electrical stimulation of the right median nerve are shown in Figure 1A. Several peaks are seen at latencies about 14, 18, 22 and 40 ms after the stimulation. These are called P14, N18, P22 and P40 according to polarity and approximate latency. The equivalent dipoles which compose each of these peaks were calculated in five subjects as shown in Figure 2. The equivalent dipole of P14 is located ipsilaterally to the stimulation, near to the midline and in the brainstem with spatial variability, which is in agreement with the report that P14 is a potential reflecting the activity of the medial lemniscus fibers (Katayama & Tsubokawa, 1987). That of N18 is located contralaterally to the stimulation and a little lower than that of P14. It seems that the equivalent dipole is located in the thalamus as suggested by Hashimoto (1984), Maugiere et al. (1983), Suzuki and Mayanagi (1984) and Tsujii et al. (1984). The equivalent dipole of P22 is located contralaterally to the stimulation and superficially to that of N18, which seems to indicate that the origin of P22 is located in the cortex as suggested by Hashimoto (1984). The equivalent dipole of P40 is located in a similar area or slightly lower than that of P22. There have been few reports on the origin of P40, but the present results seem

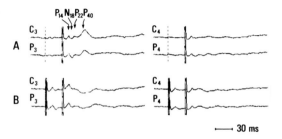

Figure 1. SEPs elicited by single shock stimulation to the median nerve (A) and by double shock stimulation (B). Four of the twenty-one recordings are shown. Recording sites are indicated on each of traces. SEPs were simultaneously recorded using band-pass filter of 3 Hz–3 kHz, and averaged 256 times at the sampling rate of 5 kHz. Single shock: electrical stimulus of 0.2 ms duration; double shock: two stimuli at an interval of 30 ms.

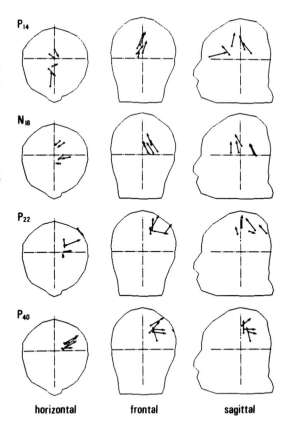

Figure 2. Equivalent dipoles of P14, N18, P22 and P40 obtained from five young healthy subjects, in the horizontal (left column), frontal (middle column) and sagittal (right column) planes.

to indicate the cortical origin of P40, which has been considered a cognitive potential by Desmedt and Robertson (1977) and Desmedt et al. (1983).

Discrimination of Double Shock

When a double shock is applied to the median nerve at an interval of less than 30 ms, the subjects cannot discriminate the shock as consisting of two successive stimuli. In this situation, no positivity at 40 ms is elicited by the second stimulus of the double shock as shown in Figure 1 B. In the present study, the equivalent dipole of P40 elicited by the single shock is called ED-control (equivalent dipole control), and that of the "P40"-corresponding potential elicited by the second stimulus of the double shock, ED-test. SEPs elicited by the single shock were mathematically subtracted from those elicited by the double shock stimulation, and the potential distribution, which corresponds to P40 of the second stimulus of the double shock, was analyzed to obtain ED-subtraction. The respective equivalent dipoles are shown in Figure 3.

As mentioned above, the origin of P40 seems to be in the cortex. The location and vector direction of the ED-test were different from those of ED-control. ED-subtraction corresponds to the component which results from the interference between the evoked potential elicited by the two stimuli and occurs at the time when the P40 of the second stimulus of the double shock would have been present. The location of ED-subtraction was different from that of the control and the vec-

tor was in the inverse direction to that of the control. This implies that as a consequence of the first stimulus, a kind of inhibitory process is generated in the cortex at approximately 40 ms after the second stimulus of the double shock.

References

Desmedt JE, Robertson D (1977) Differential enhancement of early and late components of the cerebral somatosensory evoked potentials during fast sequential cognitive tasks in man. *J Physiol* (Lond), *271*, 761–782.

Desmedt JE, Huy NT, Bourguet M (1983) The cognitive P40, N60 and P100 components of somatosensory evoked potentials and the earliest signs of sensory processing in man. *Electroenceph clin Neurophysiol, 56*, 272–282.

Hashimoto I (1984) Somatosensory evoked potentials from the human brain-stem: Origins of short latency potentials. *Electroenceph clin Neurophysiol, 57*, 221–227.

He B, Musha T, Okamoto Y, Homma S, Nakajima Y, Sato T (1987) Electric dipole tracing in the brain by means of the boundary element method and its accuracy. *IEEE Trans Biomed Eng BME, 34*, 406–414.

Homma S, Nakajima Y, Musha T, Okamoto Y, He B (1987) Dipole-tracing method applied to human brain potentials. *J Neurosci Meth, 21*, 195–200.

Katayama Y, Tsubokawa T (1987) Somatosensory evoked potentials from the thalamic sensory relay nucleus (VPL) in humans: Correlation with short latency somatosensory evoked potentials recorded at the scalp. *Electroenceph clin Neurophysiol, 68*, 187–201.

Maugiere F, Desmedt JE, Courjon J (1983) Neural generators of N18 and P14 far-field somatosensory evoked potentials studied in patients with lesion of thalamus or thalamocortical radiations. *Electroenceph clin Neurophysiol, 56*, 283–292.

Suzuki I, Mayanagi Y (1984) Intracranial recording of short latency somatosensory evoked potentials in man: Identification of origin of each component. *Electroenceph clin Neurophysiol, 59*, 286–296.

Tsujii S, Shibasaki H, Kato M, Kuroiwa Y, Shima F (1984) Subcortical, thalamic and cortical somatosensory evoked potentials to median nerve stimulation. *Electroenceph clin Neurophysiol, 59*, 465–476.

Watanabe S, Nakajima Y, Toma S, Kawamura M (1985) Double stimuli discrimination sense test and the SEP waveform. *Electroenceph clin Neurophysiol, 61*, 188.

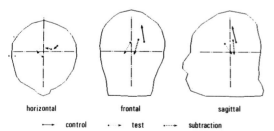

horizontal   frontal   sagittal

⟶ control   · · ▸ test   ·····▸ subtraction

Figure 3. Equivalent dipoles of P40 calculated from SEP elicited by single or double shock stimulation, and from subtracted SEP. Note that the vector direction of the control is inverse to that of the subtraction.

Topography and Model Analysis
of Auditory Evoked Potentials: Tonotopic Aspects

O. Bertrand, F. Perrin, J. F. Echallier, J. Pernier

The temporo-spatial organization of auditory evoked potentials (AEPs) was investigated between 50 and 250 ms in normal subjects. The question of the identification of the multiple brain generators responsible for these responses was adressed by means of analysis of both sequential scalp potential and scalp current density maps. Furthermore, we propose time-varying equivalent-dipoles to model the multiple bilateral generators of the auditory response.
Electrical AEPs were recorded on 24 electrodes over the scalp, after 600 ms tone-burst stimuli of 250, 1000 and 4000 Hz, delivered monaurally to the right or left ear.
Two aspects of the auditory cortical responses are emphasized:
1) The auditory cortex is known to be tonotopically organized. Several authors recently debated this topic, mainly from magnetoencephalographic topographical data. While steady-state response to amplitude-modulated tones clearly revealed a tonotopic organization within the Sylvian fissure, this property still needs to be confirmed for the transient responses. Our study shows some evidence of a frequency dependance of the electrical N1 wave topography.
2) Results concerning the left-right scalp asymmetry of the AEPs related to the ear of stimulation are presented. The question of a possible hemispheric predominance will be discussed in terms of scalp current density distribution and brain generators.

Microelectrode recordings in the primary auditory cortex of monkeys have provided an orderly representation of the cochlear partition (Merzenich & Brugger, 1973). In human, Celesia (1976) has recorded the electrical evoked responses to clicks and tone bursts from exposed cortex during surgery, exhibit-ing an activation of the primary auditory area A1 and its surroundings. However, evidence from intracranial recordings for a human tonotopic mapping are still lacking.

More recently, neuromagnetic studies by Romani et al. (1982) of the field pattern, associated with the steady-state response to amplitude-modulated tones, have revealed a tonotopic organization in which the activity occurs deeper within the Sylvian fissure for tones of higher frequency. Electric and magnetic studies on the auditory transient responses to tone bursts have provided evidence that the 100 ms component ("N1") is generated, at least in part, in or near the supratemporal plane (Vaughan & Ritter, 1970; Hari et al., 1980), but the stimulus frequency dependence of this component is still debated. Elberling et al. (1982) have reported that some brain generators of the magnetic N1 may be tonotopically organized, with the source being displaced posteriorly for higher pitch. In contrast, Tuomitso et al. (1983), Pelizzone et al. (1984) and Arthur et al. (1986) have not confirmed this finding on neuromagnetic data. These reports were focussed on the depth and the location of the equivalent current dipole generating the observed field distribution, without considering its orientation. No direct correlation has been found between these parameters and the stimulus frequency. This has been interpreted as being due either to a considerable intersubject variability of the morphology of the auditory cortex, or to a

INSERM – UNITE 280, 151 Cours Albert Thomas, 69003 Lyon, France.

greater sensibility of the N 1 component to the onset of a stimulus rather than to its pitch content.

Since, to our knowledge, the tonotopic aspects of the N1 component has not been extensively studied from scalp evoked potentials, this paper will present some preliminary results on the frequency dependence of this response, including scalp potential and scalp current density mapping as well as spatio-temporal dipole modelling. This study will provide some evidence for a tonotopic organization of some of the N1 generators, highlighting their functional properties.

Subjects and Recording Methods

Subjects were 5 right-handed adults (3 males and 2 females) without any hearing deficit. Auditory stimuli were presented monaurally in the right ear by means of a TDH 39 headphone. Stimuli were 500 ms tone bursts (10 ms rise/fall time) presented with a constant inter-stimulus interval of 2 s. Three carrier frequencies were used: 250, 1000 and 4000 Hz. The stimulus amplitudes were adjusted at the different frequencies so that they were subjectively equal in loudness (in general the amplitudes remained in the range of 70–80 dB HL). One experiment consisted of 9 runs of 100 stimuli: 3 for each stimulus frequency, randomly selected. A grand average of 300 sweeps was obtained for each frequency and subject.

Responses were recorded from 16 or 24 Ag–AgCl cup electrodes placed according to the 10–20 International System, and in additional intermediate locations: 1 subject (MT) with 16 electrodes over both hemispheres, 1 (JC) with 16 electrodes over the left hemisphere only and 3 (FL, PB, JP) with 24 electrodes over both hemispheres. The reference electrode was on the nose.

Recording parameters were sweep lengths of 1024 ms with 100 ms prestimulus baseline, digitization intervals of 2 ms, and analog filter bandpass of 0.3–160 Hz. Before analysis, signals were digitally processed with a zero-phase shift lowpass filter (0–30 Hz) to eliminate high frequency residual noise.

N100 Topography and Stimulus Frequency

Methods

In a first qualitative approach, the responses for each stimulus frequency were topographically analyzed. Scalp potential maps were generated on a color graphic terminal (TEKTRONIX 4107), connected to a mini-computer (BULL-SPS 7), using a mapping program of our own design (Giard et al., 1985). From the electrode sites, the scalp potential was computed at each pixel by a two-dimensional spline interpolation algorithm (Perrin et al., 1987 a). The advantage of this method over the classical 4-nearest neighbours interpolation is that the interpolated surfaces are smoother, their extrema are not necessarily located at electrode sites, and are generally more precisely estimated. Scalp potential maps are plane representation of an activity recorded on the scalp considered here as a spherical surface. The projection method used for the mapping system is a radial projection from Cz (for top views) or from T3 or T4 (for lateral views), which respects the length of the meridian arcs.

Moreover, the spline interpolation method, using spatially differentiable functions, allows the computation of scalp current density maps (or radial current estimate maps) by means of the Laplacian operator applied to a spherical surface, from any set of electrodes (Perrin et al., 1987 b). Scalp current density (SCD) is independent of any model, assumption about brain generators or homogeneity of the volume conduction in the head. It only assumes a constant scalp conductivity. SCD mapping has the interesting properties of being reference-free and having sharper peaks and troughs than scalp potential mapping.

Results

Scalp potential (SP) maps for subjects FL, JP, PB and JC at the three different stimulus frequencies are shown in Figure 1. In each case (subject and frequency), the map has been selected at the latency of extremum amplitude on electrode Fz during the N1 period. All maps have a polarity reversal at the temporal level. This is strongly emphasized by SCD maps, presented here for subject JC, which show a tighter sink/source pattern at the same level. Since SCDs are reference-free, this bipolar topography is not artefactually due to the location of the reference electrode. These characteristics have been observed on SP and SCD maps of all 5 subjects. Moreover, from the top view of subject FL in Figure 1, a larger frontocentral negativity and infero-temporal positivity can be noted on the left hemisphere, contralateral to the stimulated ear. Similarly, in Figure 2b, the experimental SP maps of subject MT show a larger positive activity on

the left side. A top view of the SCDs (Figure 2a), computed from the same SP data, splits the global topography into two distinct sink/source patterns, strengthening the hypothesis of an activation of both auditory cortices, with a contralateral predominance.

The way SP topography changes with increasing stimulus frequency varies with subjects, but may be roughly described by a decrease of the fronto-central negativity and an increase of the lateral positivity. However, some subjects (JP, PB) only present a decrease of the frontal negativity, without any change in positivity, sometimes accompanied by a

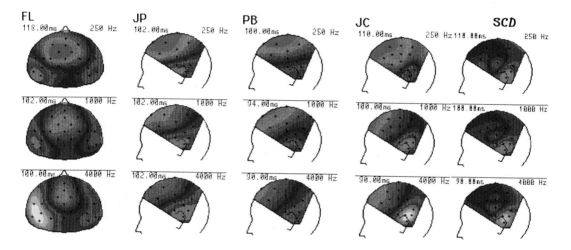

Figure 1. N100 topography of 4 subjects (FL, JP, PB, JC) at 3 stimulus frequencies (top line: 250 Hz, middle line: 1000 Hz, bottom line: 4000 Hz). The color scale is the same for the 3 conditions within each subject (yellow: +, red: −, border between blue and purple: 0 voltage). Subject FL is presented from a top view, and other subjects from the left side. SP and SCD maps are drawn together for subject JC. Black dots indicate the electrode positions.

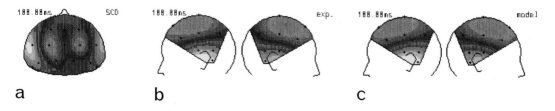

Figure 2. Dipole modelling of the N1 at a fixed latency (subject MT, 1000 Hz tone). (a) top view SCD map computed from the experimental data, (b) left and right maps of experimental potentials, (c) maps generated from the 2 equivalent dipoles found (all SP maps are average referenced and have the same scale).

frontal shift of the negativity (PB) or a post-ero-lateral shift of the positivity (JP). Similar changes of the balance between sink and source amplitudes appear on SCD maps (JC).

N1 mapping thus suggests a modification in the orientation of the underlying generators according to the stimulus frequency, with a great intersubject variability. In any case, this implies a frequency dependence of some of the N1 generators.

Dipole Modelling at a Fixed Latency

Method

Like the authors of other published works on data processing of neuromagnetic auditory N1 response, we have tried to identify the equivalent current dipoles leading to the best fit between experimental and model N1 distri-bution. A classical 3-concentric sphere head model has been used, with the same radius and conductivity values as proposed by Rush and Driscoll (1969). A quasi-Newton minimi-zation algorithm was applied for each stimu-lus frequency at the latency of maximum amplitude on electrode Fz, by seeking two equivalent dipoles, one in each hemisphere.

The relative model error was the mean square difference between data and model, divided by the mean square value of data. The goodness of fit (GOF) was evaluated by one minus the relative error, expressed as a per-centage.

Since N1 topographies showed an intersub-ject variability, this procedure was not applied to a grand average, but rather to a single indi-vidual. Data were average referenced for con-venience of the modelling procedure, without affecting the resulting dipoles. The position, the orientation and the magnitude of each dipole were thus determined (6 parameters per dipole).

Results

Figure 2b shows the scalp potential distribu-tion of the experimental data (subject MT) on each hemisphere at one frequency (1000 Hz), and Figure 2c the interpolated distribution generated by the equivalent dipoles found.

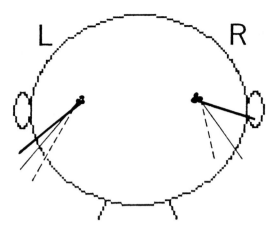

Figure 3. Frontal projection of the equivalent dipoles found from subject MT in each hemisphere for 250 Hz (hashed lines), 1000 Hz (thin lines) and 4000 Hz (thick lines) tones.

These model maps are very similar to those of Figure 2b. The GOF was greater than 98% for each frequency condition.

The positions and the orientations of the dipoles were projected on a frontal plane (Fig-ure 3). In each hemisphere, the dipoles are approximatively located at the same position for the three frequencies, and almost symmet-rically between hemispheres. They are ori-ented rather perpendicularly to the Sylvian fissure. However, their radial component seems to increase regularly with higher pitch, thus leading to a tilting effect of their global orientation. This is in agreement with what has been deduced from the frequency depen-dent changes in the positivity/negativity bal-ance observed on SP maps (Figure 1). No obvious modification in the position of the sources was noted.

Dynamic Dipole Modelling

Methods

The interpretation of the N1 topography by a single equivalent dipole in each hemisphere is an oversimplification of the brain activity during this period. Additional activity in the temporal lobes, between 70 and 150 ms, has been suggested from waveforms and sequential maps analysis (Wolpaw & Penry, 1975; Wood & Wolpaw, 1982, Peronnet et al., 1984). More recently, Scherg and von Cramon (1985, 1986) have proposed a spatio-temporal dipole model of the N1-P2 auditory responses with two bilateral sources. From a coronal chain of electrodes, four equivalent dipoles (two rather radially and two rather tangentially oriented) led to the best fit during the 60–250 ms period. Each dipole had a constant position and orientation, and a temporal course of activity (time-varying magnitude) described by a biphasic function. Although limited to a coronal plane, this methodology has proved to be able to discriminate between several sources overlapping in time. This allows new functional insight into the brain activities underlying the auditory responses.

A similar dynamic analysis has been applied to our data, in order to avoid the common arbitrary choice of a fixed latency for modelling. The main differences to Scherg's study consist, first, in 24 recording electrodes here covering the entire scalp, and, second, in an analysis restricted to the N1 period only, i.e., 25 maps from 64 to 112 ms. Each of the four dipoles has a constant position and orientation, and a magnitude varying in time according to a polynomial function defined

by three latencies (onset, peak and offset). All these parameters (9 per dipole) were found by a global fitting algorithm applied to 24 × 25 data samples. No particular constraint has been imposed to seek the sources in their respective hemisphere. A global goodness of fit was calculated as well as a GOF at each latency during the time range of study. Data from subject PB, for 250, 1000 and 4000 Hz tones, were processed with this methodology.

Results

Figure 4b shows the left SP evolution of subject PB, during the N1 period, for 1000 Hz tones. Modifications of the SP topography appear clearly between the beginning and the end of this time range, in agreement with Wood and Wolpaw's observation (1982). The positive extremum moves laterally from posterior toward lateral scalp areas. This phenomenon may also be seen on the SCD evolution (Figure 4a), showing a time varying sink source pattern. Similar changing topographies have been observed for 250 and 4000 Hz tones.

Results of the modelling procedure on subject PB are presented in Figures 4c and 5. Global GOFs are greater than 96% for all

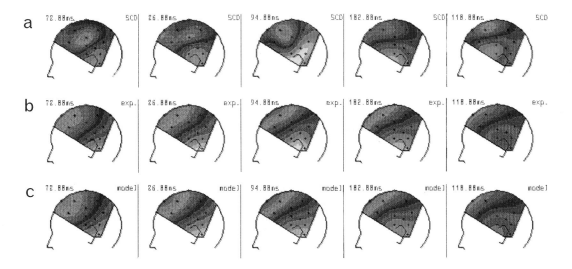

Figure 4. Sequential maps during the N1 period (subject PB, 1000 Hz tones, 78–110 ms). (a) successive SCD maps computed from the experimental data, (b) experimental SP maps, (c) successive SP maps generated by 2 dipoles in each hemisphere, overlapping in time, found by the modelling procedure (all SP maps are average referenced and have the same scale).

Generator activation

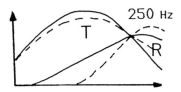

250 Hz

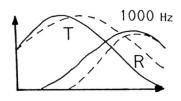

1000 Hz

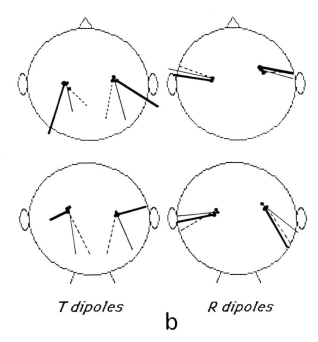

T dipoles   b   *R dipoles*

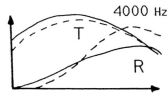

4000 Hz

a   *time (64-112 ms)*

Figure 5. Results of the dynamic dipole modelling procedure (subject PB, 64–112 ms) for 3 stimulus frequencies. (a) Time varying magnitudes of the 4 dipoles found, for each frequency condition. The earliest sources correspond to rather tangentially oriented dipoles (T dipoles), and the latest, to rather radially oriented ones (R dipoles). Full line: left hemisphere, dashed line: right hemisphere. (b) Positions and orientations of the 4 dipoles projected on horizontal and frontal planes (dotted line: 250 Hz, thin line: 1000 Hz, thick line: 4000 Hz).

stimulus frequencies, and greater than 92% at each latency. Figure 4c shows the successive interpolated distributions generated by the four equivalent dipoles found for 1000 Hz tones. These model maps are well fitted to the experimental ones in Figure 4b. Two types of dipole have been found according to their general orientation (Figure 5b) and their latency of peaking magnitude (Figure 5a). The earliest ones (T dipoles), peaking between 79 and 88 ms, are rather tangentially oriented, at least for 250 and 1000 Hz tones, while the latest ones (R dipoles), peaking between 100 and 107 ms, are rather radially oriented. The temporal characteristics of each type of dipole are quite identical between hemispheres, and similar for various pitches (Figure 5a). However, the spatial orientation of each type

shows some interhemispheric differences (Figure 5b). It should be noted that T and R dipoles have an important overlap of their time courses. This implies that modelling of the N100 at a fixed latency with a single dipole in each hemisphere leads to a localization of sources including the contribution of several brain generators.

The main point of these findings is that the T dipoles seem to have a frequency dependent orientation, while the R dipoles do not show such a change with various pitches. The variations in the orientation of the T dipoles are similar to those found by modelling the data at a single fixed latency, i.e., rotation of the T dipoles mainly due to a modification of their radial components. Again, no modification of the dipole position has been observed.

Discussion

The present topographical and model analysis of the N1 auditory response reports some preliminary evidence for a tonotopic organization of a part of the underlying brain activity.

SP and SCD maps show modifications in the positive/negative extremum locations and relative amplitudes, according to the stimulus frequency. Although N1 topography may differ between subjects, its frequency related modifications have been found to be very similar across subjects. This may imply that different sets of neural sources are activated for each pitch.

A classical dipole modelling procedure at a fixed latency has shown some differences in the orientation of both equivalent current dipoles, probably located in each Heschl's gyrus. These dipoles are regularly tilted toward the scalp surface for increasing frequencies. These quantitative changes in orientation could again be interpreted as the activation of different cortical areas. Moreover, this suggests that each one has its own equivalent neural orientation, probably reflecting the complex folding geometry of the auditory cortex.

However, dipole modelling at a single fixed latency seems to be of limited value for a realistic description of the brain activity during the N1 period. A dynamic modelling approach can take into account the overlap of several generators. Two bilateral sources, with different peaking latency and orientation, have been found with this methodology applied to one subject. In each hemisphere, the earliest sources (T dipoles) seem to involve the primary auditory cortex, or surrounding areas, because of their main tangential orientation, in agreement with the orientation of the supra-temporal plane. Moreover, these sources have a noticeable frequency dependence of their orientation, compatible with the hypothesis of a tonotopic organization of the auditory cortex. The latest sources (R dipoles) do not obviously vary with the pitch of the tones. Their positions and orientations could not be easily associated with a precise brain structure, and possibly reflect a more global activity of various cortical areas. They seem to be independent of the physical features of the stimulus. These R dipoles could be related to the temporal component of Wolpaw and Penry (1985), or to the radial source of Scherg and von Cramon (1985).

No clear relation has been found between the position of both types of dipoles and the stimulus frequency. It should be noted that scalp potential distributions seem to be more sensitive to the orientation of the sources than to their location. This is mainly due to the volume conduction effect of the head, smearing the extrema. Nevertheless, the dynamic modelling methodology permits discrimination between several overlapping activities, having different functional properties.

The present preliminary report leads to different conclusions that some previous neuromagnetic experiments on the tonotopic aspect of the N1 component. It should be recalled that magnetic fields are sensitive only to the tangential component of brain sources. Our data suggest a major frequency dependence of the radial components of the T dipoles, i.e., tonotopy of the auditory cortex, which might not be seen by magnetic recordings. This finding needs, of course, to be confirmed by an extensive analysis of several subjects, using the same methodology.

References

Arthur DL, Sullivan G, Flynn ER, Williamson SJ (1986) Source localization of the long latency auditory evoked magnetic field in human temporal cortex. In *Proceedings of the VIIIth International Conference on Event-Related Potentials of the Brain, 22—28 June 1986. Stanford, USA.*

Celesia GG (1976) Organization of auditory cortical areas in man. *Brain, 99,* 403—414.

Elberling C, Bak C, Kofoed B, Lebech H, Saermark K (1982) Auditory magnetic fields: Source location and tonotopical organization in the right hemisphere of the human brain. *Scand Audiol, 11,* 61—65.

Giard MH, Peronnet F, Pernier J, Mauguiere F, Bertrand O (1985) Sequential color mapping system of brain potentials. *Comput Methods and Prog in Biomed, 20,* 9—16.

Hari R, Aittoniemi K, Jarvinen M, Katila T, Varpula T (1980) Auditory evoked transient and sustained magnetic fields of the human brain. *Exp Brain Res, 40,* 237—240.

Merzenich MM, Brugger JF (1973) Representation of the cochlear partition on the temporal plane of the macaque monkey. *Brain Res, 50,* 275–296.

Pelizzone M, Williamson SJ, Kaufman L (1984) Evidence for multiple areas in the human auditory cortex. In Weinberg H, Stroink G, Katila T (Eds.) *Biomagnetism: Application and theory.* Pergamon Press, New York, 326–330.

Peronnet F, Giard MH, Bertrand O, Pernier J (1984) The temporal component of the auditory evoked potential: A reinterpretation. *Electroenceph clin Neurophysiol, 59,* 67–71.

Perrin F, Pernier J, Bertrand O, Giard MH, Echallier JF (1987a) Mapping of scalp potential by surface spline interpolation. *Electroenceph clin Neurophysiol, 66,* 75–81.

Perrin F, Bertrand O, Pernier J (1987b) Scalp current density mapping: Value and estimation from potential data. *IEEE Trans Biomed Eng, 34,* 283–288.

Romani GL, Williamson SJ, Kaufmann L, Brenner D (1982) Characterization of the human auditory cortex by the neuromagnetic method. *Exp Brain Res, 47,* 381–393.

Rush S, Driscoll DA (1969) EEG electrode sensitivity: An application of reciprocity. *IEEE Trans Biomed Eng, 16,* 15–22.

Scherg M, von Cramon D (1985) Two bilateral sources of the late AEP as identified by a spatio-temporal dipole model. *Electroenceph clin Neurophysiol, 62,* 32–44.

Scherg M, von Cramon D (1986) Evoked dipole source potentials of the human auditory cortex. *Electroenceph clin Neurophysiol, 65,* 344–360.

Tuomitso T, Hari R, Katila T, Poutanen T, Varpula T (1983) Studies of auditory evoked magnetic and electric responses: modality specificity and modelling. *Il nuovo cimento, 2,* (2), 471–483.

Vaughan HG, Ritter W (1970) The sources of auditory evoked responses recorded from the human scalp. *Electroenceph clin Neurophysiol, 28,* 360–367.

Wolpaw JR, Penry JK (1975) A temporal component of the auditory evoked response. *Electroenceph clin Neurophysiol, 39,* 609–620.

Wood CC, Wolpaw JR (1982) Scalp distribution of human auditory evoked potential. II. Evidence for overlapping sources and involvement of auditory cortex. *Electroenceph clin Neurophysiol, 54,* 25–38.

An Interaction of Cortical Sources Associated with Simultaneous Auditory and Somesthetic Stimulation

H. Weinberg, D. O. Cheyne, P. Brickett, R. Harrop, R. Gordon

Studies of visual, auditory and somatosensory systems have comprised a large body of MEG research. One reason for this is that the neuroanatomy and neurophysiology associated with these sensory functions is relatively well known. Therefore, initial attempts to localise sources associated with sensory evoked potentials used known neuroanatomical localisation of cortical function to validate MEG estimates of sources. However, there is relatively little known about how sensory stimulation in two or more modalities interact when stimulation is simultaneous. The experiments to be described utilise high-frequency steady-state stimulation of auditory and somesthetic systems, seperately and simultaneously in phase. Auditory stimulation was conducted by air pressure through tubes to the subject's ears; somesthetic stimulation was by mechanical pressure on the forefinger. MEG maps were constructed, and dipole location estimates were established for one equivalent dipole, and two dipoles, for each of the conditions. The data indicate that the sources estimated for simultaneous stimulation are not a sum of the sources estimated for stimulation of each modality seperately. The data are discussed in relation to the concept of current dipoles for estimates of the location of distributed systems.

Galambos et al. (1981) described what they called the 40 Hz response. This steady-state response was a sinusoidal EEG following response to repetitive auditory stimulation which was of maximal amplitude at rates between 35 and 45 Hz. Galambos suggested that the response was a superimposition of brainstem responses (waves IV and V) and thalamic mid-latency responses. Assuming that there is volume conduction of these responses, the widespread distribution of the 40 Hz response is consistent with the interpretation that the sources are primarily of thalamic or brainstem origin. Spydell et al. (1985) measured the latencies of wave V of the auditory brainstem response, assuming that they would be different in normals and patients with brainstem lesions. He came to the conclusion that there were independent generators. He also observed that the 40 Hz response appeared unimpaired in a group of patients with unilateral temporal lobe lesions. He made the conclusion that the temporal lobe was not involved in the response. Weinberg et al. (1988) reported a study in which both electrical and magnetic recordings were obtained from two healthy right-handed subjects with normal hearing. The auditory stimuli consisted of 55 db 1000 Hz sinusoidal tone bursts of 5 ms duration (non-ramped), presented binaurally at repetitition rates of 30 and 40 Hz. Electrical recordings were taken from a vertex electrode; magnetic recordings were obtained sequentially from a wide distribution. We suggested that a „source system" was active during 40 Hz auditory stimulation which included bilateral temporal cortex, and we suggested (as Borda did in 1983) that when the brain is in a steady-state as a result of being driven by repetitive auditory stimulation, it is likely that the resonance within a limited portion of the auditory pathways could account for some of the enhancement at 40 Hz stimulus rates. This interpretation is supported by current studies

Department of Psychology, Simon Fraser University, Burnaby, BC, Canada.

about the organisation of the thalamocortical auditory system in the cat. Neuroanatomy suggests a functional organisation of the auditory system by which resonance effects may account for augmentation of the steady-state response (Anderson et al., 1980; Imig & Morel, 1983).

If our speculation about the source system involved in repetitive stimulation at frequencies approximating 40 Hz is correct, the sources reported must include corticofugal-cortical modulation. The study reported here is an extension of our inital auditory experiments (Weinberg et al. 1988).

Methods

Three conditions of steady-state stimulation were examined: tactile (T), auditory (A), and simultaneous auditory and tactile in-phase stimulation (B).

Stimuli

Pressure vibration was applied to the right forefinger by means of a small plastic piston with an annular tip, 4 mm in diameter. The piston with its housing was 4 m in length allowing an electromechanical vibrator to drive the piston without magnetic artifact. The vibrator was driven by a sine wave oscillator controlling amplitude and frequency. The vibratory stimulus was applied to the tip of the right forefinger, held in place by a wooden form-fitting device, and consisted of a maximum sinusoidal displacement of 1 mm. The force was sufficient to displace 50 g over this distance measured with a force-displacement transducer (Grass Model TC10C) and was experienced by the subject as a strong fluttering sensation at the finger tip. The auditory stimuli consisted of 55 db(HL) 1000 Hz sinusoidal tone bursts of 5 ms duration (non-ramped) presented binaurally at repetition rates of 30 and 40 Hz and monaurally at 40 Hz in the combined auditory-tactile condition. In order to eliminate magnetic artifacts the sound was conducted to the subjects through plastic tubing and earpieces from a small speaker fixed to the top of the dewar. The orientation of the speaker was fixed with respect to the gradi-

ometer sensing coils so that no artifact was measured regardless of the position of the gradiometer. A steady-state paradigm was used for both tactile and auditory stimuli with a sampling rate of 1 point/ms and a time interval of 100 ms for each data record for 1000 repetitions. When auditory and tactile stimuli were presented simultaneously, onset time was adjusted such that maximal displacement of the piston coincided.with the onset of the tone burst at the earpiece.

Subjects

The data reported here are from three male subjects (U.R., R.G. and T.R.), aged between 21 and 35 years; one received only Condition A; one received only Condition T; and one received Conditions A, T and B.

MEG and EEG Recording

MEG data were collected with a 3rd order gradiometer in an automated gantry system. The subject's head shape was digitized and served as a model for automatically positioning the dewar over at least 40 preselected sites over both hemispheres. Coordinates of the positions and orientation of the sensing coil were recorded for use in dipole estimates. Configuration of the MEG system has been described elsewhere (Vrba et al., 1982). EEG was recorded from Cz referenced to linked mastoids with a bandpass of 10.6 to 70 Hz. EEG was recorded primarily for the purpose of ensuring that the 40 Hz EEG response was present but was not used in estimating sources.

Data Analysis

Fourier analysis was used to compute the amplitude and phase of the 40 Hz component from the MEG average at each recording position. These values were then plotted as vectors in polar coordinates. Since a phase difference of 180° is equivalent to a polarity reversal of the same signal, the average phase was calculated as that angle for which the root-mean square amplitude of all vectors projected onto that angle was maximal. The resulting amplitude values were used to produce isocontour maps of the field over the surface of the head.

The interpolated values for these maps were calculated as the weighted sum of all recording positions within a specified search radius; the weight for each position was proportional to the reciprocal of its distance. The topography of the phase vectors was also plotted for subject U.R. A least-squares method for estimating one or two dipole fits to the data as described by Harrop et al. (1986) was used to approximate the location of equivalent current dipole sources. The method takes into account the number, size, spatial separation and orientation of the gradiometer coils. The least-squares method utilises multiple radii defined as the distance to each recording position from an origin near the centre of the head (computed as a point on a horizontal plane defined by nasion and preauricular points). Anatomically, this origin lies in the vicinity of the brainstem at the midline of the ventral surface of the upper pons.

Results

Auditory (A)

EEG: The vertex EEG response to 30 and 40 Hz shows a clear following response, which is consistent with what would be expected from literature. The electrical response is consistent in all subjects for both unilateral and bilateral auditory stimulation.

MEG: Isofield plots of the 40 Hz component of MEG responses indicate bilateral equivalent dipole sources in the vicinity of primary auditory cortex (Figure 1 upper left side). For both binaural and monaural auditory stimulation, bilateral dipolar fields are observed over the temporo-parietal regions. For monaural stimulation (subject U.R., Figure 1 upper right side) the fields are quite symmetrical; two-dipole fits of the data estimate sources 2.0 cm posterior, 4.5 cm lateral and 4.4 cm superior to the origin placing bilateral sources roughly in the vicinity of either primary auditory cortex in superior temporal gyrus (Figure 2). The orientation of these dipoles is approximately vertical and directed toward midline indicating that such sources may comprise equivalent sources orientated vertically in the superior plane of the temporal

lobe. The strength of the current dipole estimates for the responses reported here is in the range of 2 to 3 nanoampere-meters which corresponds to values previously reported for steady-state fields by Romani et al. (1982).

Tactile (T)

EEG: The vertex EEG from tactile stimuli for 40 Hz follows the stimulus but its amplitude and phase are highly sensitive to variations in the area and position of the forefinger stimulated; it is generally lower in amplitude than the auditory response.

MEG: At maximum amplitude of the EEG response the MEG appears to be dipolar contralateral to stimulation (Figure 1 upper right side). The fields may be complex; however, if only contralateral data are used in dipole estimates, equivalent dipole fits accounting for 80% of the variance of the observed fields can be achieved. The position for this dipole in subject R.G. was 3 cm posterior, 3 cm lateral (left hemisphere), and 8 cm above the origin placing the equivalent dipole source in the area of the finger locations of somatosensory cortex (postcentral gyrus). For subject U.R. a single dipole fit to all the data from both hemispheres also places a single equivalent dipole in the same area of contralateral somatosensory cortex, accounting for over 70% of the variance. Using only observed data from contralateral hemisphere again increases this fit to account for more than 80% of the variance.

Combined Auditory and Tactile (B)

EEG: The EEG at the vertex shows a following response similar in waveform and period to tactile and auditory following responses, with an amplitude somewhat larger than that for auditory stimulation alone when the individual responses were in phase relative to each other.

MEG: The observed MEG data are shown in Figure 1 (upper right side). A complex distribution of fields appears to result in patterns of maxima and minima in both hemispheres. The arithmetic sum of the tactile and auditory fields is, however, very close to the observed field. Maxima and minima are seen to have

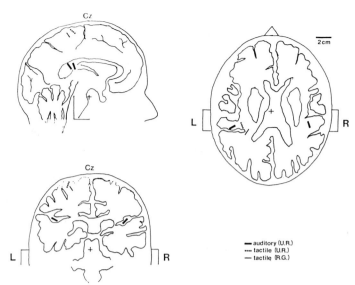

Figure 2. Three-dimensional representations of the location of equivalent dipoles source estimates fitted to the observed frequency components shown in Figure 1, using a least-squares fitting routine. Two-dipole estimates were fitted for the auditory condition (dark bars) in homologous regions of superior temporal lobe, accounting for 86.2% of the variance in the observed values. Single dipoles were fitted to the tactile data for two subjects, both in left postcentral gyrus, and account for 70% (U.R.) and 81% (R.G.) of the variance. Drawings.are taken from representative brain sections and a small cross indicates the relative position of the origin of the coordinate system used in dipole localization.

the same distribution over the head, as if the result of simultaneous stimulation is the sum of what would be expected from stimulation of each of the modalities separately. Two dipoles fit to these data accounts for 80% of the variance and results in a right hemisphere estimate very close to that of the right hemisphere auditory estimate (slightly more lateral); but the left hemisphere dipole is displaced quite laterally and above the temporal lobe (6 cm above the plane of the origin). This could possibly be expected if the left hemisphere fields were the result of the combined activity of the contralateral tactile dipole estimated near vertex, and the left hemisphere auditory dipole estimated in temporal lobe.

Distribution of Phase Differences

Figure 1 (lower left side) shows the superimposition of MEG waveforms resulting from tactile and auditory stimuli presented separately and from simultaneous stimulation in both modalities. The phase analysis to the right of Figure 1 (lower left side) shows the variability in phase for responses recorded from different locations over the head. Al-

Figure 1. Upper left side: Isofield plot of MEG response to 40 Hz auditory stimulation for subject T.R. Fields shown in red are plots of 40 Hz vectors which are 180° out of phase with respect to those shown in blue (see text for explanation).

   Upper right side: Isofield contour maps of the magnetic 40 Hz amplitude for three stimulus conditions and the sum of the tactile and auditory responses (subject U.R.). The maps are shown as equidistant projections of the head surface with vertex as the center and recording positions shown as small circles. The map border lies approximately at the level of T3/T4—indicated by the innermost circle on the inset diagram showing 10-20 system locations. Each contour level corresponds to 2.5 femtotesla and white and red lines indicate fields of opposite direction.

   Lower left side: MEG responses to tactile (T), auditory (A) and combined (A + T) in-phase stimulation of right ear and right index finger at 40 Hz. Phase vectors of the 40 Hz component are plotted to the right.

   Lower right side: Phase vector plots of the 40 Hz frequency components used to produce the isocontour maps and dipole estimates for 3 conditions in subject U.R. Direction of lines indicates the relative phase of the 40 Hz component at each recording location. Length indicates the magnitude of the 40 Hz component, the largest magnitude (left-most position for condition B) corresponding to approximately 36 fT.

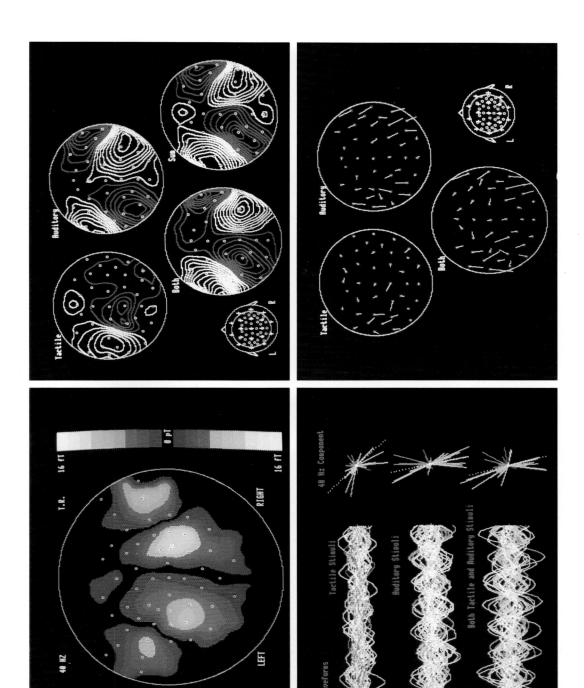

though there is variability in phase, the clusters can be easily seen; those displayed in green were arbitrarily designated as having a polarity different from those plotted in pink. Figure 1 (lower right side) shows the topography of phase vectors over the head.

Discussion

The data presented here suggest that different systems are active in response to 40 Hz tactile vibration and auditory stimulation, although the EEG response at the vertex remains quite similar. The evidence which remains to be established is the response with homologous bilateral tactile stimulation. The data from subject U.R. clearly indicated two bilaterally symmetric fields arising from sources in auditory cortex. Analysis of the fields resulting from tactile stimulation is consistent in both subjects and results in estimates of sources for tactile vibration in the expected hand and finger locations of the sensory homunculus of the postcentral gyrus.

The data from U.R. obtained during simultaneous stimulation of auditory and somesthetic modalities are instructive. The electrical responses for the auditory condition (A) appear greater than for the tactile response alone, and slightly larger for auditory-tactile combined (condition B), suggesting the possible summing of responses from deep thalamic sources at the vertex when the stimuli are in phase. Yet, the MEG data suggests a much more complex interaction of cortical sources. If only left hemisphere fields are considered the data can be seen to be a combination of the contralateral response to somesthetic stimulation and the left hemisphere response to auditory stimulation. The data from the right hemisphere of subject U.R. are similar to the right hemisphere data of subject T.R. Taken as a whole, the bilateral data from U.R. are what would be expected if the tactile and auditory stimulation were producing fields which summed on left side, and since tactile stimulation does not result in ipsilateral fields, only the auditory fields are seen in right hemisphere. This conclusion is supported by the result of summing the fields resulting from separate auditory and tactile stimulation; the sum is remarkably similar to the observed data for simultaneous stimulation in auditory and somatosensory modalities. If it is the case that the combined fields for dual modality stimulation are the sum of the fields for single modality stimulation it would seem that the 40 Hz response is confined to sensory systems related to the modality of stimulation; if there were an interaction of these modalities in the 40 Hz response the combined fields would undoubtedly not be a simple linear sum of the two. The data suggest that the two modalities may be driven independently by 40 Hz stimulation and support the interpretation that the response reflects a resonance in the sensory system stimulated.

References

Anderson RA, Snyder RL, Merzenich MM (1980) The topographic organization of corticocollicular projection from physiologically identified loci in the AI, AII, and anterior auditory cortical fields of the cat. *J Comp Neurol, 191*, 479–494.

Borda RP (1983) *The 40/sec middle latency response in Alzheimer's disease, Parkinson's disease, and age-matched controls.* Thesis, University of Texas.

Galambos R, Makeig S, Talmachoff PJ (1981) A 40-Hz auditory potential recorded from the human scalp. *Proc Nat Acad Sci, 78,* 2643–2647.

Harrop R, Weinberg H, Brickett P, Dykstra C, Robertson A, Cheyne D, Baff M, Crisp D (1986) *An inverse solution method for the simultaneous localisation of two dipoles.* Paper presented at the meeting of the Institute of Physics: Magnetism Subcommittee, Milton Keynes, England.

Imig TJ, Morel A (1983) Organization of the thalamocortical auditory system in the cat. *Ann Rev Neurosci, 6,* 95–120.

Romani GL, Williamson SJ, Kaufman L, Brenner D (1982) Characterization of the human auditory cortex by the neuromagnetic method. *Exp Brain Res, 47,* 381–393.

Spydell JR, Pattee G, Goldie WD (1985) The 40 Hz auditory event-related potential: normal values and effects of lesions. *Electroenceph clin Neurophysiol, 62,* 193–202.

Vrba J, Fife M, Burbank M, Weinberg H, Brickett P (1982) Spatial discrimination in SQUID gradiometers and 3rd order gradiometer performance. *Can J Phy, 60,* 1060–1073.

Weinberg H, Brickett P, Robertson A, Harrop R, Cheyne DO, Crisp D, Baff M, Dykstra C (1988, in press) The magnetoencephalographic localisation of source-systems in the brain: Early and late components of event related potentials. *J Alcohol.*

Source Estimation of Scalp EEG Focus

P. K. H. Wong* and H. Weinberg**

The interictal spike discharge in children with Benign Rolandic Epilepsy of Childhood (BREC) has been described as having a characteristic topographic field (Gregory & Wong, 1984). As the syndrome has well-defined and consistent ictal manifestations across patients, then perhaps the underlying neuronal mechanism is equally predictable with similar anatomy across patients. There are, as a rule, no structural lesions detected clinically or by CT scan. For these reasons, BREC is attractive as a model for the study of neuronal source generators. We wish to describe our experience with interictal spike potential field analysis and dipole localization method (DLM) in 12 children with BREC.

Monopolar reference and Hjorth source derivation were used to study the topographic configuration of each spike map sequence. DLM was implemented assuming a single generator, single-sphere model. The calculated source locations from DLM were plotted onto the scalp surface using appropriate projection procedure. The scalp-projected source locations for 12 of the 13 foci formed a tight cluster with the mean located just lateral to the C_3 or C_4 electrode position, while the standard deviation was less than a quarter of an inter-electrode distance. Despite ambiguity of the anatomic structure involved, DLM still produced credible source estimates in this homogeneous clinical group.

Accurate localization of the seizure focus in patients with epilepsy is important for proper understanding of the presenting neurological deficits, and particularly the symptomatology during ictal episodes. Ictal EEG recordings, particularly with sphenoidal or depth electrodes, provide definitive data in this respect. Interictal or routine EEG recordings, however, are more easily obtained and noninvasive. We describe the use of interictal scalp EEG discharge for localization of the discharge source in patients with benign Rolandic epilepsy of childhood (BREC), using topographic spike mapping and dipole localization method (DLM).

Material and Method

The diagnosis of BREC was made by a neurologist according to previously published criteria (Lombroso, 1967; Lerman & Kivity, 1975). These are: mid-temporal focus on EEG, seizure onset between age 4 to 14 years, normal neurological examination, absence of brain lesion and compatible seizure type. These seizures are usually nocturnal and of partial onset, although secondary generalization may occur. There is prominent oral-facial involvement, with frequent speech arrest and salivation. There is always spontaneous remission by about age 14 years, irrespective of treatment. The seizures may be very susceptible to single antiepileptic medication (Blom & Heijbel, 1982; Lerman & Kivity, 1975).

Children who had a diagnosis of BREC made and whose routine EEG recordings contained a spike focus were recruited into the study. In addition, their EEG data had to be

* Dept. of Paediatrics, University of British Columbia, Director, EEG Department, Children's Hospital, Vancouver, B.C., Canada
** Dept. of Psychology, Director, Brain Behaviour Laboratory, Simon Fraser University, Burnaby, B.C., Canada
The authors wish to thank Donna Gregory for her expert and invaluable assistance. Similarly, Mario Baff's efforts are appreciated.

sufficiently artifact-free to allow computer digitization and subsequent analysis. Surface silver-silver chloride disk electrodes were applied with collodion at the 19 International 10-20 positions. Impedance was kept below 3 kΩ. Waking and unsedated sleep recordings were obtained. Linked cheeks were used as reference. To check against contamination, ear and hand references were also used.

Signals from the 19 channels were amplified with 0.5 to 70 Hz bandwidth, and digitized at 200 Hz by a dedicated microprocessor system (Bio-Logic Systems "Brain Atlas III Plus"). In order to increase signal-to-noise ratio, up to 20 spikes from each focus were averaged together. For time alignment, the spike apex at the channel with maximum negative amplitude was used (Gregory & Wong, 1984; Thickbroom et al., 1986). Visual inspection ensured artifact-free spike segments, which were then stored on magnetic media. In addition to voltage-time plots, isopotential topographic displays were available online. These topographic maps were drawn on an idealized grid diagram, with dots representing the electrode positions. The F_{pz} and O_z positions were interpolated from the two closest real electrodes, and were included mainly for ease of display. Hjorth source derivation (Hjorth, 1976) was applied to the digital data as part of the analysis procedure.

Scalp estimation of spike focus was done by two methods: based on scalp field maxima/minima positions ("$F_{x,y}$" method), and by DLM. The former was carried out by a simple calculation using only the positions of the scalp maxima (positive) and minima (negative). The values x and y represented the abscissa and ordinate of the (flat plane) electrode grid diagram. The calculated focus, $F_{x,y}$, lay on the line joining the maxima and minima, with the distance from each extremum being weighted by the respective absolute amplitude. This method ensured that a single peak (monopolar field) had $F_{x,y}$ located at the scalp position of the electrode with the maximum spike amplitude.

DLM computations were based on the electrostatic dipole model described by Kavanagh et al. (1978). Six parameters were used (3 position and 3 magnitude) within a single homogeneous sphere. This was implemented using a

procedure similar to that described for MEG by Weinberg et al. (1986). The calculated scalp potential field was compared with the observed field and the sum square error (SSE) minimized by an iterative nonlinear algorithm (Marquardt, 1963).

The final estimate of the 6 parameters was taken as the source location only if the final SSE was less than 10% of the initial SSE. This yielded an optimized set of parameters based on an iterative algorithm (Marquardt, 1963).

For comparison with scalp field displays, the estimated generator locations were converted to polar coordinates and then projected onto the planar electrode grid diagram. This procedure plotted the point where the line defined by the center of the sphere (head) and the calculated source location intersected the surface of the sphere (scalp). In effect, this point defined the scalp position closest to the calculated source, with the only unknown being its distance from the center of the sphere (i.e., radius).

Results

The 12 patients consisted of 5 boys and 7 girls, mean age 8.6 yrs (range 4–15 yrs). One patient had bilateral independent discharges, thus yielding 13 separate foci. Figure 1 shows spike maps based on referential data from 3 different patients, plotted at the time of maximum negativity. These 3 represent all observed field patterns. The most prominent pattern was one with simultaneous temporal negativity and mid or bi-frontal positivity (Figure 1a). Ten of the 13 foci had this particular "dipolar" topography (type "a"). The mean amplitude was 72 μV for the negativity. Two others had the negativity displaced more posteriorly (type "b": Figure 1b), and the last one had a broad rolandic positivity simultaneous with separate negativity at the frontal and occipital regions ("tripolar" field pattern: Figure 1c).

Figure 2 shows Hjorth derivation maps for the same patients and time points as in Figure 1a,b. Eight foci had the typical type "a" dipolar topography (Figure 2a), four were type "b" with slightly displaced negative peaks (type

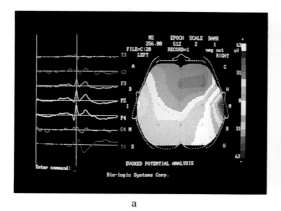

a

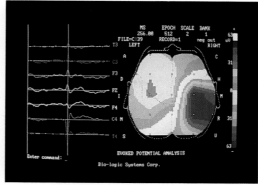

b

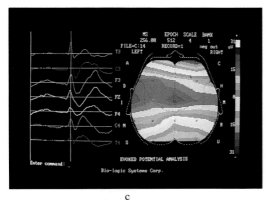

c

Figure 1. Observed spike map patterns (cheek reference). a) most common pattern (10/13 foci); b) less common (2/13); c) "tripolar field" (1/13).

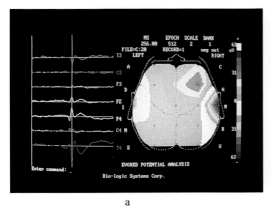

a

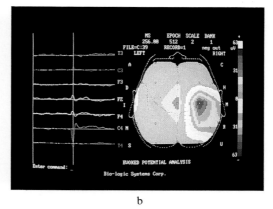

b

Figure 2. Hjorth-derived spike maps. Figure 2a,b correspond to the same data as in Figure 1a,b.

"b"), and 1 retained the complex tripolar field. For the most common type "a" Hjorth maps showed a "sharpening" of the voltage peaks, affecting the more diffuse positivity to a greater degree, and moving it generally closer to the more focal negativity. This effect is more pronounced for the type "b" cases, as shown in Figure 2b. All but the last case had the negativity entirely located over one of the three "rolandic electrodes": T_3, C_3, F_3 on the left, and T_4, C_4, F_4 on the right.

Figure 3 shows the superimposed $F_{x,y}$ and projected DLM scalp locations of all patients except that of Figure 1c. For the entire group, the $F_{x,y}$ were all within half an inter-electrode distance from the area bounded by the "rolandic electrodes." The DLM results gave a tighter clustering, with 12 of the 13 sources being within half an inter-electrode distance from the single electrode position C_4 or C_3. The remaining patient (No. 14—"tripolar" case) had the source placed near F_{p1}. As the final SSE greatly exceeded the 10% limit, this case was omitted from the calculation of the standard deviation boxes in Figure 3, on the basis of a poor DLM fit.

Figure 4 shows the three-dimensional DLM results in top and frontal views for all patients with all data plotted onto the left side. Figure 5 shows the original data. The calculated radius had a mean of 0.62, with standard deviation of 0.12.

FXY, DLM COMPARISON

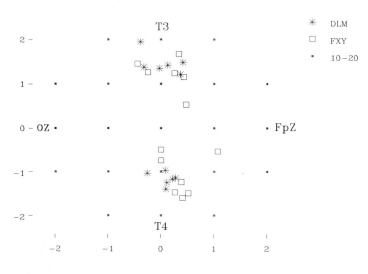

Figure 3. $F_{x,y}$ and DLM source locations of all foci except that of Figure 1c. DLM data have been projected onto the electrode grid diagram as described in text.

DLM: 12 CASES, REFLECTED TO LEFT

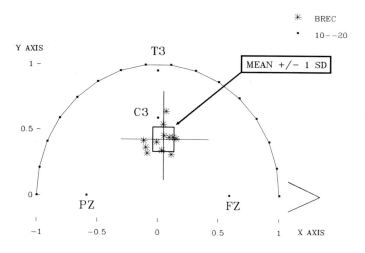

Figure 4. DLM source locations from Figure 3 replotted with right-sided results overlaid onto the left side. The mean location ±1 standard deviation is drawn as a box.

TOP VIEW OF DLM ESTIMATES: 12 BREC

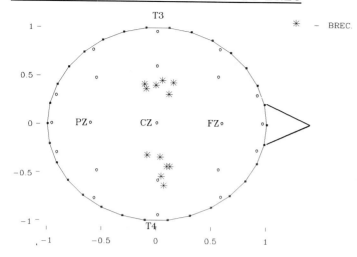

DLM: FRONTAL VIEW,   12 BREC

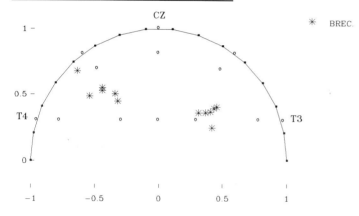

Figure 5. DLM source locations of all 13 foci from 12 patients plotted in top and frontal views from the cartesian cordinates. Selected electrode positions are overlaid for reference.

Discussion

The isopotential spike maps all showed dipolar field pattern, with 12 of the 13 having simultaneous negativity and positivity, while the remaining case showed a "tripolar" field, containing 3 spatially discrete polarities simultaneously. Hjorth-derived maps showed spatially smaller foci, generally facilitating visual estimation of the location of sources, by emphasizing voltage gradients. There was more susceptability to noise, being seen as multiple extraneous peaks of similar amplitude. These were more pronounced around the edges of the array, probably due to the absence of spatial filtering and the limited number of scalp electrodes used, and to the fact that the actual spatial Laplacian function was only approximated numerically.

In analysis of topographic EEG data, the concept of "equivalent source generator" is useful because of the degree of simplification it offers (Wood, 1982). Indeed, Kavanagh et al. (1978) have argued that sources which might be extended two-dimensional dipole sheets with irregular surfaces can be approximated by superpositions of single dipoles. The actual neuronal substrate is seldom defined anatomically, or even geometrically; however, clinical neurophysiologists often find it useful to assume hypothetical generators to help explain the pathophysiology which is responsible for the potential field under study. DLM estimation of the location, amplitude and direction of an equivalent source is a mathematical procedure which ignores nonhomogeneities of the brain and other important factors. Nonetheless, it can provide more information than visual analysis, and thus can be more useful. Therefore a model consisting of only one equivalent source may be clinically useful.

Inadequacies are known to exist in the DLM model. This would include poor geometric match of the head (children vs. adult head size and shape), mismatched skull/scalp attentuation, and most importantly the assumption of only one independent source. Geometric complexities may be present, for instance if the neuronal aggregate were curved in complex shapes (at the corner of a gyrus or depth of a sulcus). Under these conditions, the assumptions of a simple dipole vector would be invalid. Further, one can envisage a depolarization pattern spreading along tissues in a complex manner. One may expect that a two-generator model would better accomodate intricate source geometry or behaviour.

The DLM results provide an objective mathematical measure which may prove useful in spike characterization. The present results could not be interpreted easily because of the ambiguity of the radius (or depth) estimation. Without independent verification (e.g., by magnetoencephalograhy) or changes to the current source model, the only available improvement was to use Schneider's (1974) correction factor of 0.611 for the radius, in order to correct for skull attenuation. This would emulate a three-sphere model and allow for signal attenuation ignored by the single sphere model. However, such a correction factor has not been tested for children. Attempts to limit the maximum radius during the iterative solution ($R_{max} = 0.611$) produced, as expected, solutions clustered at that radius value. While this may produce a more physiologic and thus acceptable solution, it was judged inappropriate for the present purpose.

Determination of the anatomic structures involved would require complementary anatomic data from high resolution magnetic resonance imaging (MRI), putting it beyond the scope of this present paper. An important objective was to study characteristics of the spike topography of the entire BREC group. Thus, it was found useful not to place limitations upon the computation, and to use scalp-projected displays to compensate for depth ambiguity. This effectively showed the scalp location nearest to the calculated source, and allowed easy comparison with the original scalp data.

If one required an objective parameter for purposes of characterization, for instance in a classification problem involving spike data from several clinical groups, DLM produced a relatively tight clustering of the scalp projected source locations (Figure 3), in accordance with the clinical hypothesis.

Conclusion

DLM was used to estimate the source generator from scalp EEG interictal spike activity of children with clinically definite BREC. The calculated locations were projected onto the scalp surface and were found to form a tight cluster for 12 of the 13 foci studied. Despite limitations of the methodology and assumptions, a uniform finding was produced in this homogeneous group of epileptic children. Apart from its usefulness in anatomic localization, DLM may also be applied as an objective means of spike characterization.

References

Blom S, Heijbel J (1982) Benign epilepsy of children with centrotemporal EEG foci: A follow-up study in adulthood of patients initially studied as children. *Epilepsia, 23*, 629– 32.

Gregory D, Wong P (1984) Topographic analysis of the centrotemporal discharges in benign rolandic epilepsy of childhood. *Epilepsia, 25*(6), 705–711.

Hjorth B (1980) Source derivation simplifies topographical EEG interpretation. *Am J EEG Technology, 20*, 121–132.

Kavanagh RN, Darcey D, Lehmann, D, Fender DH (1978) Evaluation of methods for three dimensional localisation of electrical sources in the human brain. *IEEE Trans Biomed Eng, 25*(5), 421−429.

Lerman P, Kivity S (1975) Benign focal epilepsy of childhood. A follow-up study of 100 recovered patients. *Arch Neurol, 32,* 261−264.

Lombroso C (1967) Sylvian seizures and mid-temporal spike foci in children. *Arch Neurol, 17,* 52−59.

Marquardt DW (1963) An algorithm for least squares estimation of non-linear parameters. *J Soc Indust and Appl Math, 11,* 431−441.

Schneider M (1974) Effect of inhomogeneities on surface signals coming from a cerebral dipole source. *IEEE Trans Biomed Eng, 21,* 52−54.

Thickbroom GW, Davies HD, Carroll WM, Mastaglia FL (1986) Averaging, spatio-temporal mapping and dipole modelling of focal epileptic spikes. *Electroenceph clin Neurophysiol, 64,* 274−277.

Weinberg H, Brickett P, Coolsma F, Baff M (1986) Magnetic localization of intracranial dipoles: Simulation with a physical model. *Electroenceph clin Neurophysiol, 64,* 159− 170.

Wood C (1982) Application of dipole localization methods to source identification of human evoked potentials. *Ann NY Acad Sci, 388,* 139−155.

Section II

Analysis of Functional Topography

Functional Topography of the Human Brain

A. S. Gevins and S. L. Bressler

To represent the distributed cortical network involved in goal-directed behaviors, it is necessary to quantify event-related processing in, as well as relations between, the functional centers of the network. This paper discusses the idea that appropriately processed, scalp-recorded event-related potentials can index the activity of cortical regions involved in cognitive task performance. It also presents a set of procedures, called Event-Related Covariance (ERC) Analysis, that we use to measure patterns of statistical relationship between neuroelectric time-series recorded at different scalp sites. Applying ERC Analysis to simple cognitive tasks produced clear-cut results. These were consistent with prior neuropsychological models of the rapidly shifting cortical network accompanying expectancy, stimulus registration and feature extraction, response preparation and execution, and "updating" to feedback about response accuracy.

In studies of higher cognitive functions of the human brain, there currently is a renaissance of interest in measuring spatial aspects of brain activity. One sign of this is the reawakened concern with dipole source localization in the brain. Yet, if this resurgence is to flourish, advances in psychophysiology and the technologies of brain signal measurement and analysis will have to be utilized with a more sophisticated approach. While the localization of single equivalent-dipole generators may be quite informative in the case of sensory and motor events, it is of dubious utility in the case of higher cognitive processes. In fact, it is well known from clinical studies that even simple cognitive functions must require integrated processing in a network involving a number of distributed, specialized cortical areas (Mesulam, 1981). So, although it is convenient, it may not always be a good idea to compact all the data into a single equivalent dipole.

Rather, it seems more desirable to characterize the dynamic topology of this distributed network to determine which areas are active at any instant of time and which areas are statistically related to each other. This is an idea that has been evolving over the past four decades (Walter & Shipton, 1951; Barlow & Brazier, 1954; Adey et al., 1961; John et al., 1973; Callaway & Harris, 1974; Livanov, 1977; Tucker et al., 1986; Gevins et al., 1981, 1983, 1987; Gevins, 1987a; Bressler, 1987a,b). Our current approach is based on the hypothesis that when regions of the brain are functionally related, their event-related potential (ERP) components are related in shape and line up in time, perhaps with some delay. The idea is that the ERP waveform delineates the course of event-related mass neural activity of a population, so that if two populations are functionally related, their ERPs should line up. If

EEG Systems Laboratory, 1855 Folsom Street, San Francisco, CA 94103

The study of fatigue emerged from the collaboration of researchers from: (1) The USAF School of Aerospace Medicine, San Antonio (James Miller); (2) Systems Technology Inc., Hawthorne, California (Henry Jex and James Smith); (3) Washington University, St. Louis (John Stern); and (4) The EEG Systems Laboratory.

This research was supported by The U.S. Air Force Office of Scientific Research, The U.S. Air Force School of Aerospace Medicine, The National Institutes of Neurological and Communicative Diseases and Strokes, and The National Science Foundation. Thanks to Judith Gumbiner, Jennifer Strother and Kris Dean for manuscript preparation.

so, and if the relations are linear, this could be measured by computing the lagged covariance between the ERPs, or portions of the ERPs, from different regions—a measure we call event-related covariances (ERCs). As we shall see later, initial results of this approach have been quite promising. We must caution, however, that the hypothesis that ERCs measure functional relationships between cortical areas has not yet been proven.

The measurement of ERCs is part of a set of signal processing procedures called "Neurocognitive Pattern Analysis" (NCP Analysis) that we have developed to extract task-related spatiotemporal patterns from the unrelated electrical activity of the brain (Figure 1). In the past 10 years, these procedures have become increasingly sophisticated as the capabilities of computers have expanded. They now measure spatiotemporal task-related processes from up to 64 scalp electrodes in each of up to 25 fraction-of-a-second intervals spanning a 4—6 second period extending from before a cue, through stimulus and response, to presentation of feedback about performance accuracy. This paper describes first the basis for our approach to characterizing the functional topography of the brain, and then the current state of procedures that we are developing to carry out that characterization.

Neurophysiological Basis for the Measurement of Functional Topography

The representation of neocortex as a distributed neural network of interacting functional centers is a legacy of the Sherringtonian tradition (Sherrington, 1906). The pioneering work of Freeman (1975) has been crucial in reconciling this traditional view with more recent concepts of neural networks of individual neurons, by redefining the functional center as a cooperative domain of interconnected neuronal populations, rather than simply an anatomical pool of neurons. Freeman has demonstrated a systematic order between pulse probabilities of individual neurons and macroscopic forms of cooperative neural activity (macropotentials), showing that macro-

potentials reflect the emergence of dynamic self-organizing order in neuronal populations, lasting from tens to hundreds of milliseconds (Freeman, 1987). These ideas are consistent with the findings of Elul (1972), who concluded that extracellularly recorded cortical macropotentials result from summation of dendritic activity of the synchronized portion of a neuronal population, and of Petsche et al. (1984), who demonstrated the importance of the close relation between macropotentials and local cortical architectonics.

In laying the foundation for the concept of distributed cortical networks, studies on the emergent nature of macropotentials have been complemented by animal experiments focusing on field potential co-synchronization (Adey et al., 1961; Boudreau, 1966; Livanov, 1977). Dumenko (1970) found in dogs that correlation between extracellular potentials of visual and motor cortices increased with conditioning to a visual stimulus and was highest at the time of the conditioned stimulus and response. The finding that high correlation was specific to particular regions of motor and visual cortices was similar to the observation of Bressler (1987a,b) that high correlation between olfactory bulb and cortex in rabbits was specific to particular regions of each. Measures of similarity between field potentials have also been applied to averaged event-related potentials. John et al. (1973) measured the relatedness of waveforms recorded from different conditioned responses and demonstrated differential generalization of neural activity based on waveform similarity.

Given this view of distributed functional cortical networks, and given the sensitivity of ERPs to rapid changes in brain state associated with performance of complex behavioral tasks, we hypothesize that appropriately processed ERPs may reflect the activation of rapidly-shifting, widely distributed functional aggregates of underlying neuronal populations. In the tradition of Lashley (1958) and John (1967), we have sought to characterize the "functional topography" of distributed cortical networks by looking for consistent statistical relations between field potentials recorded over different areas of cortex during performance of highly controlled cognitive tasks.

ADIEEG IV NEUROCOGNITIVE
PATTERN RECOGNITION SYSTEM

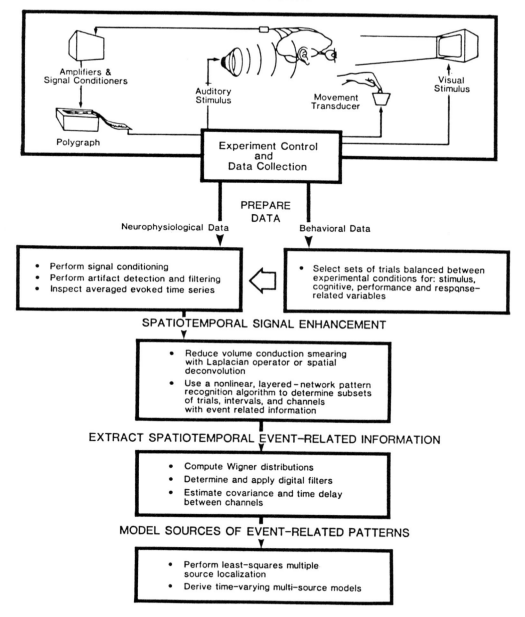

Figure 1. ADIEEG-IV system for quantification of event-related brain signals. Separate subsystems perform on-line experimental control and data collection, data selection and evaluation, signal processing and pattern recognition. Current capacity is 128 channels. Spherical-head spatial deblurring modules have been implemented, and multiple source modeling algorithms are being developed. Digital tapes of magnetic resonance images or of electrophysiological data from other laboratories are converted into the ADIEEG data format using gateway programs; they are then processed using the same program modules as data collected in the EEG Systems Laboratory. (adapted from Gevins, 1987c)

CLASSIFIER-DIRECTED ARTIFACT DETECTION

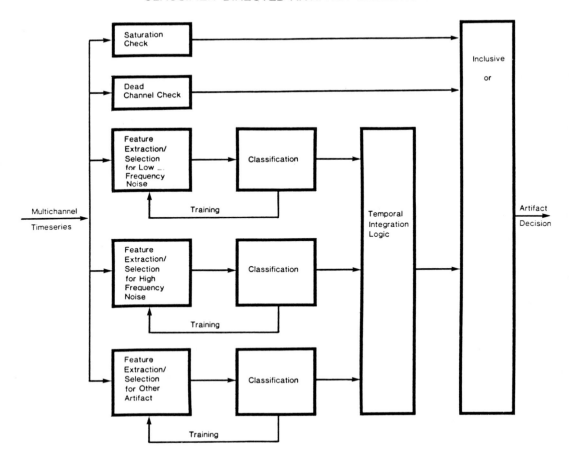

Figure 2. Classifier-directed artifact detection. A system consisting of five parallel detectors is used to find contaminants. Three of the detectors incorporate layered-network classifiers to choose and weigh feature combinations. In this way, a precise automated procedure replaces sole reliance on ad hoc waveform detectors and manually set thresholds. (adapted from Gevins & Morgan, 1986)

In practice, we have measured timeseries covariances (formerly correlations) between scalp potentials from pairs of channels, either on sets of single-trial data (Gevins et al., 1981, 1983, 1985), or on enhanced filtered averages (Gevins et al., 1987, submitted a,b, in prep). The results provide interesting new information about brain function, and suggest that these measures are worth further development. The scalp patterns we have measured have been consistent with the known functional neuroanatomy of the cerebral cortex, as determined from other lines of evidence. As predicted by neuroanatomical theory and clinical neuropsychological studies, ERC patterns corresponding to visual stimulus processing involved posterior sites that led anterior parietal sites and premotor sites, and ERC patterns at the time of a finger pressure involved the midline precentral electrode that overlies the premotor and supplementary motor cortices. Although the problem of identifying the generators of these patterns is the focus of current research, it has not yet been solved. However, the tendency of the scalp sites involved in these patterns to be spatially separated, without intervening sites, seems to rule out volume-conducted activity from just one or two cortical or subcortical generators.

Procedures for Measurement of Functional Topography

Current Computer System

The current computer system is a 32-bit multiprocessor system with 3 computing modes, a 12-MFLOP floating point capability and a 3500 megabyte on-line disk capacity. The current data acquisition system is capable of sampling up to 256 channels at up to 2 kHz sampling rates per channel. (Current amplification capabilities are 128 channels.) Trial presentation, which is performed by a PC controlled by the host computer, is automatically delayed until eye blinks, amplifier setting from eye blinks, and gross body movements have all died down. Up to 70 channels of EEG and non-EEG channels are monitored at a time on a color graphics screen for electrode problems. Other channels are bank-switchable to the monitor. Averages can also be viewed on-line to check for event-registered artifacts. Artifacts such as eye movement and muscle potential contamination are automatically marked by multiple, layered-network pattern classification programs (Figure 2) (Gevins & Morgan, 1986).

Spatial Sampling

The use of 64 scalp channels provides uniform scalp coverage with an interelectrode distance of about 3.5 cm on a typical adult head. Figure 3 shows a subject wearing a stretchable 64-channel EEG recording cap. The electrodes are placed on the cap according to an expanded version of the 10-20 system (Figure 4).

We are currently extending EEG recordings to 128 channels with interelectrode distances of about 2.25 cm. The desirability of recording from so many sites is evident since regional cerebral blood flow studies suggest that "cortical fields" of 1—3 square centime-

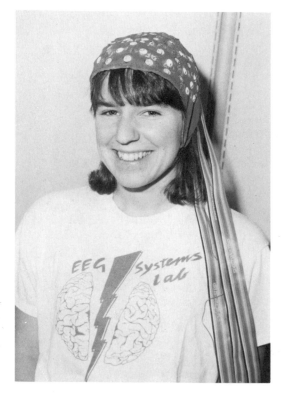

Figure 3. Subject wearing 64 channel EEG cap. (adapted from Gevins, 1988)

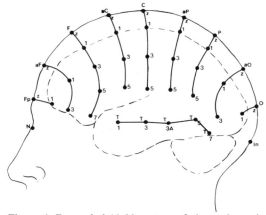

Figure 4. Expanded 10-20 system of electrode position nomenclature. Additional coronal rows of electrodes interpolated between the International 10-20 System coronal rows have the letter "a" for "anterior" added to the designation for the next row posterior, e.g., aPz for anterior parietal midline electrode. With 64 electrodes, the average distance between electrodes is about 3.25 cm. (adapted from Gevins, 1987c)

ters are activated during a wide variety of cognitive tasks (Roland, 1985a,b). Yet, while the possibility of extracting more detailed spatial information has been clearly demonstrated with the MEG (see Williamson & Kaufman, 1987 for discussion and bibliography), it is not widely appreciated that such information can be obtained from appropriately processed EEGs. Examination of spatial spectra has shown that, if information is available from the entirety of an adult's scalp, adequate sampling would require more than 128 electrodes at 2 cm intervals (Gevins, 1988).

In Figure 5, we can see the effect of an increasing number of EEG electrodes on the electric field distribution of a right index finger flexion. Note the false impression of localization with 16 electrodes, and the correct appearance of a left central focus with 27 and 51 electrodes. Although there is much current discussion about what form of interpolation is best to use in making colored EEG potential maps, it would seem that the more compelling issue is the need for more electrodes.

Rejecting Artifact-Contaminated EEG Signals

An interactive graphics trial editing program is used by an operator to check the decisions of the automatic artifact detectors (Gevins & Morgan, 1986). In practice, editors have be-

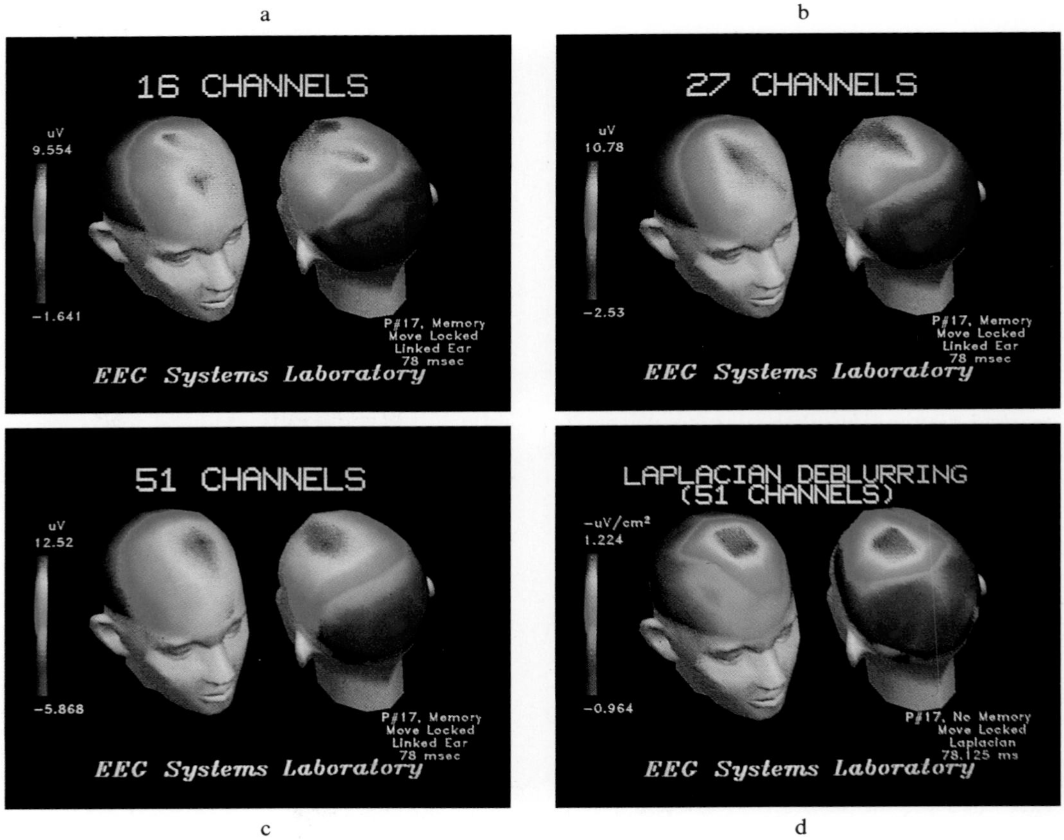

a

b

c

d

Figure 5. Movement-locked average ERPs at 78 ms after start of right-index-finger flexion, recorded against a linked-ears reference with (A) 16 channels, (B) 27 channels, (C) 51 channels and (D) after application of a Laplacian operation to the 51 channel ERPs. There is a false localization with 16 channels due to insufficient spatial sampling. The 27- and 51-channel ERP recordings show the true potential distribution with increasing resolution. Improvement in topographic localization with the Laplacian is self-evident. (adapted from Gevins, 1988)

come sufficiently skilled to check the single trials of a 64-channel recording in roughly twice the time that it takes to run the experiment. Algorithms are under development to recover trials with non-saturating artifacts. Eye blinks or eye movements, for example, can be removed using least squares noise cancellation, given EOG reference electrodes near the eyes.

Finding Trials with Discernible Event-Related Signals

We have developed a simple method for finding trials with event-related signals which does not assume that event-related signals are discernible in every trial, and which has minimal assumptions about the statistical properties of signal and noise (Gevins, 1984; Gevins et al., 1986). This method is useful for increasing the signal-to-noise ratio of average ERPs, and for accentuating the differences between averages from two conditions having subtle cognitive differences. However, it is not an essential step when these benefits are not required. First, a mild lowpass filter is applied (3 dB point at 14 Hz and 20 dB down at 32 Hz) and the data, originally sampled at 128 Hz, are decimated by a factor of 3 digitizing points. Then, a "noise" set is formed, composed of segments of single trials for each channel that are randomly timed with respect to stimulus and response events. The number of points in each segment corresponds to that of the ERP interval to be investigated, typically 3 decimated points for a 125 ms interval.

The artificially-formed "noise" data set is then compared with sets of single trial segments which are properly time-registered to stimulus or response events. This comparison produces equations characterizing the event-related signal and determines a list of trials with detectable event-related signals. A pattern classification algorithm constructs the equations that discriminate between sets of single-trial event-related and noise segments for each channel. The equations consist of weighted combinations of the filtered and decimated waveform amplitude values within the interval. Three leave-out-one-third-of-the-trials validations are used, and the average test-set classification is compared with the bi-

nomial distribution for significance. If the equations are significant on validation data, a consistent event-related signal has been found in many of the trials. ERPs that are averaged over these selected trials are called "enhanced" averages, because the signal characteristics have been accentuated (Figure 6).

Controlling for Irrelevant Between-Condition Variables

In comparing data from two conditions, it is important to balance the two data sets for stimulus-, response-, or performance-related variables that have differences unrelated to the intended comparison. For each between-condition comparison, the two sets of event-related, signal-bearing trials are statistically balanced for each subject by eliminating trials that have outlying values for these irrelevant variables (Gevins et al., 1981, 1983, 1985, 1987, submitted a,b, in prep).

First, a program automatically calculates the largest subset of trials that behaviorally balance the two conditions being compared, for a requested subset of behavioral variables. The set of about 50 behavioral variables includes response time, pressure, velocity, acceleration, duration and error, as well as stimulus parameters, indices of muscle activity and "arousal" (integrated energy in the Pz electrode, computed in 500-ms epochs before and after the onset of each event). This is followed by an interactive program that displays the means, Student's t-tests and histograms of the requested variables using a convenient, window-oriented user interface. It is used to check the automatic split of the distributions and to allow their correction if necessary. Between-condition balance is achieved when Student's t for each behavioral variable of comparison has a significance of $p < 0.2$.

Reducing Blur Distortion at the Scalp

Because potentials generated by sources in the brain are volume conducted through brain, cerebrospinal fluid, skull and scalp to the recording electrodes, potentials from a localized source are spread over a considerable area of scalp. Potentials measured at a scalp site thus represent the summation of signals from many

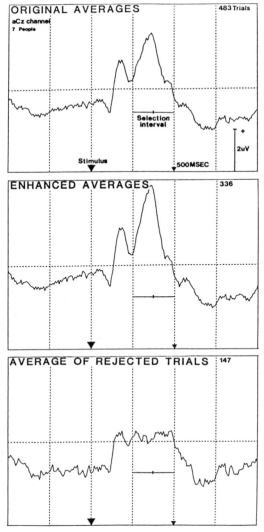

Figure 6. Use of pattern recognition analysis to remove trials without detectable task-related signals from a set of single-trial ERPs. This results in an average ERP with a higher signal-to-noise ratio obtained from fewer trials. (A) An original average ERP formed from 483 presentations of a visual numeric stimulus. (B) Average of 336 trials with consistent event-related signals in the P3 interval. Trials were selected from the original set of 483 by applying a pattern recognition algorithm to distinguish a 250 ms, P3 timeseries segment from a pre-cue "baseline" segment. Note the greatly increased size of the event-related peaks and lower frequency wave forms. (C) Average of 147 trials which did not have consistent event-related signals in the P3 interval. Note the relative lack of event-related activity in the P3 interval. (adapted from Gevins et al., 1986)

sources over much of the brain. (In the context of a 4-shell spherical head model, we have estimated the amount of spread, the "point spread," for a radial equivalent dipole source in the cortex to be about 2.5 cm—Doyle & Gevins, 1986). This spatial low-pass blurring makes source localization difficult, even for nearby cortical sources, and causes the potentials from local sources to be mixed with those from more distant generators. By modeling the tissues between brain and scalp as surfaces with different thicknesses and resistances, we can perform a deblurring operation that, in principle, makes the potential appear as it would if it were recorded just above the level of the brain surface. This operation can be performed without imposing assumptions as to the actual (cortical or subcortical) source locations. The deblurring, however, requires detailed modeling of the tissues, which is a great deal of work when the exact shape of the head is taken into account. Furthermore, there is as yet no good solution to the problem of precisely estimating the local resistances of skull and scalp. When the EEG scalp electrodes are no closer together than about 2.5–3.0 cm, a simpler, model-free deblurring method provides results comparable to the more complex procedure.

This simpler technique, called the Laplacian operator, consists of computing the second derivative in space of the potential field at each electrode. This converts the potential into a quantity proportional to the current entering and leaving the scalp at each electrode site, and eliminates the effect of the reference electrode used during recording. An approximation to the Laplacian, introduced by Hjorth (1975, 1980), assumes that electrodes are equidistant and at right angles to each other. Although this approximation is fairly good for electrodes near the midline, such as Cz, it becomes increasingly poor at the periphery. An optimal estimate of the Laplacian requires precise knowledge of the electrode positions in three dimensions, information which can be obtained by direct measurements from the head (Greer & Gevins, in prep). A properly computed Laplacian operator can produce a dramatic improvement in the spatial topographic detail of ERP components (see Figure 5D).

Choosing Filters and Analysis Windows with Wigner Time-Frequency Distributions

The ERP waveform is a function of time and does not provide explicit frequency information. Yet, the instantaneous frequency is not constant for different ERP components. For each component, the instantaneous frequency must be determined to isolate that component with digital filtering, and the duration over which that frequency is stable must be determined to define the length of the analysis interval. Power spectra of ERP waveforms provide frequency information but obscure time-dependent phenomena. A view of the spectrum as it changed over time would give a new view of the evolution of different frequency components of the ERP. A simple but ineffective approach would be to compute the spectrum over highly overlapped windows of the average ERP. A preferable method is to compute a general function of time and frequency, called the Wigner Distribution, which approximates the instantaneous energy for a given time and frequency. In practice, enhanced ERPs show strong enough energy "peaks" in the Wigner Distribution that very simple interpretations of the time and frequency locations of signal energy are valid (Morgan & Gevins, 1986; Figure 7). From visual inspection of Wigner Distributions, it is a simple matter to specify digital filter characteristics that produce optimal time-frequency resolution for a given ERP component, and to determine the frequency-stable interval for that component. This procedure need not be implemented for each experiment. For example, a filter and interval defined for the N100 in one experiment may be sufficient for analyzing the N100 in another experiment.

Computing Event-Related Covariances (ERCs) Between Channels

To summarize, these preliminary steps are followed before computing ERCs:

1. Record a sufficient amount of data using as many electrodes as possible.
2. Remove data with artifact contamination.
3. Find trials with consistent event-related signals (optional).

4. Select the pair of conditions to be compared, and eliminate trials with extreme values of behavioral variables to obtain behaviorally balanced trial sets.
5. Apply the Laplacian operator to the potential distribution of each non-peripheral scalp electrode location.
6. Compute Wigner Distribution on average ERP (optional) and determine digital filter characteristics and analysis intervals.

Once the data sets have been prepared in this way, the next step is to compute the enhanced, filtered and decimated, averaged Laplacian ERP for each condition. Then, multi-lag crosscovariance functions are computed between all pairwise channel combinations of these averaged ERPs in each selected analysis window. The magnitude of the maximum value of the crosscovariance function and its lag time are the features used to characterize the ERC. The covariance analysis interval is the width of one period of the band-center frequency of each filter. Down-sampling factors are determined by the 20 dB rejection point, and the covariance function is computed up to a lag-time of one-half period of the high frequency for each band. For example, we often use a filter with 3 dB cutoffs at 4 and 7 Hz, and with 20 dB attenuation at 1.5 and 9.5 Hz. The filtered timeseries are decimated from 128 Hz to 21 Hz for each covariance calculation. Covariance is estimated over a 187-ms window, which corresponds to one period of a 5.5 Hz sinusoid. Each window is lagged by up to 8 lags at the original undecimated sampling rate, i.e., $1/128$ s per lag.

Estimating the significance of ERCs requires an estimate of the standard deviation of the "noise" ERC. First, random intervals in each single trial of the ensemble are averaged. Then, ERC analysis is performed on a filtered and decimated version of the resulting "noise" averages, yielding a distribution of "noise" ERCs. Because of the large number of channel pairs, some spurious significant covariances may be found. Therefore, the threshold for significance is reduced according to the dimensionality of the data with Duncan's correction procedure. The number of channels is used as a conservative estimate of the number of independent dimensions. The most signifi-

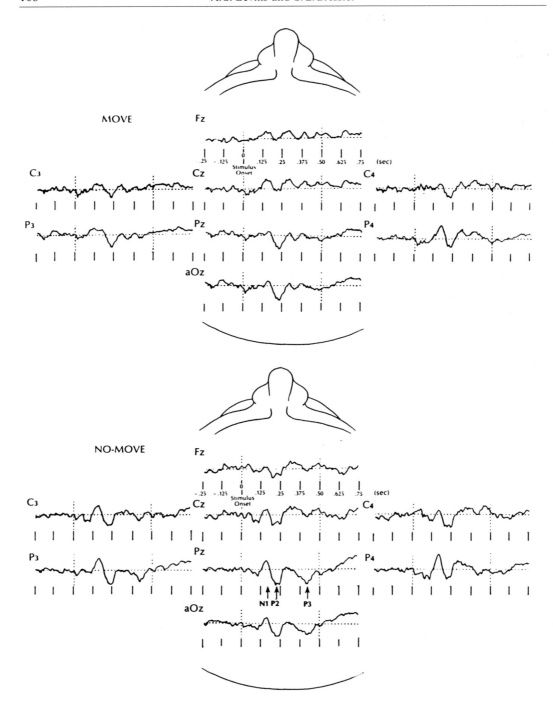

Figure 7. Two representations of eight average ERP channels for "move" and "no-move" cognitive tasks. The view is of the top of the head, with the nose at the top of each set of eight channels. (A) Average time-series of 40 no-move and 37 move trials. Three of the most commonly studied ERP peaks N1, P2, P3 are indicated on the Pz channel of the no-move task. Of these, the P3 peak is larger in the infrequently occurring no-move trials.

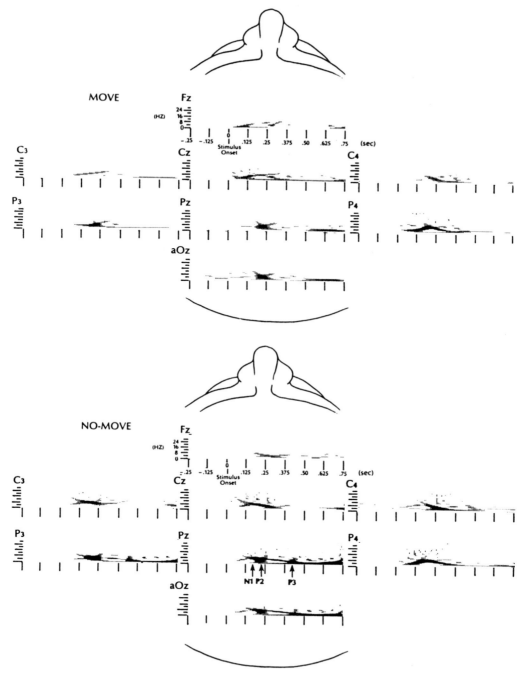

(B) The pseudo-Wigner distribution of the analytic signal of the same data. This representation shows that the event-related processes are changing rapidly in both time and frequency. The first moment along the time axis for each frequency is the group delay, while the first moment along the frequency axis is the instantaneous frequency. There is a buildup in energy after the stimulus, and a general increase in frequency until the energy concentration between the time of the N1 and P2 peaks begins to fall off (most prominent in the Pz channel). Then there is a glide down in frequency in the no-move task (most prominent in the Pz and aOz channels), which culminates in a concentration of energy around the time of the P3 peak. (adapted from Gevins 1984)

cant ERCs in each interval are graphed (Figure 8).

To compare ERC maps between conditions, the differences in means of significant ERCs between conditions are tested with an ANOVA and post-hoc t-tests. The similarity between two multivariate ERC maps is measured with an estimate of the correlation between them. The estimate comes from a distribution-independent "bootstrap" Monte Carlo procedure (Efron, 1970), which generates an ensemble of correlation values from randomly selected choices of the repeated measures. This also yields a confidence interval for the estimates.

Validating Significance of ERCs

We test the between-subject variability of ERC patterns by determining whether each pair of experimental conditions of a particular subject can be distinguished using discriminating equations generated on the other subjects. Likewise, we determine within-subject reliability by attempting to discriminate the experimental conditions for each session using equations generated on that subject's other sessions. These tests are performed on sets of single trials to quantify the extent to which the condition-specific patterns from the ERC analysis of the average ERPs are observable in each trial. Although this procedure could be done with any type of discriminant analysis, we have developed the use of distribution-independent, "neural network" pattern classification algorithms for this purpose (Gevins et al., 1979a,b,c, 1981, 1983, 1985, 1986, 1987; Gevins & Morgan, 1986; Gevins, 1980, 1984, 1987b). We have shown that this method has better sensitivity and specificity than stepwise or full-model linear or quadratic discriminant analysis (Gevins, 1980). The pattern recognition approach has the advantage of testing how well a subject's individual trials conform to those of the group in discriminating two behavioral conditions of interest. In the same way, the trials of each session of a subject are tested by conformity to trials from the other sessions of that subject. Requiring trial-by-trial discriminability is a strict condition for deciding between-subject variability and within-subject reliability.

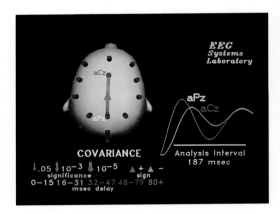

Figure 8. Schematic diagram showing the relationship of an event-related covariance (ERC) line on a top-view of a model head (left) to the theta-band-filtered, averaged event-related Laplacian derivation waveforms (right). ERCs were computed over the indicated 187-ms analysis interval from the aPz and aCz electrode sites. The width of an ERC line indicates the significance of the covariance between two waveforms, with the scale appearing above the word "significance." The color of the line indicates the time delay in ms (lag time of maximum covariance) as shown in the scale above "ms delay." The color of the arrow indicates the sign of the covariance (same color as line = positive; skin color = negative). The arrow points from leading to lagging channel, unless there is no delay, in which case a bar is shown. The covariance between aPz and aCz is significant at $p < 10^{-5}$. The aPz waveform leads the aCz waveform by about 16–31 ms (green line), and the covariance is positive (arrow also green). (from Gevins et al., submitted a)

Each subject's classification yields a score, which is the percent of trials that are correctly classified by the group discrimination equations. The score is assessed for significance by comparison to the binomial distribution (Gevins, 1980). A significant classification score for a subject indicates that the group equations are successful in discriminating the two conditions in his or her trials.

Within-subject (between-session) reliability is tested in a similar manner. The trial set (consisting of the two conditions) from each of a subject's sessions is tested with equations developed on the trial sets from his or her other sessions. The single-trial ERC values come from channel pairs that are significant in the ERC pattern formed from the average over all his or her sessions. Post-hoc comparisons are valuable in determining whether effects of learning and/or habituation are evident over sessions, by indicating which sessions are alike, and where transitions occur between sessions.

Application of ERC Analysis

Study of Visuomotor Performance

Procedure (Gevins et al., 1987, submitted a,b).

Seven healthy, right-handed male adults participated in this study. A visual cue, slanted to the right or to the left, indicated to subjects to prepare to make a response pressure with the right or left index finger. One second later, the cue was followed by a visual numeric stimulus (number 1–9) indicating that a pressure of 0.1 to 0.9 kg should be made with the index finger of the hand indicated by the cue. Feedback indicating the exact response pressure produced was presented as a two-digit number one second after the peak of the response pressure. On a random 20% of the trials, the stimulus number was slanted opposite to that of the cue, and subjects were to withhold their responses on these "catch trials." The next trial followed 1 s after disappearance of the feedback. Subjects each performed several hundred trials, with rest breaks as needed.

Twenty-six channels of EEG data, as well as vertical and horizontal eye-movements and flexor digitori muscle activity from both arms, were recorded. All single-trial EEG data were screened for eye movement, muscle potential and other artifacts. Contaminated data were discarded.

Intervals used for ERC analysis were centered on major ERP peaks. ERCs were computed between averaged Laplacian ERPs from each of the 120 pairwise combinations of the 16 nonperipheral channels in intervals from 500 ms before cue to 500 ms after the feedback.

Data sets were separated into trials in which subsequent performance was either accurate or inaccurate. Accurate and inaccurate performance trials were those in which the error (deviation from required finger pressure) was less than or greater than, respectively, the mean error over the recording session.

Results and Discussion

The ERC pattern for the interval at the peak of the finger pressure (Figure 9) closely corresponded to prior functional neuroanatomical knowledge, lending a first level of validation for the patterns associated with higher-order cognitive activity. The midline precentral electrode, overlying the premotor and supplementary motor cortex, was the focus of all movement-related patterns, and the patterns for the two hands were appropriately lateralized, clearly reflecting the sharply focused current sources and sinks spanning the hand areas of motor cortex.

ERC patterns during a 375-ms interval centered 687-ms post-cue (spanning the late Contingent Negative Variation; CNV) were distinct from those related to overt finger responses. The pattern associated with subsequently accurate right-hand performance involved predominantly left hemisphere sites, particularly left frontal and appropriately la-

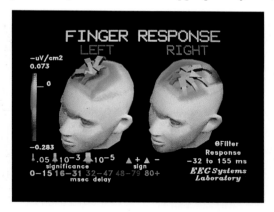

Figure 9. Most significant (top standard deviation) ERC patterns at the peak of the finger pressure for right and left hand trials from seven people, superimposed on maps of Laplacian response potential amplitude. Note that the anterior midline precentral (aCz) electrode is the focus of all covariances, with 16–31 ms time delays between aCz and Fz. The patterns are distinctly lateralized according to responding hand. The sign of the aCz covariances is positive for lateral frontal, and negative for lateral central and anterior parietal electrodes.

teralized central and parietal sites (Figure 10A). The pattern preceding accurate left-hand performance involved predominantly right hemisphere sites, in addition to the left frontal site. Inaccurate performance by the right hand (Figure 10B) was preceded by a highly simplified pattern, while inaccurate performance by the left hand was preceded by a complex, spatially diffuse pattern.

When the trials of each of the 7 subjects were classified by equations developed on the trials of the other 6 subjects, the overall discrimination was 59% (p < 0.01) for right hand and 57% (p < 0.01) for left-hand performance. For the subject with the most trials, average classification of 68% (p < .001) for subsequent right- and 62% (p < .01) for subsequent left-hand performance was achieved by testing a separate equation on each fifth of his trials, formed from the other four-fifths.

We suggest that our pre-stimulus ERC patterns characterize a distributed preparatory neural set related to the accuracy of subsequent task performance. This set appears to involve distinctive cognitive (frontal), integrative-motor and lateralized somesthetic-motor components. The involvement of the left-frontal site is consistent with clinical findings that preparatory sets are synthesized and integrated in prefrontal cortical areas, and with experimental and clinical evidence indicating involvement of the left dorsolateral prefrontal cortex in delayed response tasks. A midline precentral integrative motor component is consistent with known involvement of premotor and supplementary motor areas in initiating motor responses. The finding of appropriately lateralized central and parietal components is consistent with evidence from primates and humans for neuronal firing in motor and somatosensory cortices prior to motor responses.

Study of Incipient Fatigue

Procedure (Gevins et al., in prep)

After learning and practicing a battery of tasks until their performance was stable on one day, each of five right-handed, healthy male subjects returned to the laboratory the next morning and performed the tasks for about 6 hours. Following a dinner break, they resumed task performance for an additional 6 to 8 hours.

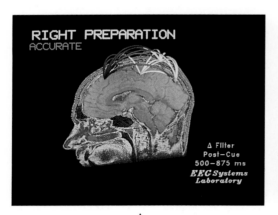

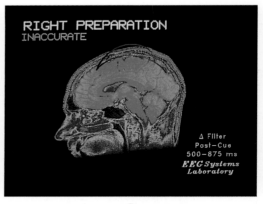

A   B

Figure 10. View of the significant (p < 0.05) Contingent Negative Variation (CNV) ERC patterns, superimposed on a mid-sagittal Magnetic Resonance Image of a subject's cranium. Measurements are from an interval 500 to 875 ms after the cue for subsequently accurate (A) and inaccurate (B) right-hand visuomotor task performance by seven right-handed men. The thickness of an ERC line is proportional to its significance (from .05 to .005). A yellow line indicates the ERC is positive, while a red line is negative. Covariances involving left frontal (F3), left central (C3), left parietal (P3), and left antero-parietal (aP1) electrode sites, all contralateral to the subsequently responding hand, are the most prominent sites in the pattern for subsequently accurate performance. Only two covariances characterize subsequently inaccurate performance: left frontal (F3) with left parietal (P3), and left frontal with left antero-parietal (aP1) sites.

There were four tasks in the battery, including easy and difficult continuous and discrete visuomotor tracking tasks, a simple numeric memory task, and a difficult visuomotor memory task (VMMT). Since we expected that early neural signs of fatigue would be most evident during demanding tasks, we analyzed the VMMT first. This task required subjects to remember two continuously changing numbers, in the presence of numeric distractors, in order to produce precise finger pressures. Each trial consisted of a warning symbol followed by a single-digit visual stimulus to be remembered, followed by the subject's finger-pressure response to the stimulus number presented two trials earlier, followed by a 2-digit feedback number indicating the accuracy of the response. For example, if the stimulus numbers in five successive trials were 8, 6, 1, 9, 4, the correct response would be a pressure of 0.8 kg when seeing the 1, 0.6 kg for the 9, and 0.1 kg for the 4. To increase the task difficulty, subjects were required to withhold their response on a random 20% of the trials. These "no-response catch trials" were trials in which the current stimulus number was identical to the stimulus two trials earlier.

Trials early in the recording session with accurate finger pressures formed the "Alert" data set. Trials from early in the evening, when performance was just starting to decline, formed the "Incipient Fatigue" data set. For each subject, trials with relatively inaccurate responses were then deleted from the Incipient Fatigue data set so that the final Alert and Incipient Fatigue data sets consisted of trials with equivalently accurate performance. This crucial step allowed measurement of neuroelectric patterns associated with incipient fatigue while controlling for those due to variations in performance accuracy.

EEGs were recorded with either 33 or 51 channels with a nylon mesh cap. Vertical and horizontal eye movements were also recorded, as were the responding flexor digitori muscle potentials, electrocardiogram and respiration. Three-axis Magnetic Resonance Image scans were made of 3 of the 5 subjects.

Grand-average (over the five pilots) ERPs were time-locked to presentation of the numeric stimulus. Incipient-Fatigue ERPs were subtracted from Alert ERPs in order to highlight changes due to fatigue. Spatiotemporal neuroelectric patterns were then quantified by measuring ERCs between all 153 pairwise combinations of the 18 nonperipheral electrodes. ERCs were measured across brief segments of grand-average Alert-minus-Incipient-Fatigue subtraction ERPs. The first ERC interval was 500 ms wide and was centered 312 ms before the numeric stimulus. The next two ERC intervals were 187 ms wide and were positioned with respect to the N125 peak elicited by the numeric stimulus, and the P380 ERP peak elicited by the infrequent, no-response catch-trial stimuli.

Results and Discussion

A number of significant Alert-minus-Incipient-Fatigue ERCs were found during the 500-ms prestimulus interval. Significance was determined by comparison to a distribution of "noise" ERCs, and corrected with Duncan's procedure, following the description above ("Computing Event-Related Covariances Between Channels"). Midline central, left parietal, left anteroparietal, right anteroparietal and right posterior parietal electrodes were the major ERC foci. There were no significant ERCs in the interval centered at 62 ms poststimulus. The ERCs computed over the P380 no-response difference ERP were focused on the midline precentral, and right anterior and posterior parietal electrodes.

The ERC changes with Incipient Fatigue suggest that dynamic functional neural networks associated with specific cognitive functions are selectively affected during early fatigue. During the prestimulus interval, when subjects were maintaining the last two visually presented numbers in working memory and preparing for the next stimulus, ERCs decreased in number in the Incipient Fatigue condition. The lack of ERC differences between Alert and Incipient Fatigue conditions during the interval centered at 62 ms suggests that the "exogenous" stages of visual stimulus processing are relatively unaffected by early fatigue. However, during the later post-stimulus interval of trials requiring an inhibition of the response, ERCs again decreased in number with Incipient Fatigue.

The results suggest that although neural systems responsible for primary visual stimulus processing are relatively unaffected by Incipient Fatigue, cortical associative areas responsible for higher cognitive functions such as working memory rehearsal, preparation, and motor inhibition are altered prior to appreciable degradations in performance.

Conclusions

The idea of distributed processing networks in the brain has been well established in the literature, dating back to Sherrington. This powerful concept has been under-utilized in neurocognitive studies, perhaps because of the difficulty of measuring activity patterns. Recent attempts at constructing "parallel distributed processing" models of cognition (Rumelhart et al., 1986) aim to derive computational principles from knowledge of the brain's own distributed processing networks. These efforts are encouraging, yet they depend on continued characterization of those networks. Measurement of the dynamic functional topography of the brain, the time-varying statistical relations among the field potentials from a distributed set of recording sites, is an empirical means of accomplishing this. It has been shown that patterns of event-related covariance, measuring functional topography, are related to cognitive processing, and thus may represent active states of a distributed processing network.

At least three major factors have contributed to our ability to begin characterizing the functional topography of the human brain. First was the use of sufficiently controlled cognitive tasks to allow inference of the cognitive processes taking place during brief analysis intervals. Along with this was the production of computer programs to choose trials from two experimental conditions that are balanced for important behavioral variables. This factor created the functional context for topographic measurements. Second was the ability to record from a sufficient number of channels to adequately sample the available recording surface of the head. Indications are that even with 64 evenly spaced scalp electrodes, there is potentially more information to be gained from greater spatial sampling. This factor allowed the topography to be represented spatially. Third was the application of sophisticated signal processing techniques to the analysis of event-related potentials. This factor was necessary to appropriately measure the inter-regional relations comprising the functional topography.

Neurocognitive Pattern (NCP) Analysis and Event-Related Covariance (ERC) Analysis should be distinguished from brain electrical activity maps, which are usually color topographic displays interpolated from 16—20 channels of averaged ERPs or EEG spectra, or the difference between such measures and a set of normative data. We use more extensive signal processing and pattern recognition algorithms to reduce volume conduction effects and to extract event-related signals from unrelated background noise of the brain, compute between-channel ERC patterns, and display their scalp distribution in 3-D perspective graphics of the head and brain. Subtle aspects of neurocognitive function, such as the measurement of preparatory sets that precede accurate performance, are revealed by these ERC patterns but are not necessarily apparent on topographic maps (Gevins et al., submitted b). ERC Analysis is currently undergoing further development. The value of scalp patterns could be greatly expanded by a more adequate understanding of their sources. The difficult problem of determining the distributed source network in the brain producing the scalp ERC patterns is crucial, and is the focus of our ongoing work.

It is a testimony to the ingenuity of cognitive psychologists, psychophysiologists, neurologists and psychiatrists that so much has been learned about the timing of neurocognitive processes using very modest recording equipment and analysis techniques. It is, therefore, almost certain that when more advanced recording methods and more powerful analytic tools are widely available, rapid advances in understanding the neural basis of human cognitive functions will take place.

References

Adey WR, Walter DO, Hendrix CE (1961) Computer techniques in correlation and spectral analysis of cerebral slow waves during discriminative behavior. *Exp Neurol, 3,* 501—524.

Barlow JS, Brazier, MAB (1954) A note on a correlator for electroencephalographic work. *Electroenceph clin Neurophysiol, 6,* 321—325.

Boudreau JC (1966) Computer measurements of hippocampal fast activity with chronically implanted electrodes. *Electroenceph clin Neurophysiol, 20,* 165—174.

Bressler SL (1987a) Relations of olfactory bulb and cortex, I: Spatial variation of bulbo-cortical interdependence. *Brain Research, 409,* 285—293.

Bressler SL (1987b) Relations of olfactory bulb and cortex, II: Model for driving of cortex by bulb. *Brain Research, 409,* 294—301.

Callaway E, Harris P (1974) Coupling between cortical potentials from different areas. *Science, 183,* 873—875.

Doyle JC, Gevins, AS (1986) *Spatial filters for event-related potentials.* EEG Systems Laboratory Technical Report-0011.

Dumenko VN (1970) Electroencephalographic investigation of cortical relationships in dogs during formation of a conditioned reflex stereotype. In Rusinov, V.S. (Ed.) *Electrophysiology of the nervous system.* Plenum Press, New York, 107—117.

Efron B (1970) *The jackknife, the bootstrap, and other resampling plans.* SIAM, Philadelphia.

Elul R (1972) The genesis of the EEG. *Int Rev of Neurobiol, 15,* 227—272.

Freeman WJ (1975) *Mass action in the nervous system.* Academic Press, New York.

Freeman WJ (1987) Analytic techniques used in the search for the physiological basis of the EEG. In Gevins AS, Remond A (Eds.) *Methods of analysis of brain electrical and magnetic signals* (Handbook of electroencephalography and clinical neurophysiology, Vol. 1). Elsevier, Amsterdam, 583—664.

Gevins AS (1980) Pattern recognition of human brain electrical potentials. *IEEE Trans Patt Analysis Mach Intell PAMI-2*(5), 383—404.

Gevins AS (1984) Analysis of the electromagnetic signals of the human brain: Milestones, obstacles and goals. *IEEE Trans Biomed Engr BME-31*(12), 833—850.

Gevins AS (1987a) Correlation analysis. In Gevins AS, Remond A (Eds.) *Computer analysis of brain electrical and magnetic signals* (Handbook of electroencephalography and clinical neurophysiology, Vol. 1). Elsevier, Amsterdam, 171—193.

Gevins AS (1987b) Statistical pattern recognition. In Gevins AS, Remond A (Eds.) *Computer analysis of brain electrical and magnetic signals* (Handbook of electroencephalography and clinical neurophysiology, Vol. 1). Elsevier, Amsterdam, 541—582.

Gevins AS (1987c, in press) Recent advances in neurocognitive pattern analysis. In Basar, E. (Ed.) *Dynamics of sensory and cognitive processing of the brain.* Springer-Verlag, Berlin.

Gevins AS (1988, in press) Analysis of multiple lead data. In Rohrbaugh J, Johnson R, Parasuraman R (Eds.) *Event-related potentials of the brain.* Oxford University Press, New York.

Gevins AS, Morgan NH (1986) Classifier-directed signal processing in brain research. *IEEE Trans Biomed Enginr BME-33*(12), l054— 1068.

Gevins AS, Zeitlin GM, Yingling CD, Doyle JC, Dedon MF, Schaffer RE, Roumasset JT, Yeager, CL (1979a) EEG patterns during "cognitive" tasks. I. Methodology and analysis of complex behaviors. *Electroenceph clin Neurophysiol, 47,* 693— 703.

Gevins AS, Zeitlin GM, Doyle JC, Schaffer RE, Callaway E (1979b) EEG patterns during "cognitive" tasks. II. Analysis of controlled tasks. *Electroenceph clin Neurophysiol, 47,* 704—710.

Gevins AS, Zeitlin GM, Doyle JC, Yingling CD, Schaffer RE, Callaway E, Yeager CL (1979c) Electroencephalogram correlates of higher cortical functions. *Science, 203,* 665—668.

Gevins AS, Doyle JC, Cutillo BA, Schaffer RE, Tannehill RS, Ghannam JH, Gilcrease VA, Yeager CL (1981) Electrical potentials in human brain during cognition: New method reveals dynamic patterns of correlation of human brain electrical potentials during cognition. *Science, 213,* 918—922.

Gevins AS, Schaffer RE, Doyle JC, Cutillo BA, Tannehill RS, Bressler SL (1983) Shadows of thought: Shifting lateralization of human brain electrical patterns during brief visuomotor task. *Science, 220,* 97—99.

Gevins AS, Doyle JC, Cutillo BA, Schaffer RE, Tannehill RS, Bressler SL (1985) Neurocognitive pattern analysis of a visuomotor task: Rapidly-shifting foci of evoked correlations between electrodes. *Psychophysiol, 22,* 32—43.

Gevins AS, Morgan NH, Bressler SL, Doyle JC, Cutillo BA (1986) Improved ERP estimation via statistical pattern recognition. *Electroenceph clin Neurophysiol, 64,* 177—186.

Gevins AS, Morgan NH, Bressler SL, Cutillo BA, White RM, Illes J, Greer DS, Doyle JC, Zeitlin GM (1987) Human neuroelectric patterns predict performance accuracy. *Science, 235,* 580—585.

Gevins AS, Bressler SL, Morgan NH, Cutillo BA, White RM, Greer DS, Illes J (submitted a) Event-related covariances during a bimanual visuomotor task, Part I: Methods and analysis of stimulus- and response-locked data. *Electroenceph clin Neurophysiol.*

Gevins AS, Cutillo BA, Bressler SL, Morgan NH, White RM, Illes J, Greer DS (submitted b) Event-related covariances during a bimanual visuomotor task, Part II: Preparation and feedback. *Electroenceph clin Neurophysiol.*

Gevins AS, Bressler SL, Cutillo BA, Morgan NH, Illes J, White RM, Greer DS (in prep.) *Neuroelectric changes precede impairment of prolonged task performance.*

Greer, DS, Gevins AS (in prep.) *Spatial deblurring of scalp recorded brain potentials using an optimal Laplacian operator.*

Hjorth B (1975) An on-line transformation of EEG scalp potentials into orthogonal source derivations. *Electroenceph clin Neurophysiol, 39,* 526–530.

Hjorth B (1980) Source derivation simplifies topographical EEG interpretation. *Am J EEG Technol, 20,* 121–132.

John ER (1967) *Mechanisms of memory.* Academic Press, New York.

John ER, Bartlett F, Schimokaochi M, Kleinman D (1973) Neural readout from memory. *J Neurophysiol, 36,* 893–924.

Lashley, K.S. (1958) Cerebral organization and behavior. *Proc Assoc Res Nervous Mental Disease, 36,* 1–18.

Livanov MN (1977) *Spatial organization of cerebral processes.* Wiley, New York.

Mesulam MM (1981) A cortical network for directed attention and unilateral neglect. *Ann Neurol, 10,* 309–325.

Morgan NH, Gevins AS (1986) Wigner distributions of human event-related brain signals. *IEEE Trans Biomed Engr, BME-33*(1), 66–70.

Petsche H, Pockberger H, Rappelsberger P (1984) On the search for the sources of the electroencephalogram. *Neuroscience, 11,* 1–27.

Roland PE (1985a) Cortical organization of voluntary behavior in man. *Human Neurobiology, 11,* 216.

Roland PE (1985b) In Solokoff L (Ed.) *Brain imaging and brain function.* Raven Press, New York.

Rumelhart DE, McClelland JL, PDP Research Group (1986) *Parallel distributed processing: Explorations in the microstructures of cognition.* MIT, Cambridge.

Sherrington CS (1906) *The integrative action of the nervous system.* Yale University Press, New Haven, CT.

Tucker DM, Roth DL, Bair, TB (1986) Functional connections among cortical regions: Topography of EEG coherence. *Electroenceph clin Neurophysiol, 63,* 242–250.

Walter W, Shipton H (1951) A new toposcopic display system. *Electroenceph clin Neurophysiol, 3,* 281–292.

Williamson SJ, Kaufman L (1987) Analysis of neuromagnetic signals. In Gevins AS, Remond A (Eds.) *Methods of analysis of brain electrical and magnetic signals* (Handbook of electroencephalography and clinical neurophysiology, Vol. 1). Elsevier, Amsterdam, 405-448.

ERD Mapping and Functional Topography: Temporal and Spatial Aspects

G. Pfurtscheller*, J. Steffan**, H. Maresch*

The short-lasting amplitude attenuation of alpha band rhythms is called Event-Related Desynchronization (ERD). ERD mapping is the topographical display of event-related desynchronization and can be used to study cortical activation patterns in space and time. The influence of reference-dependent and reference-free derivations on ERD mapping is discussed based on experimental data recorded during voluntary movement, tactile and visual stimulation. The ERD of upper alpha components can be used to study the activation of primary sensory and motor areas; lower alpha components are more widespread, desynchronize hundreds of milliseconds after upper alpha components and represent most likely neuronal processes in connection with cognitive functions.

The short-lasting amplitude attenuation or blocking of rhythmic activity within the alpha and beta bands before, during and after externally or internally paced events is called Event-Related Desynchronization (ERD) (Pfurtscheller & Aranibar, 1977). An event can either be a simple sensory stimulus, a motor action, or a complex cognitive task. The desynchronization of spontaneous EEG occurs in parallel with event-related potentials; e.g., visual stimulation results in the generation of a VEP and in "alpha blocking"; voluntary finger movement is preceded by a negative shift of cortical DC potential (Deecke et al. 1976) and blocking of the central mu rhythm (Chatrian et al., 1959). ERD in parallel with P300 was reported recently (Sergeant et al., 1987).

One of the prerequisites for the quantification of the ERD is the repetition of the "event." Therefore, EEG data must be recorded and processed before, during and after such an event. In order to express the ERD as a percentage, a short EEG segment, recorded seconds before each event, is defined as the reference interval; the power within the alpha or beta band in this reference interval is designated as 100 percent.

ERD mapping is the topographical display of event-related desynchronization with integration times varying in the range of milliseconds to seconds, and can be used to investigate cortical activation patterns in space and time (Pfurtscheller et al., 1986; Klimesch et al., 1986).

This paper focusses on some of the main aspects of ERD mapping, such as the type of derivation, the frequency band and the choice of the reference interval. EEG data recorded during visual and somatosensory stimulation,

* Ludwig Boltzmann Institute of Medical Informatics, Graz, and Department of Medical Informatics, Institute of Biomedical Engineering, Technical University of Graz, Austria
** Institute of Fundamentals and Theory in Electrical Engineering, Technical University of Graz, Austria
The research described here was supported by grants from the Austrian Ministry of Science and Research and the "Fonds zur Förderung der wissenschaftlichen Forschung," project 5240. We would also like to thank Dipl.-Ing. G. Lindinger for writing a part of the computer programs, W. Mohl for data acquisition, H. Schubert for statistical programming, and Dr. W. Klimesch and S. Toniolli for editorial assistance.

voluntary finger movement and simulated data are used to provide a better understanding of these topics.

ERD Interpretation

Berger (1930) was the first to observe a depression or attenuation of alpha waves in scalp EEG when subjects opened their eyes and were attentive. In contrast to the effect of visual stimulation on occipital alpha rhythm, there is no effect on "precentral alpha potentials." However, this precentral alpha potential (actually the mu rhythm) and the precentral beta rhythm are blocked by the preparation for or execution of movements (Jasper & Andrews, 1938).

Even these early observations indicated that the brain generates a variety of components within the alpha and beta bands, and that these components are attenuated or blocked when cortical regions become activated. Electrocorticograms in man demonstrate that the blocking of rhythmic activity due to opening and closing of the eyes or movement of the fingers is a rather localized and restricted phenomenon (Jasper & Penfield, 1949). For example, successive touching of fingers and thumb affects the rhythm of the precentral hand area but not of the precentral face area.

The new technique of ERD mapping confirms these early findings of Jasper and Penfield (1949) and others, and shows clearly that ERD is a highly specific and elementary phenomenon of intrinsic brain rhythms closely related to cortical activation. ERD can be observed in awake subjects but not in comatose patients (Pfurtscheller et al., 1983). This suggests that ERD is an electric phenomenon associated with consciousness.

Measurement and Quantification of ERD

Electrodes and EEG Recording

An "electrocap" is used for EEG recording. The electrodes are mounted according to the international 10-20 system. Additional electro-

des are used between these standard positions. The placement of the 29 electrodes is shown schematically in Figure 1. Reference electrodes are attached to the earlobes and either linked together or used separately.

Before digitizing, EEG signals are prefiltered within 1.6 to 30 Hz. An additional low pass filter with a cut-off frequency of 30 Hz (100 dB/octave) is used to avoid aliasing. The opto-coupled EEG amplifiers are designed and built in our laboratory.

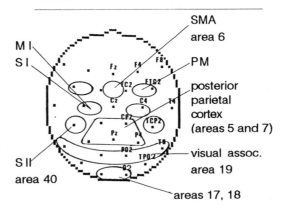

Cerebral location of electrodes

M I, SI primary sensorimotor
S II secondary somatosensory
SMA supplementary motor
PM pre motor

Figure 1. Top-down map showing electrodes' location in the "electrocap" used and the projection of a number of cerebral regions according to Homan et al. (1987).

MEG Recording

In one subject the magnetoencephalogram (MEG) was recorded from the C4 region using the same system as described by Weinberg et al. in this volume.

Data Acquisition, Processing and Display

The computer system for acquisition and processing consists of a PDP11/73 with 512 kB memory, 20 MByte magnetic disk, 32-channel

A/D converter, real time clock, 640 × 512 point resolution colour display and 3.2 GByte optical disk. A black-and-white matrix printer and an ink-jet colour printer are available for hard copy.

The technique of ERD mapping is based on triggered data acquisition from as many as 32 or even more EEG channels. The normally used 6 s epochs consist of pre-trigger, trigger and post-trigger periods. In addition, EEG can be sampled up to 20 s with a frequency of 64 Hz in each channel.

In the voluntary, self-paced action experiment, the pre-trigger period was 4 s; the voluntary finger movement started at 4 s (Pfurtscheller & Aranibar, 1979). In contrast to self-paced tasks, the pre-trigger period can be chosen within an interval of 1—3 s for externally paced tasks such as visual, acoustical and somatosensory stimulation. In the reading experiment, the pre-trigger period was 2 s, and the words were presented on a monitor for 250 ms. The visual stimulus was preceded by an acoustical warning stimulus (click).

After sampling the time series with 64 Hz and a 12-bit resolution, several artifact exclusion criteria are applied (Koepruner et al., 1984):

— A/D overflows are checked to exclude gross movement artifacts.
— The alpha band power percentage is computed: If this is less than a given threshold, movement and electrode artifacts resulting in increased activity in low frequency range are assumed.
— The beta band power percentage is computed; if a certain threshold is reached, myogenic artifacts are assumed.

In order to produce a statistically reliable result, each task has to be repeated several times. After bandpass filtering using the frequency sampling method (Rader & Gold, 1967) and squaring the amplitudes of the filtered EEG, the band power is computed. In applying this method, a time resolution corresponding to a sampling frequency of 64 Hz or 15.6 ms can be achieved. In practice, averaging is performed over 8 sampling points, reducing the time resolution to 125 ms. In this way the statistical reliability of the results is increased.

A reference interval is defined. The alpha power within this interval is the reference value. Alpha power is computed for each of the 125 ms segments of the activation interval and given as percentage of the reference value. After averaging over all trials, the probability of a given ERD value is computed by a nonparametric sign test. ERD is considered to be positive if power decreases significantly, and negative if power increases.

For computation of maps, the 4-nearest-neighbour interpolation algorithm (Buchsbaum et al. 1982) was chosen. The data processing results in two series of images, one representing the time course of the event-related power changes (ERD maps), the other that of the probabilty of these changes, both with a time resolution of 125 ms. Six or 20 maps are displayed on the colour display with 56 × 56 matrices using a scale of 20 different colours.

Frequency Band and ERD

The ERD phenomenon is dependent on the frequency components and not only observed in electric potentials on the scalp (EEG) but also in the magnetic field over the head (MEG). Simultaneous recordings of EEG and MEG during voluntary left finger movements in one subject displayed significant desynchronization in the alpha and beta bands; electric potential ERD (CZ—C1) was more affected in the beta band (Figure 2B), and magnetic field ERD (close to C4) was localized in the alpha band (Figure 2A).

For comparison two other examples of ERD measurements, one in the motor cortex of a monkey after electrical stimulation of the median nerve (Figure 2C), the other after mechanical finger vibration in a comatose patient (Figure 2D), are also displayed. Although the monkey's spectrum does not show a clear peak except in the low frequencies, a significant power decrease between 7 and 20 Hz was found. Therefore ERD does not necessarily depend on the existence of rhythmic activity. During coma, a power increase (negative ERD) can be found, which probably corresponds to the "spindling" in the EEG (Rumpl et al., 1983). This negative ERD in coma is

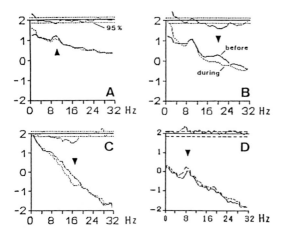

Figure 2. Logarithmic power spectra calculated for the reference interval (full line) and activity interval (dotted line) under different conditions: magnetic field (A) and electrical potential (B) recorded during voluntary finger movement; electrical potential from monkey's motor cortex during electrical stimulation of median nerve (C); electrical potential during mechanical vibration applied to the index finger in a comatose patient (D). The most significant power decrease (A, B and C) and power increase (D), respectively, are marked by black triangles. The power increase in A and B between 0—4 Hz is due to movement artifacts.

shifted to a positive ERD (blocking) after emergence from coma (Pfurtscheller et al., 1983).

The importance of the choice of the frequency band is demonstrated in Figure 3. Here, group average data from a reading experiment (see Klimesch et al., in this volume) in the lower (6—10 Hz) and upper alpha band (9—13 Hz) are displayed. Desynchronization of upper alpha components is more localized and restricted to occipital areas, whereas ERD of lower alpha components is more widespread, involving also parietal areas. This difference is particularly evident around electrode Pz overlying the posterior parietal cortex. Thus it appears that different neuronal processes are reflected in the lower and in the upper alpha band. The higher alpha band appears to reflect processes that are directly stimulus-related, while the lower alpha band most likely represents attentional and motivational processes.

The influence of the frequency band on ERD patterns is also demonstrated in a further subject during visual stimulation using a pair of goggles (Figure 4, lower panel), and during mechanical vibration of the right index finger (Figure 4, upper panel). During both stimulus modalities the ERD was more localized and closely restricted to the primary cortical area in the case of the upper alpha components. Event-related desynchronization of lower alpha components extended over a larger area and included the posterior parietal area for both modalities.

Reference Interval and ERD

Among other factors, the pattern of ERD depends on the choice of the reference interval. Two different approaches are possible: (1) intraexperimental reference and (2) extraexperimental reference. This is schematically indicated in Figure 5, upper panel.

Intraexperimental Reference

Data are recorded during such different experiments as reading, visual discrimination and voluntary movement. Each experiment requires repeated events in which event-related EEG segments are recorded, sampled and processed. The reference interval is the period of 0.2—1 s after onset of each segment and is considered to represent an intraexperimental rest condition. (B/A and BB/AA in Figure 5, upper panel).

Extraexperimental Reference

In order to discriminate between different processing stages, any experimental condition can be selected as a reference interval. As an example, let us consider the experiment described by Klimesch et al. (1986). Here, the same stimuli (words) were used in two tasks: reading alone and reading and memorizing. The data of the reading task then served as reference for the memory task. In the scheme of Figure 5, this resulted in the ERD computed as BB/B. In this way the ERD maps show only those power changes which are

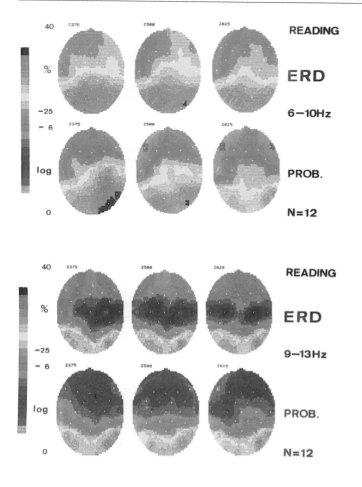

Figure 3. Group averages (N = 12) of ERD maps (upper row in each panel) and probability maps (lower row in each panel) calculated during reading of words. The maps were computed 375, 500 and 625 ms after word presentation. The power in the 6–10 Hz band is displayed in the upper panel and the power in in the 9–13 Hz band in the lower panel. The colour scale on the left hand side ranges from −25 to 40% for tne ERD maps and from 0 to 10^{-6} for the probability maps. Red (black) marks regions with the largest and, respectively, most significant alpha power decrease. Note the similarity between ERD and probability maps.

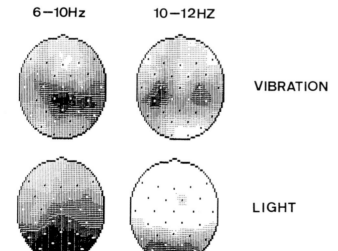

Figure 4. ERD maps calculated during 1 s mechanical vibration and 1 s light stimulation using the 6–10 and 10–12 Hz band. Note that the ERD is more localized to the primary sensory areas with the upper alpha components.

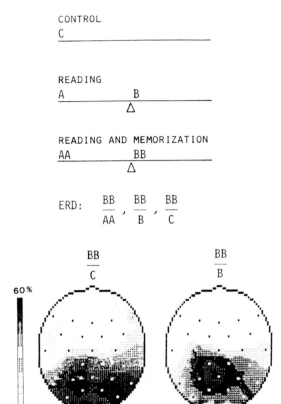

Figure 5. Upper panel: Scheme for computation of ERD. Lower panel: ERD maps calculated during word recognition (memorization) referred to control experiment (BB/C) and to reading experiment (BB/B).

caused by memory and not by reading processes.

Another extraexperimental reference may be the data recorded during a sustained rest period. This is called the extraexperimental rest condition (C in Figure 5, upper panel). Provided that the experimental paradigm and experimental setup are carefully designed, the extra- and intraexperimental rest conditions should show similar results. In fact, however, attention, interest, involvement, arousal, etc. of the subjects change throughout a recording session and can result in changes of the reference within different experiments.

ERD maps calculated during a visual recognition task using different reference intervals are shown in Figure 5, lower panel. The

use of an extraexperimental test condition (BB/C) results in an ERD map similar to that of an intraexperimental reference (not shown). The ERD data referring to the reading experiment (BB/B), however, results in a different topographical display of the ERD. Whereas the ERD was more diffusely distributed over the right and left parietal and occipital regions during visual recognition (Figure 5, BB/C), the ERD was more focussed on the posterior parietal region when it referred to the reading experiment (Figure 5, BB/B). This can be taken as evidence that activation due to sensory processing is subtracted from the activation due to more complex sensory *and* cognitive processing, with the resulting map showing the area related to the cognitive component.

Experiments with monkeys have shown that a visual stimulation changes the neuronal activity not only in the primary visual cortex, superior colliculus and frontal eye fields, but also in the posterior parietal cortex (Brodmann's area 7). Neuronal activity in area 7 increases when the animal addresses its attention to a visual stimulus (Bushnell et al., 1981). The ERD map displayed in Figure 5 with the ERD focus over the posterior parietal region thus apparently has something to do with visual attention, which is certainly greater during visual recognition than during reading alone.

During visual imagination the largest increase in regional cerebral oxidative metabolism (rCMRO$_2$) in normal, healthy volunteers was found in the posterior superior parietal cortex (Roland & Widen, this volume). These authors suggest that the posterior parietal cortex is a visual association area and used for the recalling of visual information. These observations obtained with positron emission tomography correspond very well to our results obtained with measurements of electrical potentials from the scalp.

Derivation and ERD

Two different types of EEG recordings can be used: the reference-dependent and the reference-independent or reference-free recordings. In the reference-dependent recording, each amplifier is connected with an active electrode and the reference electrode. The reference electrode is called common reference and placed such that it minimizes the possibility of picking up potentials from the brain (e.g., one earlobe, linked earlobes, noncephalic, mastoid, etc.). Because there is no reference point with zero potential, each map depends on the choice of the common reference, and the maps are not unique.

The term reference-independent recordings comprises bipolar derivations, common average reference derivations and the "Laplacian operator." It should be emphasized that bipolar derivations display local potential gradients or first spatial derivatives whereas the Laplacian operator can be interpreted as local current source density or second spatial derivative (Nunez, 1981).

Bipolar Derivation

The bipolar method is used in clinical EEG to display "phase reversal." Slow potentials and artifacts that occur synchronously at a number of electrode sites are diminished in amplitude. This attenuation of slow frequency components is a desired effect in ERD measurements, because only alpha and beta band activities are quantified.

Two types of bipolar derivations are calculated from referential recordings, namely a transverse and a longitudinal montage. With the transverse montage, changes due to eye movements are extremely small, and electrode movement artifacts are better attenuated because of the highpass filter effect. Compared to an earlobe reference, the transverse montage can enhance and localize the ERD better during voluntary movement.

Recording over the sensorimotor cortex with reference to the earlobe (or mastoid) may result in the masking of event-related changes of central recorded potentials by large potentials at the reference electrode. Therefore, monopolar recording with an earlobe reference can even demonstrate that there is no blocking reaction due to voluntary movement; bipolar derivations, however, can display a significant ERD in the central region (Figure 6, first and second map in the upper row).

The difference in ERD maps between monopolar and bipolar derivations during visual stimulation is less pronounced but also evident, as can be seen in Figure 7. The bilaterally symmetric representation of the ERD over the occipital region with the bipolar montage seems to be more realistic than the lateralized ERD with the earlobe reference.

Because of this enhancement of the ERD with bipolar derivations and the better suppression of movement artifacts due to the spatial highpass filtering, a transverse bipolar montage is recommended for measurements

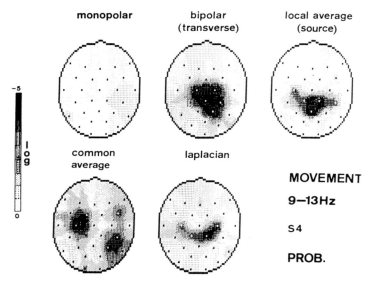

monopolar   bipolar
(transverse)

local average
(source)

common
average   laplacian

MOVEMENT

9–13Hz

S4

PROB.

Figure 6. Influence of the type of derivation on the topographical display of ERD during voluntary finger movement. Displayed are the probabilities calculated by a sign test; scale from $p = 0$ to $p = 10^{-5}$. Note the differences in the maps and the complete masking of ERD with common ear reference (monopolar).

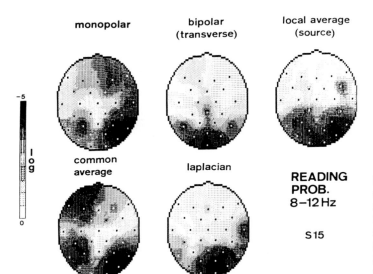

monopolar   bipolar (transverse)   local average (source)

common average   laplacian

READING PROB. 8–12 Hz

S 15

Figure 7. The same as Figure 6, but data from a reading task. Note the similarity in the probability maps between bipolar, local average reference and Laplacian operator and the significant left frontal ERD with the common average reference derivation.

in patients with unilateral cerebral ischemia (Pfurtscheller et al., 1984, 1988; Pfurtscheller 1986).

Common Average Reference

In this method, first described by Goldman (1950), either all electrodes on the scalp are connected with the help of equal resistors, or the potentials recorded from each electrode are averaged. The common average reference for EEG mapping is strongly recommended by Lehmann (1977).

The EEG maps obtained by this method are reference independent and unique. However, a disadvantage of this method is that the occipital alpha band activity may appear in frontal derivations, and eye movement artifacts may appear posteriorly. Examples of reference power maps for different types of derivation are displayed in Figure 8.

The ERD can also be enhanced with a common average reference, but the localization is very often different from the bipolar montage. In contrast to the bipolar montage, the ERD is more widespread and can also be evident over frontal areas (compare Figures 6 and 7). Obviously, care must be taken in interpreting maps obtained with common average reference.

Laplacian Operator

The Laplacian operator is a mathematical, differential operator that can be viewed as a mapping of one function (the electrical field of the scalp surface) onto another function

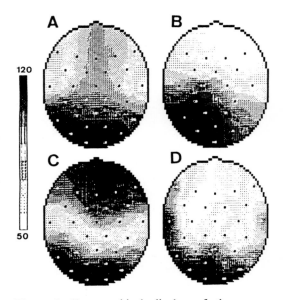

Figure 8. Topographical display of the power (6–10 Hz) within the reference interval with monopolar (A), bipolar (B), local average (C) and common average reference derivations (D). Scale in μV^2 for A and in arbitrary units in B, C and D.

(current source density). On the one hand, this technique has the advantage of improving the spatial resolution in local features of the electroencephalogram (Nunez, 1981); on the other hand, it provides a function that is not as smooth as the original function because second-order differences have to be calculated and higher frequencies exert a large influence on the result. The Laplacian operator method can be calculated for any electrode distance and angle and gives good results for electrodes near the vertex.

So far the results indicate that the Laplacian operator gives the best gross localization of the parts of anatomical structures activated during voluntary movement or reading (compare Figures 6 and 7). However, the method is very time consuming and sensitive to higher frequency components in the primary data; furthermore, the quality of the results deteriorates at the periphery.

Local Average Reference

When the interelectrode distances are equal, the use of the Laplacian operator is mathematically equivalent to the arithmetic mean of the four nearest electrodes, provided that they are positioned along 2 perpendicular lines. This approximation is known as "source derivation" (Hjorth, 1975) in electroencephalography and named "local average reference," in contrast to the "common average reference," where not only four but all electrodes are averaged. Examples of the local average reference are displayed in Figures 6 and 7. Here the results also deteriorate at the periphery.

Using Simulated EEG Data to Compare Different Derivations

Simulated EEG data can be used to make evident the influence of different EEG derivations. With this aim we developed a program package to simulate EEGs.

In the example given in Figure 9, four different kinds of derivations are compared with each other by using the same synthetic data; the activity source is always in the same position (the electrode in the third row and in the fourth column), and has identical characteristics of activity in the alpha band. The maps

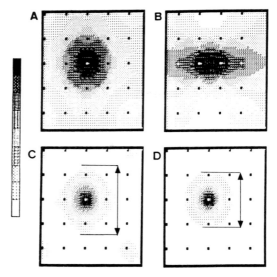

Figure 9. Simulated data with a source localized to the electrode in the third row and third column. Distribution for monopolar (A), bipolar transverse (B), common average reference (C) and Laplacian operator method (D). In B, instead of marking the electrodes, the interspaced points for computing the maps are marked. Note that the best localization of the source is obtained with the Laplacian method. The maximal value in each map is taken to be 100. Scale 0–100; black indicates largest values, white smallest values.

were obtained by using a 30-electrode matrix with an orthogonal order of electrode positions.

Figure 9A represents a monopolar recording; the area of activity is relatively large in comparison to the common average reference (Figure 9C), the bipolar derivation (Figure 9B) and the Laplacian operator method (Figure 9D). The common average and the local average derivations (not displayed) result in a similar resolution and the best localization of the activity (source).

The Laplacian operator method, in which the eight electrodes nearest to a point are used to calculate the second spatial derivative at that point, produces the map shown in Figure 9D. This map has the best local resolution. As mentioned before, the local average reference and the Laplacian operator method should be in good agreement if and only if the interelectrode distances are equal and the electrodes are positioned along perpendicular lines.

Local and Temporal ERD Criteria

Visual Information Processing

Two electrophysiological signals can be recorded after visual stimulation: the visual evoked potential (VEP) and the change in spontaneous EEG, known as alpha blocking or visual ERD. Both electrical phenomena are evoked by visual afferences, but demonstrate three fundamental differences:

1) different topographical distribution over the scalp,
2) different duration and time course,
3) different dependence upon the state of consciousness.

ad (1): Long-latency VEPs—and all other stimulus modality EPs—are largest over the vertex (Keidel, 1971); visual ERD is strongly localized to occipital and parietal areas (see Figures 3 and 4).

ad (2): Mid- and long-latency VEP components last no longer than approximately 200 ms. With respect to these results, the VEP can therefore be interpreted in terms of an on-effect. However, the ERD reaches its maximal magnitude about 200 ms after stimulus onset and has a duration of some seconds. This latency of the visual ERD is confirmed by studies of alpha blocking after single flash stimulation (Kawabata, 1972; Nogawa et al., 1976; Aranibar & Pfurtscheller, 1978). The current interpretation implies that the low frequency components of visual ERD are not so much related to the activation of primary visual cortex, but rather to the activation of visual association cortex and other extrastriate cortical areas. The ERD of upper frequency components within the alpha band, however, seems to be more related to activation of primary and secondary visual areas as demonstrated in Figure 4. There is also some evidence that the ERD of upper alpha components starts before the ERD of lower alpha components, which means that the time course of the ERD depends on the frequency band analyzed.

ad (3): Whereas occipitally recorded VEPs of normal and comatose subjects are to some ex-

tent comparable, the effect of ERD is either less pronounced or even not found (negative ERD) in comatose patients (Pfurtscheller et al., 1985). These results suggest that the usual, positive ERD is more linked to processes of the conscious state than the VEP.

Processing of visual information depends not only on physical properties of the stimulus and its information content, but also on the initial state of the brain, that is, the degree of activation, arousal, attention, interest and engagement of the subject. Furthermore, the ERD pattern is different during reading of words and classification of words (Klimesch et al., 1986). This means that cognitive factors and memorization processes do indeed affect and modulate the ERD.

ERD maps obtained during reading can be contaminated by VEPs and lambda waves in the first 250 ms after stimulus onset. Lambda waves are potentials related to oculo-motor-visual integration resulting from interaction between oculomotor and visual afferences, and demonstrate the largest energy in the lower alpha band (Chatrian & Lairy, 1976). These components have latencies of 40–340 ms in response to eye movements and are therefore maximally represented in the first hundreds of milliseconds after stimulation onset.

Voluntary Movement

Neuronal structures such as the association cortex, basal ganglia, cerebellum, thalamus, supplementary motor area (SMA) and motor areas are involved in planning and performing voluntary movements (Deecke et al., 1976; Roland, 1985). The rhythmic EEG activity generated in one part of these regions is known as mu rhythm; it is attenuated or blocked before and during a motor action (Chatrian et al., 1959). The ERD of central mu rhythm was studied extensively in normal subjects (Pfurtscheller & Aranibar, 1980) and patients with cerebrovascular insufficiency (Koepruner et al,. 1984) using a transverse bipolar montage across the vertex in six channels. The most interesting result of these studies was that ERD patterns demonstrated a relatively high degree of bilateral hemispheric symmetry in normal subjects and were very often suppressed or attenuated over the affected hemisphere in patients with unilateral cerebral ischemia. These hemispheric asymmetries can be explained by assuming the existence of two relatively independent hemispheric rhythm-generating systems in the central region (Storm van Leeuwen et al., 1978). The bilateral, symmetrical desynchronization during planning and execution of unilateral movements in normal subjects is confirmed by a bilateral increase of regional cerebral blood flow in premotor and supplementary motor areas (Roland, 1985).

Localization, magnitude and distribution of movement-related desynchronization depend on the frequency band and the type of derivation used. In general, the ERD is more widespread and of larger magnitude in the lower alpha band, similar to the results found during visual stimulation. In the upper alpha band the ERD is less widespread and more localized to the central region, and depends very much on the type of derivation used (compare Figure 6).

In order to demonstrate both the spatial and the temporal resolution of ERD patterns, a sequence of maps computed during planning and initiation of a left-thumb movements is shown in Figure 10. The ERD pattern calculated from the local average reference for 10−12 Hz components corresponds closely to neuroanatomical knowledge, since it was maximal at electrodes C4, overlying the primary sensorimotor hand area, and TCP2 (see Figure 1), overlying the secondary somatosensory area (Brodmann's area 40). In addition an ERD was found at electrode TCP1 over the ipsilateral side. This type of ERD pattern, predominantly involving the contralateral right hemisphere, was already present 1750 ms (map 2250) prior to movement onset. These data gives clear evidence that primary sensorimotor hand areas seem to be activated more than 1 s before the movement is made. A similar ERD pattern with a left hemisphere dominance was found with right finger movement.

Tactile Stimulation

Repetitive mechanical vibration (100 Hz, 1 s duration, interstimulus interval 10 s) of the first digit of the right index finger demon-strates an ERD pattern similar to that of voluntary movement. The upper alpha band ERD is very localized to primary sensorimotor areas (electrodes C3 and C4), and is already present contralaterally in the first hundreds of milliseconds before stimulus application (Figure 11, lower row, first map). After stimulation the ERD pattern is bilaterally symmetrical, but still localized to the electrodes C3 and C4. A quite different time-dependent behaviour is found with the lower alpha components. There is no ERD before stimulus presentation, and the ERD increases gradually in the first hundreds of milliseconds (Figure 11, upper row). Furthermore, the ERD is more widespread and maximal over posterior parietal areas. The early contralateral ERD before stimulation is presumably a part of a specific, selective, preparatory process. The contralateral sensorimotor cortex seems to be activated before the stimulus is applied.

Conclusion

Grey Walter, the discoverer of the Contingent Negative Variation (CNV) (Walter, 1964), made an important remark at an International Conference on Attention in Neurophysiology (Mulholland, 1969):

"We've managed to check the alpha band rhythm with intracerebral electrodes in the occipital-parietal cortex; in regions which are practically adjacent and almost congruent one finds a variety of alpha rhythms, some of which are blocked by opening and closing the eyes, some are not, some are driven by flicker, some are not, some respond in some way to mental activity, some do not. What one sees on the scalp is a spatial average of a large number of components, and whether you see an alpha rhythm of a particular type or not depends upon which component happens to be the most highly synchronized process over the largest superficial area; there are complex rhythms in everybody."

This helps us to explain one of the most interesting findings, namely that lower and upper

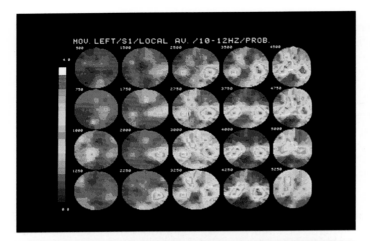

Figure 10. Serial probability maps from a time period of 3500 ms before (maps 500–3750) to 1250 ms after movement (maps 4000–5250). EEG data recorded during left finger movement with right ear reference, maps with computed local average reference. Scale displays probabilities from p = 0 to p = 10^{-4} for the power decrease in the 10–12 Hz band; most significant (p < 0.001) ERD is marked by colours white and red, respectively, and blue indicates regions with non-significant ERD.

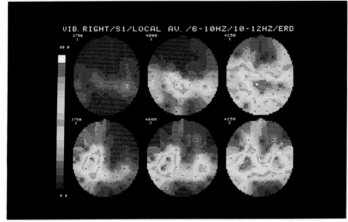

Figure 11. ERD maps computed 250 ms before (map 3750) and during 1 s vibration of the right index finger (maps 4000 and 4250). Data recorded with right ear reference, maps with computed local average reference. ERD is displayed for the 6–10 Hz (upper row) and 10–12 Hz band (lower row). Scale displays power decrease from 0–60%. Colours red and white mark regions with largest ERD.

alpha components behave differently during sensory stimulation. Desynchronization of upper alpha components seems to be linked more with visual or somatosensory afferences, whereas desynchronization of lower alpha components appears to be a sign of sensory association, attention and expectancy in the human brain. In general, lower alpha components demonstrate larger ERD than upper alpha components. In terms of Grey Walter, this means that the synchronized and desynchronized generator volume is larger for lower than for upper alpha components. Upper alpha components also show a more localized desynchronization pattern whereas lower alpha components exhibit more widespread desynchronization. This difference between lower and upper alpha components holds not

only for sensory stimulation but also for sensorimotor activation during planning and execution of voluntary movements.

It is of interest to note that electrodes C3 and C4 overlie the primary sensorimotor hand area, and electrodes TCP1 and TCP2 (see Figure 1) overlie the secondary somatosensory areas (Homan et al., 1987). These electrodes demonstrate significant ERD in the upper alpha band during tactile finger stimulation and voluntary finger movement.

During visual stimulation upper alpha band ERD is focussed on the electrodes O1 and O2 overlying the primary and secondary visual areas. These data give evidence that upper alpha components and event-related desynchronization are related to the activation of primary and secondary cortical areas.

Another interesting cortical region is the superior parietal area (Brodmann's areas 5 and 7) which corresponds to electrodes CP1, CP2, P3, P4 and Pz (see Figure 1). In this region lower alpha components are desynchronized with visual and tactile stimulation as well as with voluntary movement. Measurements of cerebral regional oxidative metabolism (rCBRO$_2$) and regional cerebral blood flow (rCBF) give evidence that the lobus parietalis superior is activated during motor and nonmotor activities (Roland & Widen, in this volume).

Measurement of ERD suggests that this parietal area seems to be one of the last structures to be activated and linked with conscious experience (compare Figure 11).

The ERD pattern calculated preceding self-initiated voluntary motor acts often displays a mid-frontally localized ERD at Fz and sometimes also at FC1 and FC2 about 2000 ms before movement onset. The electrodes Fz, FC1 and FC2 overlie the premotor and supplementary motor areas (SMA). These data suggest that about 2000 ms preceding movement onset the SMA is active first, followed by activation of the contralateral primary sensorimotor area and bilateral activation of secondary somatosensory areas.

These results are partially confirmed by the studies of Gevins et al. (1987), reporting dominance of the contralateral hemisphere during the preparatory process of finger movements (see also Gevins & Bressler, this volume). Unlike us, Gevins et al. used another method of data processing, namely the event-related covariance (ERC) technique.

Further research has to be done to confirm the findings of mid-frontal ERD more than 1 s before movement onset. Movements of different quality and complexity have to be studied by the ERD mapping technique.

In summary, we can speculate that different cortical structures have their own intrinsic rhythms; this rhythmicity decreases (desynchronization) when the neuronal mass becomes activated. This fact is shown by means of the ERD mapping technique. With this simple technique the spatial and temporal patterns of local cortical activation can be studied not only during externally paced stimulation, but also preceding internal, self-paced events.

References

Aranibar A, Pfurtscheller G (1978) On and off effects in the background EEG activity during one-second photic stimulation. *Electroenceph clin Neurophysiol, 44,* 307–316.

Berger H (1930) Über das Elektrenkephalogramm des Menschen. II. *J Psychol Neurol (Lpz), 40,* 160–179.

Buchsbaum MS, Rigal F, Coppola R, Capelletti J, King C, Johnson J (1982) A new system for gray-level surface distribution maps of electrical activity. *Electroenceph clin Neurophysiol, 53,* 237–242.

Bushnell MC, Goldberg ME, Lee Robinson D (1981) Behavioral enhancement of visual responses in monkey cerebral cortex, I: Modulation in posterior parietal cortex related to selective visual attention. *J Neurophysiol, 46,* 755–772.

Chatrian GE, Lairy GC (1976) The lambda waves. In Remond A (Ed.) *Handbook of EEG and clinical neurophysiology.* Elsevier, Amsterdam, 123–149.

Chatrian GE, Petersen MC, Lazarte JA (1959) The blocking of the rolandic wicket rhythm and some central changes related to movement. *Electroenceph clin Neurophysiol, 11,* 497–510.

Deecke L, Groezinger B, Kornhuber HH (1976) Voluntary finger movement in man: Cerebral potentials and theory. *Biol Cybernetics, 23,* 99–119.

Gevins AS, Morgan NH, Bressler SL, Cutillo BA, White RM, Illes J, Greer DS, Doyle JC, Zeitlin GM (1987) Human neuroelectric patterns predict performance accuracy. *Science, 235,* 580–585.

Goldman D (1950) The clinical use of the "average" reference electrode in monopolar recording. *Electroenceph clin Neurophysiol, 2,* 209.

Hjorth B (1975) An on-line transformation of EEG scalp potentials into orthogonal source derivations. *Electroenceph clin Neurophysiol, 39,* 526–530.

Homan RW, Herman J, Purdy P (1987) Cerebral location of international 10-20 system electrode placement. *Electroenceph clin Neurophysiol, 66,* 376–382.

Jasper HH, Andrews HL (1938) Electroencephalography III. Normal differentiations of occipital and precentral regions in man. *Arch Neurol Psychiat, 39,* 96–115.

Jasper HH, Penfield W (1949) Electrocorticograms in man: Effect of the voluntary movement upon the electrical activity of the precentral gyrus. *Arch Psychiat Z Neurol, 183,* 163–174.

Kawabata N (1972) Nonstationary power spectrum analysis of the photic alpha blocking. *Kybernetik 12,* 40–44.

Keidel WD (1971) What do we know about the human cortical evoked potential after all? *Arch klin exp Ohr-, Nas- u Kehlk Heilk, 198,* 9—37.

Klimesch W, Pfurtscheller G, Lindinger G (1986) Das kortikale Aktivierungsmuster bei verbalen Gedächtnisaufgaben. *Sprache und Kognition, 5,* 140—154.

Koepruner V, Pfurtscheller G, Auer LM (1984) Quantitative EEG in normals and in patients with cerebral ischemia. In Pfurtscheller G, Lopes da Silva F, Jonkman J (Eds.) *Brain ischemia, quantitative EEG and imaging techniques* (Progress in Brain Research, Vol. 62). Elsevier, Amsterdam, 29—50.

Lehmann D (1977) The EEG as scalp field distribution. In Remond A (Ed.) *EEG informatics.* Elsevier, Amsterdam, 365—384.

Mulholland T (1969) The concept of attention and the electroencephalographic alpha rhythm. In Evans CR, Mulholland TB (Eds.) *Attention in neurophysiology.* Butterworth, London, 100—127.

Nogawa T, Katayama K, Tabata Y, Ohshio T, Kawahara T (1976) Changes in amplitude of the EEG induced by a photic stimulus. *Electroenceph clin Neurophysiol, 40,* 78—88.

Nunez PL (1981) *Electric fields in the brain: The neurophysics of EEG.* Oxford University Press, New York.

Pfurtscheller G (1981) Central beta rhythm during sensory motor activities in man. *Electroenceph clin Neurophysiol, 51,* 253—264.

Pfurtscheller G (1986) Event-related desynchronization mapping. Visualization of cortical activation patterns. In Duffy F (Ed.) *Topographic mapping of brain electrical activity.* Butterworths, Boston, 99—111.

Pfurtscheller G, Aranibar A (1977) Event-related cortical desynchronization detected by power measurements of scalp EEG. *Electroenceph clin Neurophysiol, 42,* 817—826.

Pfurtscheller G, Aranibar A (1979) Evaluation of event-related desynchronization (ERD) preceding and following self-paced movement. *Electroenceph clin Neurophysiol, 46,* 138—146.

Pfurtscheller G, Aranibar A (1980) Voluntary movement ERD: Normative studies. In Pfurtscheller G, Buser P, Lopes da Silva F, Petsche H (Eds.) *Rhythmic EEG activities and cortical functioning.*

Elsevier/North-Holland Biomedical Press, Amsterdam, 151—177.

Pfurtscheller G, Schwarz G, Pfurtscheller B, List W (1983) Quantification of spindles in comatose patients. *Electroenceph clin Neurophysiol, 56,* 114—116.

Pfurtscheller G, Ladurner G, Maresch H, Vollmer R (1984) Brain electrical activity mapping in normal and ischemic brain. In Pfurtscheller G, Jonkman J, Lopes da Silva F (Eds.) *Brain ischemia—Quantitative EEG and imaging techniques* (Progress in Brain Research, Vol. 62). Elsevier, Amsterdam, 287—302.

Pfurtscheller G, Schwarz G, Gravenstein N (1985) Clinical relevance of long-latency SEPs and VEPs during coma and emergence from coma. *Electroenceph clin Neurophysiol, 62,* 88—98.

Pfurtscheller G, Lindinger G, Klimesch W (1986) Dynamisches EEG-Mapping—Bildgebendes Verfahren fuer die Untersuchung perzeptiver, motorischer und kognitiver Hirnleistungen. *Z EEG-EMG, 17,* 113—116.

Pfurtscheller G, Maresch H, Koerner E, Lechner H (1988, in press) ERD mapping: Basis, normal values and clinical results. In Gerstenbrand F (Ed.) *The present state in clinical neuroimaging.* G. Fischer, Stuttgart.

Rader CM, Gold B (1967) Digital filter design techniques in the frequency domain. *Proc IEEE, 55,* 149—171.

Roland PE (1985) Cortical organization of voluntary behavior in man. *Human Neurobiol, 4,* 155—167.

Rumpl E, Prugger M, Bauer G, Gerstenbrand F, Hackl JM, Pallua A (1983) Incidence and prognostic value of spindles in post-traumatic coma. *Electroenceph clin Neurophysiol, 56,* 420—429.

Sergeant J, Geuze R, Van Winsum W (1987) Event-related desynchronization and P300. *Psychophysiology, 24,* 272-277.

Storm van Leeuwen W, Wieneke G, Spoelstra P, Versteeg H (1978) Lack of bilateral coherence of mu rhythm. *Electroenceph clin Neurophysiol, 44,* 140—146.

Walter WG (1964) The convergence and interaction of visual, auditory, and tactile responses in human nonspecific cortex. *Ann NY Acad of Sciences, 112,* 320—361.

ERD Mapping and Long-Term Memory: The Temporal and Topographical Pattern of Cortical Activation

W. Klimesch*, G. Pfurtscheller**, W. Mohl***

It is widely accepted that different regions of the limbic system play an important role in short-term memory processes. In contrast to short-term memory, however, it is not clear which areas of the brain contribute to long-term memory processes. It may be assumed that widespread rather than particular cortical areas are involved in long-term memory processes. This assumption is in accordance with more recent memory theories, which hold that memory codes are not represented by clearly defined holistic units but by a structure of different components or features. Thus the different components of a code might well be represented not only in different, but also in widespread cortical areas.

In the present study the issue of interest is whether or not expectancy and attention affect search and retrieval processes in long-term memory. Dynamic ERD mapping was used to examine this question. Being a topographic method, the dynamic ERD mapping is able to portray the regional brain activity in the form of maps. Its most outstanding feature is that maps can be computed for time intervals of 125 ms or even less. This method was applied for studying the topographical pattern and time course of cortical activation in three different tasks: a reading, a semantic and a numerical classification task. A sample of twelve right handed male subjects participated in the present study. In the semantic task subjects had to indicate the various categories to which a series of words belonged. In the numerical task they had to judge whether or not a presented number was odd or even. Attention was manipulated by means of expectancy: the words and numbers were presented either blockwise or in random order. Only if the material was presented blockwise did the subjects know in advance which type of task they were to perform in the next trial. Under the random presentation condition, subjects could not prepare themselves for a particular type of task.

The results show that attention affects the pattern of cortical activation in two different ways. First, in the blockwise and random presentation condition, different cortical areas were activated in the interval preceding the presentation of a word or number. Secondly, the activated cortical areas differed in size in both the interval preceding and the interval following the presentation of a word or number. Furthermore, the results show that large brain areas including occipital, parietal and parietotemporal areas of both hemispheres are significantly activated when subjects perform a long-term memory task. Comparing the magnitude of activation in the reading and in the memory tasks, it can be observed that in the memory task occipital regions show a much higher level of activation than in the reading task. In agreement with earlier work, we may therefore conclude that not only parietal and parietotemporal, but also occipital regions are involved in long-term memory processes. In addition, the results show that attention and long-term memory processes do interact.

* Dept. of Physiological Psychology, Institute of Psychology, University of Salzburg, Austria
** Ludwig Boltzmann-Institute of Medical Informatics, Graz, Austria
*** Dept. of Medical Informatics, Institute of Biomedical Engineering, Technical University of Graz, Austria
The authors wish to thank Dipl. Ing. Gerald Lindinger for the development of software and Michael Nigitz for data recording and photography.
This research was supported by the Austrian "Fonds zur Förderung der wissenschaftlichen Forschung," projects 5240 and 5844 as well as the Austrian Ministry of Science and Research.

The Localization of Memory Processes: Theoretical Considerations

Theories of memory distinguish between encoding and retrieval processes as two fundamental aspects of memory. When attempting to explain encoding processes, the crucial question is how a memory trace is established and consolidated. This issue is closely related to studies of short-term memory. Theories of long-term memory, on the other hand, focus on the question of how stored information is accessed and retrieved. Both the encoding and the retrieval aspects relate to yet another important aspect: the format that represents information in memory. It may be assumed, e. g., that memory codes can be best characterized by a propositional, sensory specific, holistic or componential format. As more elaborate memory theories show, the type of coding format interacts with the way information can be retrieved (Anderson, 1983; Klimesch, 1986, 1987). Accordingly, assumptions regarding the coding format and retrieval processes must be considered together.

Are short-term and long-term memory processes localizable in the brain? Here, it is generally accepted that short-term memory depends on the integrity of the hippocampus and on other regions of the limbic system as well (Irle & Markowitsch, 1982; Markowitsch, 1985; Murray & Mishkin, 1985). In contrast to short-term memory, it is less clear which areas of the brain contribute to long-term memory processes (Thompson, 1983; Markowitsch, 1985).

One possible reason for the difficulty in localizing long-term memory processes may be misleading assumptions about the format of memory codes. In the traditional view, memory codes were considered as clearly definable holistic units. According to this view, it was tempting to assume that a holistic code must be represented in a single and clearly definable area of the brain or even in individual neurons. A completely different picture arises if we assume that memory codes are not represented by holistic codes but instead by a structure of different components. Because the different components of a code might well be represented not only in different but also in widespread cortical areas, the assumption of a componential coding format leads to the prediction of a distributed memory system. Thus, whether we expect that long-term memory is clearly localizable or not depends at least partly on those assumptions of a memory theory that define the format of long-term memory codes.

The difficulty in localizing long-term memory might also be due to a close interaction between short- and long-term memory processes. Short-term memory most likely serves as the basis for selecting and initiating a search process in long-term memory as well as for evaluating its results. Retrieval and search processes may spread automatically in long-term memory without requiring the processing capacity or attention provided by short-term memory. The selection, initiation and evaluation of long-term memory processes does require short-term memory capacity and attention. It is thus not surprising that in some studies, brain regions such as the limbic system, which are typical for short-term memory processes, were found to be involved in long-term memory tasks (John et al., 1986; see also the review in Thompson, 1983). This possibly interactive nature of long-term memory gives us an important clue for the way in which an experiment must be designed: some strategy must be found to separate the short-term from the long-term memory component of a task.

Finally, it will be helpful for the following discussion to point out the close relationship between attention and short-term memory. Attention refers to the way in which capacity of short-term memory is allocated to the processing of the various components of a complex task. Because the capacity of short-term memory is limited, the allocation and distribution of its capacity is an important aspect of human information processing.

Brain Imaging and Long-Term Memory

As a result of recent advances in brain imaging technology, many techniques are available for diagnostic purposes (see Holder 1987 for a review). Some of these brain imaging techniques such as the rCBF technique and methods monitoring the uptake of glucose have been applied successfully to the study of cognitive processes (Ingvar & Risberg, 1967; Risberg & Ingvar, 1973; Wood, 1983; Roland, 1984) and long-term memory processes (Maximilian et al., 1978; Wood et al., 1980a; Mubrin et al., 1985; John et al., 1986; see also Roland, this volume). The results of these studies seem to indicate that large cortical areas are activated during long-term memory processes. Thus, these results agree with the assumption of a distributed memory system.

The results are less clear if we ask in which regions of the brain long-term memory is represented. Whereas some studies show that occipital and parietal regions are involved in long-term memory (cf. Maximilian et al., 1978; Mubrin et al., 1985), other studies indicate that frontal, frontotemporal and temporal regions show the highest level of activation in long-term memory tasks (Wood et al., 1980a, 1980b). One obvious reason for these divergent results is the variety of different tasks (recognition, free recall and discrimination tasks) and stimuli (e.g., visually and aurally presented words), which are used to study long-term memory processes. Another and probably more important reason is that in some studies, no attempt was made to separate the memory-specific processes from the sensory and motor components of a task. The results of those studies thus do not permit a distinction between brain regions involved in memory processes and brain regions involved in sensory and motor processes.

Major Methodological Problems

Wood et al. (1980a) brought attention to the fact that brain imaging studies focusing on the investigation of the relationship between brain and memory processes must fulfill the requirement of distinguishing between the different components of a task. Two different strategies can be used to do this.

One strategy, which involves the design of an experiment, is to separate different processing stages by holding perceptual and response processes constant and varying the instructions only. As an example, let us consider a within subject design in which the same set of words is used as stimulus in three different tasks, a reading, recognition, and semantic memory task (for a more detailed description, see Klimesch et al., 1986). Because the three tasks differ with respect to the instructions only, any difference obtained in the pattern of cortical activation may be due to cognitive, but not to perceptual, responses or motor processes.

Another strategy is to distinguish different processing stages by studying the time course of cortical activation with short integration intervals. To illustrate this strategy, let us consider a semantic memory task in which a subject has to decide whether or not a word (e.g., "eagle") belongs to a previously specified category (e.g., "bird"). Here, a sequence of the following four processing stages may be assumed: first, the presented word must be perceived; second, its meaning must be accessed in semantic memory; third, the meaning of the perceived word and the category have to be compared; fourth a response must be made. As the results from typical experiments show, the average reaction time in semantic memory tasks of the type described above is about 800 ms. Thus, we have to assume that any of the four processing stages lasts only for a few hundred milliseconds. Consequently, brain imaging techniques with a temporal resolution of a second or more cannot be used to distinguish between the different processing stages of a memory task. The objection may be made that a low temporal resolution is not disadvantageous as long as the experiments are designed in accordance with the first principle discussed above. This argument holds only if the different processing stages are independent from each other and do not interact with the type of task or instruction. Subjects may adapt their encoding and/or response strategies to the type of task or instruction. Thus, even a competently controlled and designed experiment is no guarantee that the results will differ with respect to the cognitive processing stage only. These considerations make it clear that studying the temporal pattern of cortical activation is then the only way to identify and finally to discriminate between the different processing stages of a task.

Because of their low temporal resolution, brain imaging techniques such as the rCBF method and related techniques make the latter strategy unacceptable here. The same holds true for methods imaging the glucose uptake in the brain. The ERD mapping, as a topographic EEG method, is one of the few brain imaging techniques which allows portrayal of regional brain activity with a high temporal resolution of 125 ms or even less. This outstanding feature renders ERD mapping eminently suitable for studying cognitive processes, and memory processes in particular (Pfurtscheller et al., 1986).

ERD Mapping and the Study of Memory Processes

In earlier work, ERD mapping was applied to study the pattern and time course of cortical activation in two different memory tasks, which were designed according to the two principles discussed above (Klimesch et al, 1986). The results of this study indicate that parietal and occipital regions are involved in long-term memory processes. The most interesting result, however, involves the time course of cortical activation. A striking similarity was found between the pattern of cortical activation preceding and following stimulus presentation. In the prestimulus interval, maximal activation was observed at about 300 ms before a stimulus was presented. Then, shortly before the stimulus actually appeared, cortical activation dropped to the baseline or reference level and reached its second maximum at about 400 ms after stimulus onset. Whatever the meaning of this phenomenon, we will refer to it as the phenomenon of "preactivation" in the following. By preactivation we mean that a few hundred milliseconds before a stimulus is presented, primarily those brain regions are activated which later are involved in the processing of that stimulus.

It seems plausible to assume that—similar to the CNV—the phenomenon of preactivation is due to expectant attentional processes. However, one of the most intriguing questions is how expectancy and attention influence the processing of a stimulus or memory processes in particular.

With respect to the second strategy discussed above, these preliminary results show that it is the high temporal resolution that gives us new insights into the relationship between brain and memory processes.

Hypotheses and Experimental Design

The purpose of the present study is to show whether or not there is an interaction between those processing stages preceding and those following the presentation of a stimulus. In particular, the experiments were designed to study the relationship between attention and long-term memory. If all other variables—including task type, stimulus and response variables—are kept constant, in which way does attention affect search and retrieval processes?

Our subjects had to perform a semantic and a numerical classification task. Whereas in the semantic task subjects had to indicate the category to which each of a series of words belonged, in the numerical task they had to judge whether or not a presented number was odd or even. Because both classification tasks can be performed on the basis of preexperimental knowledge only, they were considered pure long-term memory tasks.

As will be illustrated below, attention was manipulated by means of expectancy. The words and numbers to be classified were presented either blockwise or in random order. When the material was presented blockwise, subjects knew which type of task they would have to perform in the next trial. When words and numbers were presented randomly, subjects did not know in advance whether a word or a number would be presented in the next trial. Under this condition, subjects could not prepare for a particular type of task. The random presentation of words and numbers can thus be considered to be more difficult than the blockwise presentation.

The issue of interest here is whether or not expectancy and attention affect search and retrieval processes. According to the distributed memory model outlined above, we have to assume that search and retrieval processes are of a complex nature and require considerable processing capacity. It is thus plausible to suppose that specific access and/or retrieval strategies must be selected before the search process is initiated. If words and numbers are presented blockwise, subjects are able to select a particular strategy even before a stimulus is presented. However, presenting words and numbers in random order prevents subjects from choosing a particular strategy.

We therefore expect that in the period preceding the presentation of a stimulus, the pattern of cortical activation will differ between both presentation conditions. The crucial question is whether or not, in the period after the presentation of a stimulus, the pattern of cortical activation will also differ between the two presentation conditions. If this is the case, we may conclude that the two processing stages, referring to the pre- and poststimulus interval, do interact: the way in which a subject prepares for a task determines the way in which he performs that task.

Method

Our subjects were 12 right-handed males. Handedness was checked with a questionnaire. All subjects were students at the University of Graz and were paid for their participation in the experiment.

The stimuli were 48 words and 48 numbers. Both sets of stimuli were chosen to be divisible into two categories of 24 items each. Half of the 48 words belonged to the category "tools," the other half to the category "animals." Half of the 48 numbers were odd, the other half even. All of the numbers consisted of two digits.

Two stimulus conditions (words and numbers) and two presentation conditions (blockwise and random presentation of words and numbers) were orthogonally combined and administered in a within subject design. The experimental session was preceded by a control condition, in which the subjects had to read first the 48 words and then the 48 numbers.

With the exception of the control condition, the subjects had to perform a semantic or numerical classification task. They were instructed to indicate to which of the two categories (animals/tools or odd/even numbers)

an item belonged. Subjects had to respond with "yes" if a word denoted an animal and to respond with "no" if a word denoted a tool. When a number was presented, the subject had first to subtract three and then to decide whether the resulting number was odd or even. If the resulting number was even, the subject responded "yes," otherwise "no." As an example, consider the number 67. First, the subject performs the subtraction ($67-3 = 64$) and then decides that the result is an even number. Accordingly, the subject gives a yes-response. Since the subtraction of three always turns an even number into an odd number and vice versa, subjects could also use an alternative strategy, which consists of responding "yes" to an odd number and "no" to an even number. However, regardless of the strategy used, the purpose of this procedure was to increase cognitive load.

The stimuli (words or numbers) were exposed for 250 ms and presented via a computer-controlled video terminal. A warning signal appeared 1 s before stimulus presentation. The interstimulus interval was 4 s in the reading task and 5 s in the classification tasks. A single trial was defined by the time period beginning 2000 ms before the presentation of a stimulus and ending either 2000 ms (in the reading task) or 3000 ms (in the classification tasks) after stimulus presentation. The period between the warning signal and the presentation of a stimulus is termed "prestimulus interval," the period following stimulus presentation is termed "poststimulus interval." The procedure underlying the acquisition and processing of EEG data as well as the computation of ERD maps is described in Pfurtscheller et al. in this volume (see also Pfurtscheller et al., 1986).

The letters of the words and the digits of the numbers were 3 cm in height. The longest word was 30 cm in length. Subjects sat at a distance of 1.6 m from the video terminal. All responses were given verbally and were recorded by the experimenter. Erroneous trials were excluded from data analysis. Computed for each of the four experimental conditions, error rates range from 3.99% to 5.90%. The mean percentage of errors in the random presentation condition was 4.95% as compared to 4.43% in the blockwise presentation condition.

Results

According to the ERD technique applied in earlier studies, the colors of a map indicate the extent to which the percentage of alpha power values changes with respect to a reference interval. In interpreting ERD maps, one of the crucial requirements is the use of a criterion which defines a significant alpha power increase or decrease. We computed probability maps to meet this requirement. Instead of showing the percentage alpha power increase or decrease, probability maps show the probability with which an alpha power decrease or increase occurs. The computation of the probabilities is based on the sign test, a non-parametric statistical procedure. Furthermore, in order to guarantee that only those changes in alpha power are considered which are of primary importance, a high significance level of $p < .0001$ was adopted.

For the sake of simplicity the results will be described and discussed simply in terms of different levels of cortical activation in the following manner: low probability values (hot colors in Figure 1) indicating a large and highly significant decrease in alpha power are interpreted in terms of a high level of cortical activation. High probability values (cool colors in Figure 1) on the other hand indicate only a small and insignificant decrease in alpha power and are interpreted in terms of a low level of cortical activation. Because words and numbers showed similar results, the data were pooled for both stimulus conditions. The maps discussed below show the mean probability of an alpha power change for the averaged data of 12 subjects.

The Topographical and Temporal Pattern of Cortical Activation in the Poststimulus Interval

One of the basic issues of the present study is the question as to which cortical areas are involved in longterm memory processes. The relevant results for both expectancy conditions consistently show that, 375 ms after stimulus presentation, large cortical areas including primarily occipital, parietal as well as temporal regions are activated significantly (cf. the respective maps in Figure 1 b). However,

the two expectancy conditions differ with respect to the amount of activation, which is much larger for the condition in which words and numbers were presented in a random sequence. The difference between these two conditions is more pronounced for the upper alpha band than for the lower alpha band (cf. the first and second row of maps in Figure 1 d and 1 f). The reading task, which is not shown here, yields similar results. Here also, occipital parietal and temporal regions are activated, but as compared to the memory tasks, the magnitude of activation is much smaller in the reading task.

The temporal activation pattern also differs between the two expectancy conditions and the control condition (i. e., the reading task). The duration of cortical activation was defined as follows: First, the entire set of 12 maps representing the poststimulus interval was inspected and the highest level of activation was recorded. Then, the time period between the first and the last occurence of maximal activation was determined. Thus, the duration of cortical activation was defined on the basis of sustained maximal activation. As defined in this way, the results show that the onset of activation occurs—with one exception only—at the same time in all of the three experimental conditions. The duration of sustained maximal activation in the random presentation condition is, however, about 200 ms longer as compared to both the control and the blockwise presentation condition.

The Effect of Expectancy on Memory Processes

Expectancy was varied in two steps. When words and numbers were presented blockwise, subjects knew that the same type of stimulus would be presented in the next trial. But with random presentation, subjects could only guess whether a word or number would appear.

Figure 1 a shows the results for the prestimulus interval in the range of 1500—1750 ms. As all three maps in the first row in Figure 1 a indicate, parietotemporal and occipital regions of the left hemisphere—but not those of the right hemisphere—are significantly activated when word and numbers

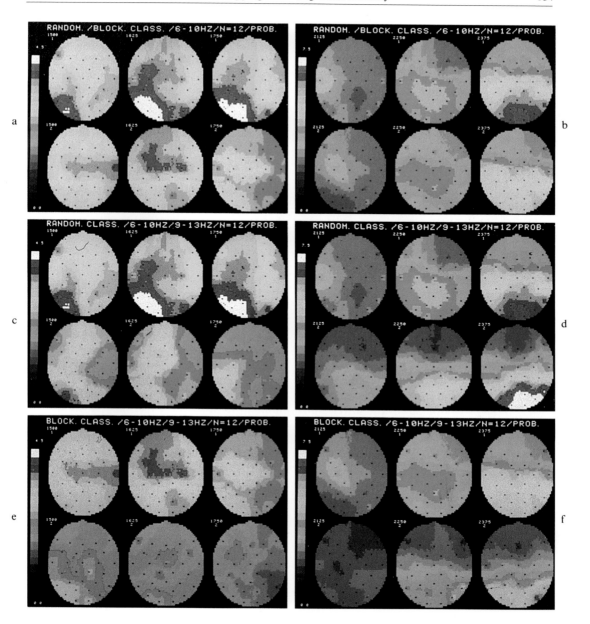

Figure 1a—f. Probability maps showing the significance with which an alpha power decrease occurs when words and numbers are presented blockwise (second row of maps in Figure 1a,b and both rows in Figure 1e,f) or in random order (first row in Figure 1a,b and both rows in Figure 1c,d). The results for two frequency bands (6—10 Hz; 9—13 Hz) are shown in the first and second row of Figures 1c—f. The three maps on the left side (Figure 1a,c and e) show the results of the prestimulus interval (1500—1750 ms), the three maps on the right side (Figure 1b,d und f) show the results of the poststimulus interval (2125—2375 ms). The stimulus appeared at 2000 ms. Each map represents a time period of 125 ms. Hot colors indicate highly significant, cool colors only small and insignificant alpha power changes. Note that different color scales—ranging from 0 to 4.5 in the pre- and from 0 to 7.5 in the poststimulus interval—were used to display the results. The scale value is the negative exponent of 10. As an example, a scale value of 3 refers to a probability of 1/1000.

are presented in random order. When presented blockwise, a completely different activation pattern can be observed (cf. the second row in Figure 1 a). Here, central regions instead of parietal and occipital regions are activated. The results further show that the two conditions also differ with respect to the extent to which brain areas are significantly activated. Whereas large areas are activated when words and numbers are presented in random order, only small areas reach the .0001 significance level when words and numbers are presented blockwise.

Figure 1 b presents the most important results for that part of the poststimulus interval when a significant increase in cortical activation occurs. A comparison of the maps in the first and second rows of Figure 1 b indicates that parietal and occipital areas are significantly activated in both conditions no sooner than 375 ms after stimulus presentation. The only difference between the two conditions here is that cortical activation is much more extensive under the random presentation condition (cf. the first row in Figure 1 b).

All of the results reported thus far are based on maps computed for the lower alpha band.

The Results for the Lower and Upper Alpha Band

The EEG data were analyzed with respect to two different but partly overlapping alpha bands, a lower alpha band ranging from 6–10 Hz and an upper alpha band ranging from 9–13 Hz. Comparison of the respective maps computed for the lower and upper alpha bands provides highly significant differences with respect to the prestimulus interval and with respect to the overall extent of cortical activation.

First, in the prestimulus interval, a significant increase of cortical activation was found—with a single exception—for the lower alpha band only. Figure 1 c shows the results for the random presentation of words and numbers. Here, all three maps referring to the lower alpha band (cf. the first row of Figure 1 c) exhibit a strong increase in cortical activation. As the respective maps indicate, large areas of the left hemisphere are activated sig-

nificantly. In contrast to the maps in the first row, only one map in the second row shows a small and significantly activated brain area representing the results for the upper alpha band. As for the random presentation, similar results were obtained for the blockwise presentation of words and numbers (cf. Figure 1 e). Whereas a significant activation was found for the lower alpha band (first row of Figure 1 e), none of the maps reflecting the upper alpha band reached significance.

Second, with respect to the overall extent of cortical activation, the results show that larger brain areas reached significance, if the lower alpha band was chosen for data analysis. This is not only true for the prestimulus interval (Figure 1 c and 1 e) but for the poststimulus interval (Figure 1 d and 1 f) as well. A good example is Figure 1 f, which shows the results for the blockwise presentation of words. Here, the lower alpha band reflects an extensive activation covering large cortical areas (cf. the first row in Figure 1 f). The upper alpha band shows activated cortical regions which are—compared to the lower band—much smaller in size. The results were similar in all four experimental conditions (the pre- and poststimulus interval for the random and blockwise presentation of words and numbers), as a comparison of the first and second row in Figure 1 c, 1 d, 1 e and 1 f shows.

General Discussion

Our results show that expectancy affects the pattern of cortical activation in two different ways. First, different cortical areas were activated in the prestimulus interval. Second, the activated cortical areas also differ in size in both the prestimulus and the poststimulus intervals.

With respect to the prestimulus interval, the data show that occipital and parietal regions of the left hemisphere showed maximal activation when subjects did not know whether a word or number would be presented in the next trial. When subjects did know which type of stimulus would be presented, primarily central but not occipital and parietal regions were activated. Obviously, under the latter condition subjects did not need to put much effort into preparing for the task. As a consequence, those brain regions needed to perform the task were not preactivated. According to this interpretation it is not surprising that occipital and parietal regions which proved to be involved in performing the memory tasks failed to reach a significant level of activation in this condition. In contrast to the blockwise presentation of stimuli, subjects may have had to put considerably more effort into preparation for the task if words and numbers were presented randomly. Because of this effort, the task-related occipital and parietal regions were significantly activated even before a stimulus was presented. In addition to these regions, central areas were activated as well. Thus, as with the blockwise presentation of words and numbers, the activation of these central regions may again reflect the readiness or preparation for a verbal response.

For the pre- and poststimulus interval the results show that—compared to the blockwise presentation—cortical activation was much more widespread when words and numbers were presented in a random sequence. Thus, expectancy not only affects the cortical processes preceding but also those following stimulus presentation. Because of this result and because—with the exception of expectancy—all of the other experimental variables were exactly identical for both presentation conditions, it can be concluded that different processing stages are not independent from each other but instead do interact: the greater the activation of cortical regions during the prestimulus interval, the greater the involvement of cortical regions in the processing of a stimulus.

All of the considerations discussed above are based on the implicit but fundamental assumption that the brain regions which are significantly activated during the poststimulus interval are those regions in which the stimulus is actually processed. Though a tempting conclusion, we must also consider the possibility that cortical activation—as infered by the ERD mapping technique—reflects not only stimulus specific processes but attentional, motivational or general arousal effects as well.

In order to explain this hypothesis let us discuss the results outlined above in terms of task difficulty. Because subjects could not prepare for a particular type of task when words and numbers were presented in a random sequence, this experimental condition can be considered to be more difficult than the blockwise presentation of words and numbers. The more difficult a task is, the more attention a subject must pay to performance of the task. As a consequence, the extent of cortical activation should increase as task difficulty increases. This is exactly what was found: for the random presentation of stimuli cortical activation was more widespread than for the blockwise presentation. Furthermore, the cortical activation in the reading task, which can be considered the easiest of the present study, is less widespread than in the two memory tasks. The late onset of cortical activation at about 250 ms after stimulus presentation may also be considered as good evidence for the hypothesis that ERD mapping does not primarily reflect stimulus-specific processes. As can be infered from the results of other studies (e.g., Klimesch & Pfurtscheller, 1987), the visual perception and identification of a single word usually does not last longer than about 200 ms. The late onset of cortical activation may be partly due to lambda waves generated by eye movements and causing an artificial increase of power in the lower alpha band. Because the onset of cortical activation does not differ between the lower and upper alpha band, lambda waves most likely are not the reason for the late ERD onset.

In evaluating the above-mentioned arguments, we also have to consider the different results which were found for the lower and upper alpha band. Because expectancy and attention effects were found primarily for the lower alpha band, we may assume that the lower band shows attentional processes more sensitively than the upper alpha band. This assumption is in good agreement with the fact that under all of the conditions observed in this study, the lower alpha band shows a pattern of cortical activation which is consistently more widespread than that of the upper alpha band.

With these precautions in mind, we may finally turn to the question of the cortical areas involved in long-term memory processes. In trying to answer this question we have to consider the upper alpha band, which most likely is less sensitive for attentional and more sensitive for stimulus-related memory processes. Here, the results for the two memory tasks still showed that large brain areas including occipital, parietal and parietotemporal areas of both hemispheres are significantly activated. Because occipital region were also activated in the reading task, which served as a control condition, one might object that occipital regions are involved in reading but not in memory processes. Comparing the magnitude of activation reveals that in the memory task, occipital regions show a much higher level of activation than in the reading task.

Moreover, there is yet another fact which suggests that even in the reading task, occipital regions may be involved in long-term memory processes: as in the memory task, the onset of cortical activation in occipital areas in the reading task does not occur earlier than 250 ms after stimulus presentation. We already have pointed out that the process of perceiving a word or number has long been completed before ERD rises to a significant level after about 250 ms. If we consider the fact that a word must be perceived before its meaning can be accessed in semantic memory, we may assume that the onset of cortical activation as observed in this study signals the beginning of semantic memory processes. Taken together, the results are in good agreement with the assumption of a distributed memory system: long-term memory codes are represented by a structure of different components, which are localized in widespread cortical areas. According to this view, the extent to which cortical areas are activated reflects the complexity of a memory task. The more memory codes there are to be processed and the more widely distributed they are, the more complex search and retrieval processes will be and the more processing resources a task will require. This view shows how closely memory processes and attention are related. The more difficult a memory task is, the more attention will be required to perform that task.

The late onset of cortical activation occurring at about 250 ms and reaching its maximum at about 375 ms leads one to speculate that ERD onset and P300 may be considered as related phenomena. And indeed, Sergeant et al. (1987) demonstrate in their interesting study that ERD and P300 are different cortical indices of the same attentional (cf. van Winsum et al., 1984) or memory processes. They found that with increasing task difficulty or cognitive load, the amount of ERD increased whereas the amplitude of the P300 decreased. Furthermore, ERD duration and P300 latency increased as task difficulty was increased. Thus, with respect to ERD and task difficulty, this is almost exactly what the present study shows: compared to the blockwise presentation of words and numbers, which can be considered the easier of the two tasks, cortical activation is more widespread and lasts longer if words and numbers are presented in a random sequence.

If we keep this relationship between ERD and P300 in mind, the results of the following studies provide further evidence for the assumption that both cortical indices may reflect attentional rather than memory or storage related processes. First of all, it is well established that P300 is elicited by unexpected events, and that the lower the subjective probability of an event is, the larger the amplitude of the P300 will be (cf. Duncan-Johnson & Donchin, 1977). With respect to memory in particular, several studies show that words which were later recalled had elicited larger P300s on their initial presentation than words not recalled (Fabiani et al., 1986; Karis et al., 1984). These results, however, provide more insight into attentional than into memory processes. Most likely, they simply show that without a certain level of attention, no memory trace will be established: those words which received more attention elicited larger P300s and consequently were better remembered. A similar interpretation holds true for the results of Chapman (Chapman et al., 1978; Chapman et al., 1981) who identified a memory-related evoked potential component with a poststimulus maximum at about 250 ms.

The results presented in this study serve to illustrate the way in which different processing stages may be identified. In particular, the results show that attentional and stimulus related memory processes do interact. The higher the level of attention is, the more widespread memory processes are.

References

Anderson JR (1983) *Architecture of cognition.* John Wiley, New York.

Chapman RM, McCrary JW, Chapman JA (1978) Short-term memory: The "storage" component of human brain responses predicts recall. *Science, 202,* 1211–1214.

Chapman RM, McCrary JW, Chapman JA (1981) Memory processes and evoked potentials. *Can J Psychol, 35,* 201–212.

Duncan-Johnson CC, Donchin E (1977) On quantifying surprise: The variation of event-related potentials with subjective probability. *Psychophysiology, 14,* 456–467.

Fabiani M, Karis D, Donchin, E (1986) P300 and recall in an incidental memory paradigm. *Psychophysiology, 23,* 298–308.

Holder DS (1987) Feasibility of developing a method of imaging neuronal activity in the human brain: A theoretical review. *Med Biol Eng Comput, 25,* 2–11.

Ingvar DH, Risberg J (1967) Increase of regional cerebral blood flow during mental efforts in normals and in patients with focal brain disorders. *Exp Brain Res, 3,* 195–211.

Irle E, Markowitsch HJ (1982) Connections of the hippocampal formation, mamillary bodies, anterior thalamus and cingulate cortex. *Exp Brain Res, 47,* 79–94.

John ER, Tang Y, Brill AB, Young R, Ono K (1986) Doublelabeled metabolic maps of memory. *Science, 233,* 1167–1175.

Karis D, Fabiani M, Donchin E (1984) P300 and memory: individual differences in the von Restorff Effect. *Cogn Psychol, 16,* 177–216.

Klimesch W (1986) The structure of memory codes. In Klix F, Hagendorf H (Eds.) *Human memory and cognitive capabilities.* Elsevier, Amsterdam, 245–252.

Klimesch W (1987) A connectivity model for semantic processing. *Psychol Res, 49,* 53–61.

Klimesch W, Pfurtscheller G, Lindinger G (1986) Das corticale Aktivierungsmuster bei verbalen Gedächtnisaufgaben. *Sprache und Kognition, 5,* 140–154.

Klimesch W, Pfurtscheller G (1987, in press) The decomposition of semantic processing times:

Studied with the dynamic EEG-mapping, evoked potentials and reaction time experiments (abstract). *J Psychophysiol.*

Markowitsch HJ (1985) Gedächtnis und Gehirn. *Psychologische Rundschau, 36,* 201–216.

Maximilian VA, Prohovnik I, Risberg J, Haakonsson K (1978) Regional blood flow changes in the left cerebral hemisphere during word pair learning and recall. *Brain and Language, 6,* 22–31.

Mubrin Z, Knezevic S, Barac B, Gubarev N, Lazic M, Liscic R, Vidosic S (1985) Distinct rCBF pattern during different types of short-term memory activation. In Hartmann A, Hoyer S (Eds.) *Cerebral blood flow and metabolic measurement.* Springer-Verlag, New York, 170–176.

Murray EA, Mishkin M (1985) Amygdalectomy impairs crossmodal association in monkeys. *Science, 228,* 604–606.

Pfurtscheller G, Lindinger G, Klimesch W (1986) Dynamisches EEG-Mapping – bildgebendes Verfahren für die Untersuchung perzeptiver, motorischer und kognitiver Hirnleistungen. *Z EEG-EMG, 17,* 113–116.

Risberg J, Ingvar DH (1973) Patterns of activation in the grey matter of the dominant hemisphere during memorization and reasoning. *Brain, 996,* 737–756.

Roland PE (1984) Metabolic measurements of the working frontal cortex in man. *Trends in Neurosciences, 7,* 430–435.

Sergeant J, Geuze R, van Winsum W (1987) Event-related desynchronization and P300. *Psychophysiology, 24,* 272–277.

Thompson R (1983) Brain systems and long-term memory. *Behav Neural Biol, 37,* 1–50.

van Winsum W, Sergeant J, Geuze R (1984) The functional significance of event related desynchronization of alpha rhythm in attentional and activating tasks. *Electroenceph clin Neurophysiol, 58,* 519–524.

Wood F (1983) Laterality of cerebral function: Its investigation by localized indicators of metabolism. In Hellige J (Ed.) *Cerebral functional asymmetry: Method, theory and application.* Praeger, New York, 255–278.

Wood F, Taylor B, Penny R, Stump D (1980a) Regional cerebral blood flow response to recognition memory versus semantic classification tasks. *Brain and Language, 9,* 113–122.

Wood F, Armentrout R, Toole J, McHenry L, Stump D (1980b) Regional cerebral blood flow response during rest and memory activation in a patient with global amnesia. *Brain and Language, 9,* 129–136.

Noninvasive Mapping of Motor-Evoked Potentials in Humans

L. G. Cohen and M. Hallett

It is possible to stimulate the human motor cortex through the intact scalp using short duration, high voltage electrical stimulation. This technique has been used to measure motor conduction velocities in the central nervous system in normal volunteers and patients with different disorders such as multiple sclerosis. We modified this technique and found it possible to map the locations of face, hand and leg areas of the motor cortex.

Constant voltage stimuli were delivered through a bipolar surface stimulator with anode at multiple sites over the scalp and the cathode 2.5 cm anterior to the anode. Recordings were bilateral from abductor pollicis brevis (APB), tibialis anterior (TA) and depressor labii inferioris (DLI) or risorius. We averaged the amplitudes of three muscle responses after stimulating each scalp position and the value obtained was assigned to represent that point over the scalp.

Similar and reproducible results were obtained in eight normal volunteers. Maximal responses of the right APB were obtained to stimulation of C3, of the left APB to stimulation of C4, of the right and left TA to stimulation of Cz, of the left DLI to stimulation of T4 and of the right DLI to stimulation of T3. These motor maps were compared to maps of somatosensory evoked potentials to median, tibial and trigeminal nerve stimulation in order to demonstrate the relationship to primary sensory cortex.

Noninvasive electrical stimulation of human motor cortex has been used for several years (Merton & Morton 1980; Rossini et al. 1985). This methodology has opened the possibility, for the first time, of studying central motor conduction times in intact humans. Different groups have reported abnormalities in central motor conduction velocities in patients with multiple sclerosis (Cowan et al., 1984; Mills & Murray, 1985), tumors in the central nervous

system (Levy, 1987) and hemispheric infarction (Berardelli et al., 1987). We have studied the different possible methodologies for noninvasive mapping of the human motor cortex using electrical stimulation (Cohen at al., 1987 a, b). The best technique for this purpose involves delivering constant voltage stimuli through a bipolar surface stimulator with 2.5 cm between anode and cathode. The anode is positioned over the desired scalp location and the cathode 2.5 cm anterior to the anode. Maintenance of a low impedance between anode and cathode is required. The stimulus intensity is increased over the theoretical motor representation area (C3 for right upper limb, Cz for lower limbs, etc.) until a muscle response of 500–1,000 µV is achieved. The same stimuli are delivered over the different scalp locations corresponding to the same represention area. Three muscle responses are recorded at each scalp position. The average of the three amplitudes is assigned to characterize that scalp position. Locations stimulated should be less than 2.5 cm apart in order to maximize the sensibility of the map.

Hand motor areas in normals map maximally close to C3 or C4 (for right and left hand respectively) (Cohen et al., 1987 b; Cohen & Hallett, submitted). Figure 1 shows an example of the muscle responses recorded when mapping the left hand (left abductor pollicis brevis, APB) and stimulating different

Human Motor Control Section, Medical Neurology Branch, National Institute of Neurological and Communicative Disorders and Stroke, National Institutes of Health, Bethesda, MD 20892, U.S.A.

scalp positions. The maximal muscle response was obtained when stimulating over C4 and its size faded when moving the stimulator in the sagittal and coronal axis. The latency of the response recorded from APB was 20 ms.

Leg motor areas map maximally close to the midline (Cohen et al., 1987b; Cohen & Hallett, submitted). Figure 2 shows an example of the muscle responses recorded when mapping the left leg (left tibialis anterior, TA) and stimulating different scalp positions. The maximal muscle response was obtained when stimulating positions 2.3 cm to the right and 2.3 cm behind Cz. The latency of the response recorded from TA was 33 ms.

We have also compared motor and sensory maps of the same areas. For this purpose, somatosensory evoked potentials (SEP) were recorded after electrical stimulation of the median nerve at the wrist and the tibial nerve immediately behind the internal malleolus. Stimulus intensity was chosen to evoke a visible twitch of thenar muscles and foot flexor muscles when stimulating median nerve and tibial nerve respectively. The number of stimuli delivered was that necessary to evoke SEP resulting in 20% or less amplitude difference of repeated trials. SEP's were recorded with 29 electrodes positioned according to the 10—20 system, plus two intermediate rows of electrodes anterior and posterior to the critical line crossing C3—T3—Cz and referenced to linked earlobes. Electrode impedances were maintained below 5 KΩ. Potentials were amplified with a gain of 200,000 using a band-pass of 30—1,000 Hz and sampling rate was 4,000 Hz.

Motor maps were constructed by quantifying the size of the muscle responses (recorded from APB and TA upon stimulation of differ-

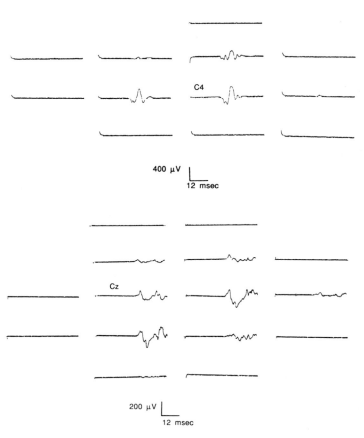

Figure 1. Representative muscle responses recorded from left abductor pollicis brevis (APB) when stimulating different scalp position with the same stimulus duration and intensity. The distance between stimulating positions was 2.3 cm. Note that the largest muscle responses from left APB were obtained when stimulating over C4 (550 µV) and 2.3 cm medial to C4 (450 µV) and that the responses faded abruptly when stimulating farther in any direction in the coronal or sagittal axis.

Figure 2. Representative muscle responses recorded from left tibialis anterior (TA) when stimulating different scalp position with the same stimulus duration and intensity. Note that the largest muscle responses from left TA were obtained when stimulating scalp positions 2.3 cm to the right and 2.3 cm behind Cz and that the responses faded when stimulating farther in any direction in the coronal or sagittal axis.

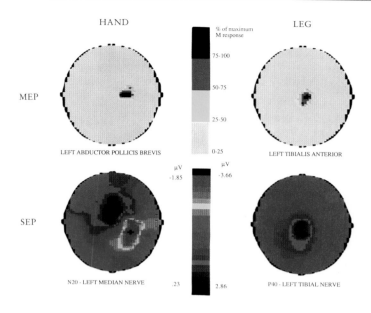

Figure 3. Comparison of left hand and leg motor (MEP) and sensory (SEP) maps. Motor maps, constructed by quantifying the amplitudes of M responses (recorded from left APB and left TA with stimulation of different scalp locations) relative to the maximum M response. The left hand motor area was localized to C4 and 2.3 cm medial to C4 (black area, left upper map). The left leg motor area was localized more medially in positions 2.3 cm to the right and 2.3 cm behind Cz (black area, right upper map) The other colors represent the areas in which stimulation evoked smaller M responses from APB and TA. Sensory maps, obtained by recording the SEP elicited by left median and tibial nerves stimulation. The maps were constructed by analyzing the first cortical component of the left median nerve SEP (parietal negativity N20, which was recorded 19 ms after electrical stimulation of the left median nerve) and of the left tibial nerve SEP (scalp positivity P40, which was recorded 38 ms after stimulation of the left tibial nerve). The amplitude of the N20 component of median nerve SEP was maximal 3.5 cm behind C4. The amplitude of the P40 component of tibial nerve SEP was maximal over Cz and 2.3 cm behind Cz and its scalp distribution was slightly ipsilateral to the side stimulated.

ent scalp positions) relative to the maximum M response recorded from that muscle. Black areas in the motor maps show the scalp positions which, upon being stimulated, generated muscle responses of 75 to 100% of the maximum M obtained from that muscle. Red and yellow areas show scalp positions which, upon being stimulated, generated muscle responses of 50–75% and 25—50% of the maximum M, respectively. Sensory maps were constructed by quantifying the amplitudes of the N20 and P40 components of median nerve and tibial nerve SEP in μV on a 22-color scale. Values at intermediate pixels of both the motor and sensory map images were computed using the following second order interpolation algorithm:

$$V(x,y) = \sum_{n=1}^{4} V(En) / r(En)^2$$

$V(x,y)$: Value of pixel (x,y)
$V(En)$: Voltage at nearest neighbor n
$r(En)$: Distance from pixel (x,y) to electrode n

Figure 3 shows the scalp distribution of sensory and motor maps for the left hand and leg in the same normal volunteer depicted in Figures 1 and 2. Note that the hand motor map localized maximally slightly anterior to the sensory map (as defined by the N20 component of left median nerve SEP). Motor and sensory representations for the hand are in the convexity, relatively close to both recording and stimulating scalp electrodes. The situation is different for the leg. The leg motor map localized very close to the sensory map in the midline. The reason for the apparent superimposition of leg sensory and motor maps lies perhaps in the deep localization of the leg representation areas in the interhemispheric sulcus.

The technique described allows noninvasive mapping of different representation areas in human motor cortex and its comparison with sensory cortex. This study can be completed in relatively short sessions with only moderate discomfort for the patient.

References

Berardelli A, Inghilleri M, Manfredi, M, Zamponi A, Cecconi V, Dolce G (1987) Cortical and cervical stimulation after hemispheric infarction. *J neurol Neurosurg Psychiat, 50,* 861–865.

Cohen LG, Hallett M (submitted) Methodology for non-invasive mapping of human motor cortex with electrical stimulation. *Electroenceph clin Neurophysiol.*

Cohen LG, Hallett M (submitted) Noninvasive mapping of human motor cortex. *Neurology.*

Cohen LG, Hallett M, Johnson L (1987a) Methodological considerations for mapping of human motor cortex. *Electroenceph clin Neurophysiol, 66,* 72.

Cohen LG, Hallett M, Johnson L (1987b) Noninvasive mapping of human motor cortex. *Neurology 37* (Suppl. 1), 219 ff.

Cowan JMA, Dick JPR, Day BL et al. (1984) Abnormalities in central motor pathway conduction in multiple sclerosis. *Lancet, 2,* 304–307.

Levy W (1987) Clinical experience with motor and cerebellar evoked potentials monitoring. *Neurosurgery, 20,* 169–182.

Merton PA, Morton HB (1980): Stimulation of the cerebral cortex in the intact human subject. *Nature* (London), 285, 227.

Mills KR, Murray NMF (1985) Corticospinal tract conduction time in multiple sclerosis. *Ann Neurol, 18,* 601–605.

Rossini PM, Marciani MG, Caramia M, Roma V, Zarola F (1985) Nervous propagation along "central" motor pathways in intact man: Characteristics of motor responses to bifocal and unifocal spine and scalp non-invasive stimulation. *Electroenceph clin Neurophysiol, 61,* 272–286.

Section III

Brain Electrical Activity Mapping

Issues Facing the Clinical Use
of Brain Electrical Activity Mapping

F. H. Duffy

There has been a recent resurgence of interest in the use of topographic mapping for both research and clinical applications. This has been coupled with an ever increasing availability of commercial instruments capable of mapping. These events require a careful look at principals underlying the mapping methodology. There is general agreement that maps may provide useful spectral-spatial summation of EEG and spatial-temporal summation of EP data. However, details of the methodology remain more controversial. Should color be used or is it inherently deceptive? How important is the interpolation algorithm? How many electrodes should be used and to what should they be referenced? Should one approach the detection of abnormality through statistics and, if so, by what specific means? How can one avoid "capitalization on chance" given the many unique univariate significance tests that are often performed? If control groups are needed how should the subjects be selected? Is there a danger in the creation of "super controls"? It is unlikely that all these issues can be easily resolved by a review of work done to date. Considerable new research may be required to reach solutions for these important problems. These and other issues are discussed.

The mapping of brain electrical activity, also referred to by such other names as EEG topography, electrocartography, and BEAM, has seen increasing application in the practice of clinical neurophysiology. Over the past five years many manufacturers have commenced production of topographic mapping units, providing neurophysiologists not only research, but also clinical capabilities. Twelve major and several minor firms now produce such equipment, with costs that range from a few thousand to over $300,000. Functional levels of these units range from the simple PC-based units, capable of making colored images of data imported via floppy disk, to complete laboratory systems. The latter may incorporate any or all of the following: polygraph and stimulators, minicomputer with megabyte memory and hard disk, normative data base, and discriminant (diagnostic) functions.

Penetrance of mapping into clinical neurophysiology has met with a wide spectrum of interest ranging from immediate uncritical acceptance to instant rejection with all in-between viewpoints represented. If all manufacturers are included, we estimate 350 units now in place in the USA performing clinical studies, with one or more neurophysiologists at each site. Unfortunately, some few manufacturers eager to capitalize on new markets, have produced equipment capable of little more than making colored images, to meet the demand of some few clinicians whose only desire appears to be the use of colored images to attract new business and augment income. This unfortunate development has produced a negative reaction, "confirming" the suspicions of those already negatively disposed to clinical mapping.

There is intense interest in brain electrical activity mapping, spawning a series of seminars on the topic at national meetings. Basic and important issues have arisen out of these seminars. In this brief chapter I shall attempt to enumerate the salient issues and formulate

Harvard Medical School, Developmental Neurophysiology, The Children's Hospital, 300 Longwood Avenue, Boston, MA 02115, USA.

constructive responses based upon our five years' experience in clinical mapping at Boston Children's Hospital, with over 1500 topographic mapping or BEAM studies to date.

Questions and Answers

What Role Does Mapping Play in Neurophysiology?

The demonstration of the spike and wave by Gibbs et al. (1935) established a major role for EEG in the diagnosis and management of epilepsy. Over the ensuing years EEG has continued to fulfill its promise vis-à-vis epilepsy and certain other clinical conditions, but has failed to become a universal tool for neuroscientific investigation. Most normal and many abnormal brain states fail to produce an EEG signature as characteristic and/or as distinct as the discharge of epilepsy. When characteristic discontinuities are not seen in an EEG, the next traditional step is to analyze the remaining background activity. This process involves an estimation of frequency content (e.g., delta, theta, alpha and beta), its consistency or lack of consistency over time, its spatial extent, and its deviation from "normality." Success in the extraction of information from EEG background has been limited by difficulties inherent in the performance of such spectral, temporal, spatial and statistical analyses by simple, unaided visual inspection. Thus while many clinical conditions may affect EEG background, subtle changes can be difficult for the neurophysiologist to "see."

During the past 10 years, techniques of quantified EEG (QEEG) have been developed, allowing these four analytic modes to be performed by computer, thereby relieving the neurophysiologist of these burdensome tasks. Computerized spectral analysis has been available for some time (Cooley & Tukey, 1965) and has been extensively used for EEG analyses. This technique not only summarizes frequency content, but may be applied to EEG epochs of differing lengths, thereby summarizing spectral content over time (Bickford et al., 1973). To facilitate analysis, relatively long EEG segments are usually broken down into shorter segments ranging from one to ten seconds. Results of spectral analyses on these subsegments are then typically averaged to represent the mean EEG spectral content. The standard deviation (sd) of each spectral band can also be derived. In addition, the coefficient of variation (standard deviation divided by the mean) constitutes a useful parameter of spectral variability that can readily be calculated via computer. It can be thought of as a measure of paroxysmal activity within a spectral band (Duffy, 1986) and a measure of spectral consistency over time. Results of the above analyses can be spatially mapped and conveniently displayed on color graphics terminals (Duffy et al., 1979; Duffy, 1986). Finally, comparisons can be made to an age appropriate normative data base, results re-expressed in units of standard deviation, and resulting Z scores reimaged as Significance Probability Maps (SPM) (Duffy et al., 1981) which are maps of regional deviation from normal. Thus computer techniques have been developed which perform all four analytic functions in analyzing EEG data, and in so doing, relieve the neuropsychologist of the difficult burden of analysis via visual inspection of EEG tracings.

For long latency evoked potential (EP) data it is sometimes difficult to define components across subjects, a limitation which has served to restrict clinical utility. Jeffreys and Axford (1972) were the first to suggest that in defining a component one must take into account not only amplitude and latency, but also spatial extent. With this in mind, it seems the next step is to create a series of maps from sets of multichannel EP data so as to define spatio-temporal relationships more carefully by viewing the resulting cartooned images (Duffy, 1982; Duffy et al., 1979). The SPM process can then be applied to EP, as described above for EEG data.

The justification for mapping comes from the hypotheses that the factor limiting maximal extraction of information from EEG and EP data is the inherently limited nature of the human visual system. EEG and EP data contain not too *little* information about brain function, rather they contain too *much* to be easily assessed by unaided visual inspection. Mapping—and the quantified techniques that underly its utility such as spectral analysis, SPM, and cartooning—augment the very analytic processes where visual inspection is weakest.

Are Color Maps Inherently Deceptive?

Just as the proper use of color scaling can be used to enhance the visibility of data in topographic maps, its improper use can create false and misleading impressions. The proper choice of color scale should provide an immediate sense of gradient, i.e., which direction of color change represents "more" and which "less." Typically a rainbow scale is used for maps of spectral-analyzed EEG, with the blue to black color group representing the lowest values and the red to white end of the spectrum highest values. Some personal computer (PC)-based color displays lack a sufficient number of color steps to achieve the desired number of scaling steps. As a solution some manufacturers have repeated colors with a slightly different saturation or with a superimposed pattern. By such techniques, greater resolution is achieved but at the sacrifice of a sense of gradient. Resulting maps may appear quite confusing.

For EP data, zero microvolt readings should be encoded black, with red representing positive readings and blue negative. Changes of hue and saturation within red and blue may then provide incremental steps. Blue-white and red-white represent maximal values of negative and positive activities, respectively. Inversions with negative red and positive blue may be used in some laboratories that display EP waveforms where negative is upgoing. This convention can prevent confusion if used consistently. Occasionally white is used to represent 0 μV and black maximal value. Once again, if consistent, this use is acceptable. However, the use of rainbow scaling for EP data by some systems creates confusing imaging. The color value representing zero may not stand out, the gradient is unidirectional (least to most) rather than bidirectional (zero to plus maximum and zero to minus maximum), and the distribution between negative and positive data is not visually distinct and meaningful.

The color sequence should be so chosen that sequential contour line crossings are associated with the appearance of equally distinct color steps. The use of color scales where certain steps are dramatic (i.e., yellow to red) but comparable steps of equal magnitude are much less distinct (i.e., blue to green-blue) may deceptively highlight certain spatial regions, such as those in bright red. Once again this color convention problem is most often encountered in simple systems where graphics capabilities limit the number of possible colors. The intentional use of an abrupt color transition to signal the passage of an important threshold (e.g., Z or t reaching statistically significant levels) is, of course, appropriate.

Color scales are not inherently deceptive; however, improper usage can lead to confusion and false conclusions. To suggest that color should not be employed for mapping because it can be abused would be much like saying that one ought not have children because they can be abused. In our opinion, color adds much to a topographic image, much as it does to ordinary vision. The point is to use color judiciously.

Does the Large Amount of Data Analyzed in Clinical Studies Lead To False Findings by Capitalization on Chance?

In our laboratory, clinical studies utilize spectral analyses of EEG data in the "eyes-open" and "eyes-closed" state, and EP data based on separate flash and click stimulation. These result in approximately 680 observations. The spectrally analyzed EEG data from 20 channels, in two states, and over six spectral bands produce 240 variables ($20 \times 2 \times 6$). The EP data from 20 channels, for two modalities, and over eleven 40 ms latency ranges produce 440 variables ($20 \times 2 \times 11$). For the resulting 680 total variables, it is virtually certain that at least one variable will appear significant by chance alone (Maus & Endresen, 1979). At the 0.05 probability level, 19 to 35, and, at the 0.01 level, 2 to 10 variables are expected to reach significance by chance alone. Critics of topographic mapping may ask how one is to discriminate "real" results from "chance" results.

However, this data-related problem is not limited to topographic mapping. If we apply the same research approach to classic electroencephalography, similar difficulties also result. Given a 20-minute 16-channel recording and the assumption that an EEG reader can estimate spectral content in four spectral bands every four seconds, then 19,200 variables are produced ($[20 \times 60]/4 \times 16 \times 4$). Since EEG is of clearly established clinical value, this statistical quandary must be manageable in some way.

In a concise review of such issues, Maus and Endreson (1979) suggest either limiting the number of variables used and/or adjusting significance levels upward as a function of the number of variables. Unfortunately, reduction of variable number presupposes advance knowledge of those variables which could be omitted. This constitutes an unattractive option, since useful variables might be inadvertently discarded. Raising the significance level could prove equally restrictive. Based upon the binomial theorem for a 10% level of significance for all tests combined and for 680 variables, one would have to demand a significance level of .00016 for each variable: $p = 1. - (0.9)^{**}(1/680)$. At the $p < 0.00016$ level, few variables would be likely to attain statistical significance. Should one wish to retain the individual criterion level at $p < 0.05$, then one would have to limit oneself to two variables at most. On the surface, it would seem to be an unsolvable problem.

Again, such issues are not limited to the analyses of topographic maps. Indeed the interaction between number of variables and significance levels is a classic statistical problem of importance to all comparisons involving multiple observations. It is generally agreed that it is difficult, if not impossible, to distinguish "chance" from "real" findings unless the variable number is small and the significance level high. A solution to this apparent enigma is derived from the observation that the hallmark of *chance* findings is their randomness and that of *real* results is their reproducibility. Accordingly, a repeated study should yield the same results as a first study if the results are real and differing results if they are due to random chance. Clearly this is what an electroencephalogra-

pher does when he reads an EEG. Every few pages, he forms an "opinion" and matches it against what he finds in the next few pages. Eventually, changes that occur by random chance stand out against patterns that remain constant and are presumed to be real. This same technique applies to the use of SPM in clinical mapping studies. One searches for spatial patterns that are constant across states, for involvement of more than one electrode, and for high levels of statistical significance. Conversely, scattered spatial patterns of low significance involving only a single electrode are to be ignored. If the reader is in doubt, testing on a given state or all states should be repeated. These overall statistical issues are part of a branch of statistics known as Exploratory Data Analyses, or EDA. In his excellent text, Tukey advises on the use of separate exploratory (first step) analyses to develop hypotheses and confirmatory (second step) analyses to test these hypotheses (Tukey, 1977). It is a demanding task to repeat analyses, but this is the only way to be sure. Figure 1 illustrates the value of repetitive study.

It is true that the large number of variables in a mapping study may yield falsely "significant" findings; however, only by recognizing those that are constant across states and that stand up under repeated study can the real be separated from the spurious.

Is the Construction of a Normative Data Base Composed of Optimally Healthy Subjects (Super Normals) Inappropriate? Can This Lead to False Detection of Abnormality?

Experience indicates that a reliable normative data base is critical for clinical mapping studies. For example, while asymmetry of data constitutes abnormality in most neurophysiological studies, no normal subject has absolutely symmetrical data. The only way to tell whether an apparent asymmetry in a map excedes the normal bounds of variation is to maintain a normative data base for comparative purposes. Accordingly, the manner in which control groups are selected and analyzed becomes an important issue.

Recruitment is a pivotal issue. Ideally, one should follow procedures employed for the

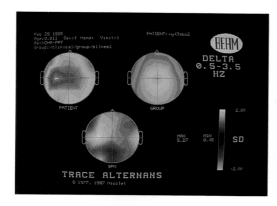

TRACE ALTERNANS

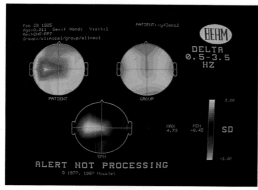

ALERT NOT PROCESSING

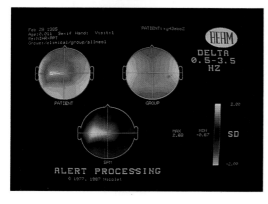

ALERT PROCESSING

Figure 1. This figure shows nine BEAM images in three groups of three from one patient. Each image shows the head in vertex perspective, equal area projection. The nose is above, right ear to the right, left ear to the left, and occiput below. For each group of three the patient data are shown to the upper left, normative control data to the upper right, and SPM below. All images reflect spectral-analyzed EEG data in the delta range. Plots of subject- and mean-group spectral energy are shown from each group of three in the same scale (rainbow: minimum dark color, maximum red-white). The SPM are shown below in bipolar color scale with red representing regions where the EEG data of the patient exceed the group mean data, and blue signifying regions where they are below mean. A vertical scaling bar is shown to the right for the SPM data only. Between the scale bar and the SPM the maximum positive and maximum negative deviations from normal are shown.

The patient is a premature neonate, studied at 42 weeks post conception, who had been born at 30 weeks gestation. He suffered a grade II intraventricular hemorrhage affecting the left hemisphere. A BEAM study was performed to search for evidence of electrophysiological abnormality as his classic neurological examination was surprisingly normal. The study was conducted in three segments, with the baby brought to full alertness "alert processing (AP)," allowed to become slightly drowsy "alert not processing (ANP)," and in quiet sleep "trace alternans (TA)." Note the consistent augmentation of delta centered about the left central electrode (C3) for all three states, reaching 2.68 sd for AP, 4.73 sd for ANP, and 5.27 sd for TA.

Note the virtually identical change seen in all three states. The key to detection of clinically important abnormalities is the finding of repetitive deviations from normal in the same location. Spurious or chance deviations from normal would not be expected to show the spatial consistency produced by real brain abnormalities. It is of particular interest that the classic EEG was interpreted as normal in waking and probably normal in sleep by a trained neurophysiologist.

determination of characteristics of large populations. For example, in the USA it is usual to forecast election results by programmed voter sampling such that accuracy within a few percent error can be obtained from samples as low as several thousand. This requires a specific pre-planned sampling schedule and acquiescence on the part of all polled. Unfortunately, this approach is impractical for the

collection of electrophysiologic data. Not only would the collection of such large amounts of data require several years, by no means would everyone recruited respond positively when asked to spend a half a day away from their normal daily responsibilities to have paste smeared in their hair and to endure a series of benign but boring procedures for a minimal reimbursement. It would be hard to imagine many successful businessmen agreeing to take time away from work for such a study. On the other hand, it is not hard to imagine someone who is out of work due to drug, emotional, alcohol, or intellectual problems readily agreeing to be studied. Often, such individuals have concerns about the state of their brain, find the study a welcome change in their otherwise boring routines, and value the small financial reimbursement. By such unintentional mechanisms, the recruited population could become skewed away from a truly representative or "normal" sample. One might attempt to avoid this bias by selecting from among resulting data that which "looks normal," as some investigators have done. However, this only results in the immortalization of someone's preconceived notion of normality. Such selection procedures result in data with very small variance, with resulting control groups that become too "sensitive." When compared to such groups many truly normal subjects show electrophysiological "abnormalities." Screening neurophysiologic data is no substitute for screening subjects prior to gathering data. The goal should be to accept all data that comes from subjects considered "normal" by other criteria. Data should be screened only to ensure technical quality. Resulting control groups then reflect the variance that really exists within such a "normal" population. In our experience there are a surprising number of truly normal subjects with technically perfect data who demonstrate unusual asymmetries. It is important to include these subjects.

For the reasons given above we have turned away from the "large random sample approach" toward a more practical one. Rather than attempt to establish a "representative" subsample of the entire population, we have instead turned to a "benchmark approach" based upon medical health. Subjects are recruited from as wide a population base as practical and then carefully screened for "health." Our experience has been that the tighter one's exclusionary criteria, the more stable the population. The goal is to choose subjects to be as "healthy as we ourselves would like to be." All subjects receive medical, neurological, psychiatric, and psychological screening examinations. Their body chemistries (liver, renal, hepatic) and blood pressure are carefully evaluated. Subjects with abnormalities on examination, with history of disease affecting the CNS (hypertension, epilepsy, head injury, alcoholism, etc.), or who are taking medications are eliminated. For those who pass these stringent criteria, final say is given to the EEG technologist at the time of electrophysiological examination. Subjects have been known to confide to the technologist how they "fooled the doctors" and concealed crucial historical details.

As expected, the ratio of subjects accepted to those recruited declines as one recruits control subjects from those in their elder years, reflecting the higher ambient disease level in those groups. Thus, there are far fewer subjects in their 70s and 80s who fulfill our criteria than subjects in their 20s and 30s. Such a population of "optimally healthy" subjects has been termed "super controls." It is certainly true that optimally healthy 70-year-old subjects are not representative of the "national norm." However, such a healthy population establishes a reliable age group benchmark against which comparisons can be made.

It has been suggested that such criteria are too strict and should be "loosened." A problem with relaxation of exclusionary criteria is that what gets "loosened" could be a function of the characteristics of the local population source. One center may wish to include patients with asymptomatic hypertension; another, past history of alcoholism; another, depression; etc. Not only would such loosening increase the group standard deviation (or covariance) and thereby reduce sensitivity, but resulting groups would not be comparable among centers and would be difficult to reproduce elsewhere.

Clinical experience shows that if one forms a normative data base of "optimally healthy" subjects where only technically flawed data are excluded and all other data, despite the appearance of unusual features, are included, few, if any, false positives are obtained when normal subjects are compared to this data base. In our laboratory, we originally screened and analyzed a normative group (n = 45) for the age-group decade 40 to 49 years. Subsequently, we compared 27 newly studied normal subjects from the same age group, and no clinical abnormalities at all were demonstrated (manuscript in preparation).

Although not ideal, basing control group formation on "optimal health" results in a reproducible benchmark measure that has demonstrated its usefulness here and at other centers.

How Many Electrodes Are Necessary for Mapping?

Typically overlooked when considering this frequently asked question is the necessary qualifying phrase "for what purpose?" That is, what is the objective or condition being tested for in a given situation? For example, generalized encephalopathies ordinarily produce diffuse EEG slowing. Accordingly, one should be able to follow the course of a patient with a metabolic encephalopathy with from one to four electrodes. In contrast, if one undertakes the more refined task of topographically discriminating by EPs between stimulation of adjacent digits on the hand, then a much denser electrode array of 81 electrodes overlying one somatomotor area is required (Duff, 1980). Much more theoretical and practical work needs to be done in this area. For some time we have based our mapping on the standard 10—20 electrode placement (Jasper, 1958) augmented by additional artifact monitoring placements. In our experience, the transition from 16 to 20 scalp electrodes provided more definition for our clinical studies. We have tried, but are not yet convinced that an increase from 20 to 28 or more scalp electrodes is desirable for routine clinical screening of adults.

Theoretically, the number of scalp electrodes should be based upon a three dimensional extension of the better known Nyquist sampling theorem which tells us how rapidly we should sample single channel EEG data. The problem with this approach lies in the establishment of a basic map of spatially varying brain signal information density. As previously mentioned, such requirements will vary from one pathology to another, and can be expected to show differences among scalp regions, between differing states of alertness, and between EEG and EP data. One approach is simply to use lots of electrodes. Unfortunately, the time and discomfort involved in accurate electrode placement, the cost of the many amplifiers and display devices needed to monitor amplifier output, and the large amounts of memory and disk space that would be required place practical constraints on this notion.

Surprisingly, there has been little emphasis in the topographic research literature on the number and placement of *artifact* electrodes. In our opinion, this is a crucial issue to aid in the detection and elimination, or reduction, of eye and muscle activity contamination. The issue deserves as much or more consideration than the question of the number of scalp electrodes.

Until more theoretical and practical information becomes available, we recommend a minimum of 19 scalp electrodes placed in the 10—20 format and at least four additional artifact electrodes placed so as to monitor vertical eye movement, horizontal eye movement, and muscle activity in the temporal and occipital regions.

How Does One Ensure Trustworthy Discrimination Between Real and Artifactual Data in Topographic Images?

In our experience, the most common errors in the clinical interpretation of topographic mapping studies stem from mis-reading of artifact. Just as mapping makes the underlying spatial structure of neurophysiologic data more visible, so it enhances the visibility of artifact. Just as SPM images highlight brain-generated deviations from normal, so they delineate artifact. Indeed, artifact may produce some of the largest Z values. Accordingly, reduction of artifact assumes great importance in mapping studies. Each electrode must be properly positioned by measurement-spot placement. Further, the uncritical use of electrode caps leads to inaccuracy. All electrodes must have comparable low impedance and remain securely attached and free of motion effects; collodion application is recommended. Muscle activity should be reduced by proper patient positioning and the calming effect of a competent technologist. Eye movement and eye blink are to be reduced by the use of fixation targets accompanied by relaxation periods (blink hol-idays) in the "eyes-open" states and by light gauze pads placed on the eye lids during "eyes-closed" states. Ironically it is often harder to control eye movement in "eyes-closed" than in "eyes-open" states. Control of a patient's state of alertness is a crucial responsibility of the technologist. To accom-plish this he/she should monitor the EEG carefully, relying upon EEG signs of drowsi-ness (Santamaria & Chiappa, 1987), frequent patient interrogation, occasional breaks with walks and, as a last resort, allowing the sub-ject a cup of coffee or tea. Patients who seem exceptionally fatigued should be allowed to sleep for periods of up to 30 minutes. Ulti-mately, alertness must be maintained during EP as well as EEG states.

The use of appropriately placed artifact electrodes greatly facilitates recognition of artifact as it occurs, allowing the technologist to implement the appropriate strategy for its reduction. Moreover, inspection and/or auto-matic analyses of data from these channels permits segments containing residual artifact to be omitted from subsequent spectral ana-lyses or signal averaging.

Laboratory experience has nonetheless demonstrated that despite our best efforts, artifact has a way of persisting. Fortunately, there are two key advantages of topographic mapping in the recognition of artifact. The *FIRST* are the characteristic spatial signatures that most artifacts produce. For example, eye blink-induced delta and time locked eye blink during the flash and VER produce crescentic abnormality in the prefrontal region. Tem-poral muscle beta artifact produces abnormal-ity in the characteristic distribution of that muscle. Electrode artifact demonstrates abnormalities graphically limited to one elec-trode position. Horizontal eye movement pro-duces abnormalities maximal simultaneously in both anterior temporal regions. The *SEC-OND* involves the valuable contribution arti-fact electrodes make to the SPM process. Data from these electrodes are subjected to the same statistical comparisons (t or Z) as scalp derived data. Comparisons between the degree of statistical abnormality in scalp regions and in adjacent artifact electrodes are most useful in discriminating artifact contami-

nation. For example, if abnormal levels of frontal delta are found in an SPM, one must decide whether this is attributable to eye movement artifact or to brain activity. If due to vertical eye movement, there should be equal or greater abnormality in electrodes spe-cifically placed so as to be maximally sensitive to such movement. If, however, the delta is due to brain activity much lesser abnormality should be found in the eye movement chan-nels.

Experience has shown that topgraphic maps highlight the spatial structure of under-lying data, making both real and artifactual deviations from normal more visible. Fortu-nately, the spatial and spectral signature ʻof artifact is usually distinct and, in concert with artifact channel data analyses, permits recog-nition by the trained neuroscientist. It should be remembered that all artifacts affecting maps derive from artifact in the underlying EEG or EP derived data. The act of mapping, if properly done, does not create artifact. Nonetheless, the increased visibility of artifact in maps demand more stringent procedures to recognize and reduce artifact than ordinarily used for classic EEG and EP recordings. Only by such measures is the full potential of map-ping realized.

What Reference Electrodes Should Be Used For Mapping?

As is true for EEG and EP data, there is no ideal and no universally accepted electrode reference location for topographic mapping studies. Every known anatomical location (e. g., ears, mastoid, face, chin, chest) has dem-onstrated advantages and disadvantages. Indeed, the question of the ideal reference electrode has been a longstanding issue in electroencephalography. Most mapping labo-ratories employ linked ear or linked mastoid placement. By referencing one common point, it is possible to recalculate bipolar linkages by suitable subtraction of recorded data. Another common approach is to record other reference sites to linked ears. By this means, if the linked ear reference should prove active (e. g., midtemporal slowing) then a new reference can be recalculated offline. Nunez (1981) has argued theoretically that linked ears may distort the scalp field by passing current from one hemisphere to another. Our investigations have not found this to be a problem (unpublished data).

Two techniques which have been used in mapping have recently gained increased attention. The first is the "common average" reference (Lehmann, 1986; Offner, 1950). Its biggest disadvantage is seen in the testing of clinical patients with focal pathology. Electrode values from the abnormal region will influence values from uninvolved regions yielding unreliable results. The second technique is the "source derivation" or Laplacian method, where data are replaced by their second spatial derivative (Hjorth, 1975, 1986). This truly reference-free approach has the advantage of visualizing current sources and sinks. In certain circumstances, this approach may provide important new information as to source localization, especially in the auditory brainwaves of the newborn infant (Vaughn, work in progress). However, the process of mathematical differentiation inherently increases noise as well as signal. In our limited experience with the Laplacian, we have found it produces more complex, more confusing, and less intuitive images than produced by mapping unprocessed data. Nonetheless, the average reference and the Laplacian methods of reference are valid and important additions to mapping and should be available on all systems. Only experience will clarify their value relative to more conventional reference electrode placements. Until this is established, most mapping systems used for clinical work should allow many or all of these reference options.

How Does One Deal with the Fact that Electrophysiological Data from a Single Subject Is Unstable over Time?

It is certainly a valid observation that electrophysiological data from a given subject can change randomly over time. One cannot expect data from a single subject to remain absolutely stable over time, even when care is taken to ensure comparable recording conditions. But that is not, in itself, the real issue. The real question is whether change due to an evolving pathology exceeds the change due to such random variation. Experience demonstrates that in most circumstances pathological change outpaces random change. For example, as shown in Figure 2, spectral delta from one subject recorded from two studies four months apart shows significant change by t-test SPM only over the left temporal lobe produced by a slow growing tumor.

Random differences among normal subjects and random change with repeated measures are major factors influencing the statisti-

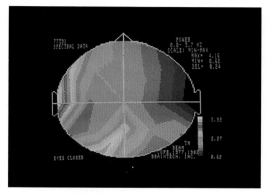

Figure 2. This figure shows a t-statistic SPM comparing the EEG delta activity recorded from one subject on two separate occasions, four months apart. An older display convention is shown, with t data displayed in rainbow color scale. The color key is to the right with white representing a t of 3.92 or above. At each study point, at least three minutes of artifact-free data were collected. Average spectra were formed by summation of individual spectra, each derived from two-second EEG epochs. At each electrode, both mean and standard deviations were calculated, allowing calculation of the t statistic for that electrode.

The patient was a young adolescent who presented with migraine headaches, but a normal neurological examination. A CT scan, however, demonstrated an apparent tumor in the left posterior temporal-parietal region. The patient remained stable for a year with no change in the CT scan, a normal examination, and resolution of headaches on a mild medication. The neurosurgeon declined to operate in the absence of evidence of progression.

As can be seen in the t-SPM, there was significant change in delta over the left temporal region ($-t = 4.16$ max) but not elsewhere. On the basis of this demonstrated change a surgical procedure was performed, revealing an oligondendroglioma. The topographic mapping results were instrumental in establishing the progressive nature of the lesion, thereby confirming the suspicion of tumor which lead to a timely medical response.

cal variance of any electrophysiological measure. In a sense these factors place a limit on the threshold for detection of abnormality. Fortunately most pathologies of interest and concern appear to excede these thresholds and thus facilitate detection.

What is the Role of Mapping in the Formation of a Clinical Diagnosis? What Is the Role of Group Comparison Studies?

The relationship between a study showing significant difference between two populations and the ability to correctly classify individual members of the groups is quite complex (Bartels & Bartels, 1986). Group difference concentrates on the separation between the multivariate means (centroids) of the two groups. Subject classification, however, depends upon the actual distribution of subjects in the two groups, especially the presence or absence of population overlap. Although centroid separation and population overlap are clearly related, it is possible with real data to have a significant group centroid difference, but with non-trivial population overlap. Thus the fact that electrophysiological difference can be reliably demonstrated between two populations does not necessarily mean that this information can be used for diagnostic purposes.

The issue is even more complex. Even if one can establish a statistical function accurately discriminating individual patients with disease X from normal subjects, one is not assured of how that function would classify patients with other illness (Y and Z). These are issues of sensitivity (ability to discriminate disease X from normality) and specificity (ability to separate disease X from Y from Z) (Ransohoff & Feinstein, 1978). It is not enough for a diagnostic classifier to demonstrate sensitivity; the specificity issue must be dealt with.

Among our research publications are papers showing topographic difference between normals and patients with dyslexia (Duffy et al., 1980; Duffy & McAnulty, 1985), schizophrenia (Morihisa et al., 1983; Morstyn et al., 1983a, 1983b), Alzheimer's disease (Duffy et al., 1984), and poorer functioning premature newborn infants (Duffy & Als, 1983). These studies were intended to advance our understanding of the basic neurophysiology of these important clinical problems. They were not, however, intended to establish "diagnostic" criteria and were not intended to demonstrate that one can diagnose these conditions on the basis of neurophysiologic data alone. Although our findings may speak for the sensitivity of neurophysiologic data in recognizing these disease entities, they were not designed to say anything about diagnostic specificity. To develop useful discriminant functions to diagnose dyslexia, for example, one would also need to develop separate classifiers of children with all other forms of learning disability, alone and in combination. Such an effort would require many person-years of work at very high costs. Moreover, even if successful, it would not be obvious that neurophysiologic classifiers would be any better than more common neuropsychologically based classifiers. Accordingly, our research efforts have been more organized to provide basic information about disease processes than to provide information of immediate value to the process of automated classification.

If, then, clinical mapping studies are not intended to be "diagnostic," of what clinical value are they? It is our opinion that the goal is not to diagnose patients solely on the basis of topographic data, but to provide important pieces of information useful in establishing a diagnosis. It is commonly taught that one does not diagnose epilepsy by the EEG but by the entire clinical picture of which EEG-derived data play an important part. In this same spirit we feel that mapping data are not necessarily diagnostic but may be diagnostically useful.

Will Mapping Studies Replace EEG?

Visual inspection of traditional polygraphic tracings stands as the primary method for the accurate detection and classification of the epileptic discharge. Even the better quantified methods of spike detection use visual confirmation as the ultimate benchmark (Gotman & Gloor, 1976). Moreover, there are other facets of the EEG which remain best appreciated by eye and are poorly recognized by techniques of quantified EEG. From this perspective it would be a great waste should EEG data gathered during a mapping study not be clinically evaluated by a skilled electroencephalographer.

EEG tracings serve another crucial function during mapping. They provide continuous, online indications of level of consciousness, attention, and degree of artifact. Any neurophysiologist reading topographic maps in a clinical setting must have first read the accompanying EEG, if only to ensure that he/she does not interpret artifact as real data.

For these two important reasons, EEG must remain a part of all mapping studies. Far from replacing electroencephalography, mapping will enlarge the field, increasing its complexity and placing new demands upon clinician training. Electroencephalographers have spent years extracting information in the time domain. Now tools are available to examine data in space as well.

Final Comments

The field of clinical mapping of neurophysiologic data is now in its formative stages. As discussed above, many issues and many unanswered questions remain. Despite these uncertainties, we have found topographic maps to greatly enhance the clinical value of scalp recorded data. To quote a pioneer in the field of exploratory data analyses: "The greatest value of a picture is when it forces us to notice what we never expected to see" (Tukey, 1977).

References

Bartels PH, Bartels HG (1986) Classification strategies for topographic mapping data. In Duffy FH (Ed.) *Topographic mapping of brain electrical activity.* Butterworths, Boston, 225-253.

Bickford RG, Brimmer J, Berger L (1973). *Application of a compressed spectral array in clinical EEG.* Raven Press, New York.

Cooley JW, Tukey JW (1965) An algorithm for the machine calculation of Fourier series. *Math Comput, 19,* 297-301.

Duff TA (1980) Topography of scalp recorded potentials by stimulation of the digits. *Electroenceph clin Neurophysiol, 49,* 452-460.

Duffy FH (1982) Topographic display of evoked potentials: Clinical applications of brain electrical activity mapping (BEAM). *Ann NY Acad Sci, 388,* 183-196.

Duffy FH (1986) *Topographic mapping of brain electrical activity.* Butterworths, Boston.

Duffy FH, Als H (1983) Neurophysiological assessment of the neonate: An approach combining brain electrical activity mapping (BEAM) with behavioral assessment (APIB). In Brazelton, TB, Lester BM (Eds.) *New approaches to developemental screening of infants.* Elsevier, New York, 175-196.

Duffy FH, McAnulty G (1985) Brain electrical activity mapping (BEAM): Search for a physiological signature of dyslexia. In Duffy FH, Geschwind N (Eds.) *Dyslexia: A neuroscientific approach to clinical evaluation.* Little, Brown and Co., Boston, 105-122.

Duffy FH, Burchfiel JL, Lombroso CT (1979). Brain electrical activity mapping (BEAM): A method for extending the clinical utility of EEG and evoked potential data. *Ann Neurol, 5,* 309-321.

Duffy FH, Denckla MB, Bartels P, Sandini G (1980) Dyslexia: Regional differences in brain electrical activity by topographic mapping. *Ann Neurol, 7,* 412-420.

Duffy FH, Bartels PH, Burchfiel JL (1981) Significance probability mapping: An aid in the topographic analysis of brain electrical activity. *Electroenceph clin Neurophysiol, 51,* 455-462.

Duffy FH, Albert MS, McAnulty G (1984) Brain electrical activity in patients with presenile and senile dementia of the Alzheimer's type. *Ann Neurol, 16,* 439-448.

Gibbs FA, Davis H, Lennox WG (1935) The electroencephalogram in epilepsy and in conditions of impaired consciousness. *Arch Neurol Psychiatry, 34,* 1133-1135.

Gotman J, Gloor P (1976) Automatic recognition and quantification of interictal epileptic activity in the human scalp. *Electroenceph clin Neurophysiol, 41,* 513-529.

Hjorth B (1975) An on-line transformation of scalp potentials into orthogonal source derivations. *Electroenceph clin Neurophysiol, 39,* 526-530.

Hjorth B (1986) Physical aspects of EEG data as a basis for topographic mapping. In Duffy FH (Ed.) *Topographic mapping of brain eletrical activity.* Butterworths, Boston, 175-193.

Jasper (1958) The ten-twenty system of the International Federation. *Electroenceph clin Neurophysiol, 10,* 371-375.

Jeffreys DA, Axford JG (1972) Source locations of pattern-specific components of human visual evoked potentials. *Exp Brain Res, 16,* 1-40.

Lehmann D (1986) Spatial analysis of EEG and Evoked Potential data. In Duffy FH (Ed.) *Topographic mapping of brain electrical activity.* Butterworths, Boston, 29-61.

Maus A, Endresen J (1979) Misuse of computer-generated results. *Med Biol Eng Comput, 17,* 126–129.

Morihisa JM, Duffy FH, Wyatt RJ (1983) Brain electrical activity mapping (BEAM) in schizophrenic patients. *Arch Gen Psych, 40,* 719–728.

Morstyn R, Duffy FH, McCarley RW (1983a) Altered P300 topography in schizophrenia. *Arch Gen Psych, 40,* 729–734.

Morstyn R, Duffy FH, McCarley RW (1983b) Altered topography of EEG spectral content in schizophrenia. *Electroenceph clin Neurophysiol, 65,* 263–271.

Nunez PL (1981) *Electric fields of the brain.* Oxford University Press, New York.

Offner FF (1950) The EEG as potential mapping: The value of the average monopolar reference. *Electroenceph clin Neurophysiol, 2,* 215–216.

Ransohoff DF, Feinstein AR (1978) Problems of spectrum and bias in evaluating the efficacy of diagnostic tests. *N.E.J.M., 299,* 926–930.

Santamaria J, Chiappa K (1987) The EEG of Drowsiness in Normal Adults. *Journal of Clinical Neurophysiology, 4,* 327–382.

Tukey JW (1977) *Exploratory data analysis.* Addison-Wesley, Reading, MA.

Sex Differences in the Ongoing EEG: Probability Mapping at Rest and during Cognitive Tasks

H. Petsche, P. Rappelsberger, H. Pockberger

The study was performed on 33 male and 35 female right-handed students.

Data acquisition: common reference recordings from 19 electrodes (10-20 system) vs. connected ear lobes; EEG recording before, during and after 1 min silent reading and mental arithmetic, respectively; computation of averaged power and cross power spectra—between adjacent electrodes and between electrodes in homologous places of both hemispheres; extraction of broad-band parameters for power and coherence for 5 frequency bands between 4 and 32 Hz.

For the statistical evaluation of differences between males and females in the chosen parameters the Fisher permutation test was used to obtain error probabilities for the rejection of the null hypothesis. The error probabilities are colour coded and presented in topographic probability maps.

Among the subjects examined in this study, females distinctly differ from males in the two parameters, power and coherence, in both the eyes-closed and eyes-open conditions. In particular, females display higher power in the beta range and lower coherence than males. There are also differences between males and females as to the changes of the EEG parameters due to silent reading and due to mental arithmetic.

This work is actually a byproduct of EEG studies on cognitive processing involving groups of young people. The aim was to obtain some insight into strategies the brain may use in the solution of cognitive tasks. Discrepancies encountered in these studies, particularly with the mental cube rotation test (Rappelsberger et al., 1988), encouraged us to study each sex separately. The present study not only explained these discrepancies, but also produced plentiful new data on sex differences in the EEG recorded at rest, as well as on the ways the two sexes may process information.

Method

The method used in this study was originally developed to study EEG changes that may occur during perception of music (Petsche et al., 1985, 1986). It centers on the essential question of whether and how an EEG at rest may differ from an EEG during a cognitive task. Thus we were looking for differences between the EEG recorded for one minute during which the subject had to perform a certain cognitive task and the two minutes of control before and after this task. A detailed description of the method is found in Rappelsberger et al. (1986).

EEGs were recorded simultaneously from 19 electrodes (10/20 system) with connected ear leads as reference and stored on analog tape for off-line processing.

After digitization at 256/s, eye and muscle artifacts were eliminated by visual inspection. For spectral analysis, 15 sections of 2s each were chosen for computation. After Fourier transformation of the 2s epochs, averaged power and cross-power spectra were computed, the latter between adjacent electrodes and between electrodes on homologous sites on both hemispheres. The amount of data was

Institute of Brain Research, Austrian Academy of Sciences, and Institute of Neurophysiology, University of Vienna, Austria.

reduced by extracting broad-band parameters for five frequency bands: theta (4—7.5 Hz), alpha (8—12.5 Hz), beta1 (13—18 Hz), beta2 (18.5—24 Hz) and beta3 (24.5—31.5 Hz). The broad-band parameters are *absolute power* and *coherence*. Being aware of the still unknown physiological meaning of power and coherence, we focused mainly on their changes.

In order to increase the reliability of the results, the data obtained during the minute of cognitive activity were compared to two periods of the EEG at rest, one before and one after task performance. Only when changes emerged during the cognitive task and vanished afterwards, did we consider them as likely to have been caused by the task in question. We call these changes "significantly reversible."

The data were evaluated statistically with the Fisher permutation test (Edgington, 1980; Lebart et al., 1982). The results are presented in topographic maps. The colours indicate the error probabilities for the rejection of the null hypothesis: "red" means low error probability (2P ≤ 0.10) or that the respective parameter is significantly larger; "blue" also means low error probability but the respective parameter is significantly smaller, and "green" means no significant difference.

The results to be represented may be either:

1) a comparison between 2 1-min EEG periods in one group of subjects, for example: if "b" is the period during which a certain cognitive task is performed, and "a" and "c" are the periods of control before and afterwards, the following question arises: Are there significant differences between "a" and "b" and "c" and "b," respectively? This is tested by the paired Fisher permutation test. A mean of these two test results yields some hints of the significant reversible changes of the parameters that are most likely caused by the involvement of the brain in the task in question.

2) Or, the EEG differences between two groups of subjects may be examined under the same condition, either at rest ("a" or "c") or during a certain task ("b"); in this case the question is: how does the EEG at rest or under a certain task differ between these two groups, in the present case, between males and females?

3) A third possibility is an examination of the EEG changes of two groups of subjects ("a—b" or "c—b"), in our case males and females, while they are performing the same cognitive task. This third type of analysis yields the significant differences between males and females in their brain strategies while performing the task in question. It serves to combine items (1) and (2).

Results

EEG at Rest

In Figure 1, the EEG differences between male and female students (ages: males 23.5 ± 3.0, N = 33; females 22.7 ± 3.8, N = 35) are shown during the eyes-closed and the eyes-open conditions (see item 2) above). "Red," in this presentation, means that the parameter in question is significantly larger in females than in males, "blue," that it is smaller in females.

The figure presents quite a number of remarkable sex differences in the spontaneous EEG.

As far as *power* is concerned, females with eyes closed (Figure 1, upper diagram) have less alpha and theta power in the anterior parts of the head; beta power, on the other hand, is greater than in males in the rear parts of the head and, in the beta3 band, also greater in the left frontal and occipital areas.

As regards *local coherence* (the middle column in Figure 1), females exhibit lower values than males in all frequency bands and over larger regions of the head , particularly in the frontal parts. In the beta bands, coherence is noticeably lower in the left frontal region, whereas, on the right side, it reaches farther parietally. On the other hand, larger coherence values than in men are found in the occipital regions in the entire frequency range between theta and beta2.

The *interhemispheric* coherence values are also generally lower in females than in males, particularly in the alpha band in the frontal region.

With opened eyes (Figure 1, lower diagram), there is some change of this pattern of differences, particularly as far as *power* is concerned: in contrast to the eyes-closed condition, there is now hardly any sex difference in the theta and alpha bands, whereas, in the beta bands, the region of higher power with respect to males is much larger than with eyes closed: now it extends over almost the entire head with the exception of the anterior temporal regions.

The differences in *local coherence* do not change as much as power changes while the eyes are kept open, with the exception of the alpha band, in which the distribution of the zones of lower coherence with respect to males has changed from frontal to posttemporal and parietal. The distribution of the zones of lower local coherence in females in the beta bands is not changed at all by eye opening but the lateralization to the left becomes more distinct.

As far as *interhemispheric coherence* is concerned, the most remarkable differences are seen in the alpha and in the beta bands: occipitally, interhemispheric coherence is higher in females in beta1 and beta2 upon eye opening. In beta3, on the other hand, the coupling between the two occipital regions, already weaker than in males during eyes closed, is also weaker than in males.

Silent Reading

A text was presented on a DIN A 4 page (a popularized scientific article from a newspaper). The subjects were asked to read carefully for 1 min and to prepare to be asked to recall what they had read.

The upper part of Figure 2 presents the probability maps containing the data of 68 students (33 males and 35 females), when reading was compared to the two control EEGs before and after reading (see (1) above).

As to *power,* an increased beta3 power is most noticeable especially in the posterior part of the head, with a left-side accentuation (the left temporo-occipital area also being in-

volved while the right one remains unaltered). The alpha reduction involves the greater part of the head with the exception of the two temporo-anterior regions and the right frontal area.

The changes of the *local coherence* pattern with reading are by far more complex, as in most frequency bands local increases and decreases are observed in different areas of the head. The increase of local coherence almost exclusively involves the parietal and central regions of the head. In the alpha band as well as in the theta band a decrease of local coherence during reading is preponderant. It mainly involves the temporo-occipital areas on both sides and also the frontal areas (more extensively on the left than on the right side).

Interhemispheric coherence exhibits a far more uniform pattern of changes during reading than local coherence; generally, in all frequency bands, the coupling decreases in the frontal regions and increases in the rear parts of the head.

This finding seems to be characteristic of silent reading; it was previously observed with a much smaller number of subjects (N = 19) (Petsche et al., 1987).

As regards sex differences during reading, they are shown in the lower part of Figure 2 (see (3) above under "Methods").

As to *power* changes, females seem to produce more lambda waves than males while reading, as may be concluded from the larger amount of theta in the occipital area. In the alpha range, females and males behave equally in their power reduction during reading. The most distinct differences are seen in the beta1 range, where females produce less power than males in the left occipito-temporal area and also in O2. In CZ and PZ in the beta3 range, on the other hand, females produce even more power than males during reading.

Sex differences in *local coherence* changes during reading are most pronounced in the beta3 range centro-parietally, where females surpass males in coherence increases during reading.

The same holds true for *interhemispheric coherence* changes. In females this parameter also shows the same tendencies in the beta bands occipitally and partly parietally and centrally.

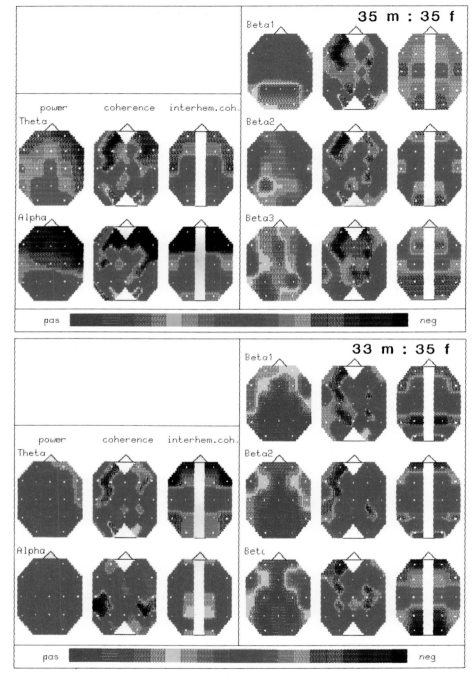

Figure 1. Significant probability mapping of power and coherence differences between males (N = 33) and females (N = 35) in the EEG at rest (1 min), with eyes closed (upper part) and eyes open (lower part) (Fisher permutation test for independent variables). The three columns from the left to the right are power, local and interhemispheric coherence. The five frequency bands theta, alpha, beta1, beta2 and beta3 are arranged horizontally. "Red" means the parameter in question is significantly larger in females. "Blue" means it is lower in females, "green" means no significant difference.

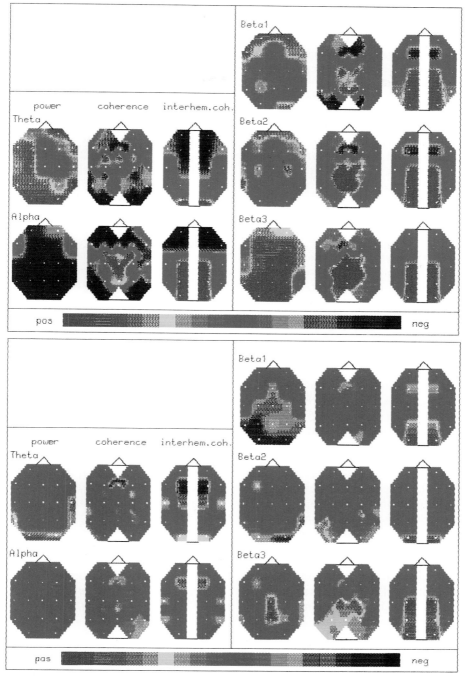

Figure 2. Upper part: Probability maps for power and coherence differences during *silent reading* for 1 min as compared with 1 min EEG at rest recorded immediately before and afterwards (Paired Fisher permutation test for 68 subjects, 33 males and 35 females). Lower part: Probability maps for power and coherence changes between males and females while reading (Fisher permutation test for independent variables).

Mental Arithmetic

The task to be performed consisted of adding, for one minute, subsequent numbers, beginning with 1. Again the EEG during this period was compared to two periods of 1min each before and after the task. Eyes were closed during the whole time. Of the 64 subjects undergoing this test, 30 were males, 34 females.

As Figure 3, upper part, demonstrates, *power* was reduced in the greater part of the frequency spectrum and over wide regions of the head, and most extensive in the alpha range.

In this test as well, the *coherence* changes are most impressive. There are clear asymmetries as far as the increase of coherence is concerned: in the theta range mainly the left hemisphere is involved, in the beta range almost only the right. In the former, the increase of coherence involves the left parieto-occipito-temporal areas; in the latter, the right precentral to parietal areas (beta2 and beta3) are mainly affected by mental arithmetic. In the same frequency bands, there is also an increased interhemispheric coherence, meaning an increased coupling of the two hemispheres that involves, in the theta band, the entire rear half of the head, in the beta1 and beta2 bands only the posterior temporal regions, and in the beta3 range, the precentral and parietal regions.

A decrease of local coherence during mental arithmetic takes place in the alpha and theta range over both frontal regions (in the alpha range also over both occipital regions) and, in the beta ranges, almost only over the right frontal region.

The lowering of *interhemispheric coherence* over the frontal part of the head in the alpha range is similar to that during silent reading.

The differences in *power* changes between the two sexes when doing mental arithmetic are almost negligible (Figure 3, lower part).

During mental arithmetic, *local coherence* is even more reduced in females than in males in the frontal areas in the alpha band. In the beta bands, there is a more localized reduction in females in the left precentral area, mainly in beta2.

Females also exhibit still more decrease of *interhemispheric coherence* than men during mental arithmetic in the frontal area and temporo-occipitally in the alpha range.

Discussion

Differences in brain electric activity between males and females have been reported sporadically. As early as 1962, Vogel and Götze observed in a large number of normals and patients (2907 males and 2063 females) a preponderance of beta activity in females as the most remarkable finding. With their data they confirm an earlier report by Mundy-Castle (1951) established in a much smaller group of patients. Smith (1954), in a study on healthy females and males, comes to the same conclusion. In their studies on the developing EEG, Petersen and Eeg-Olofsson (1971) and Matousek and Petersen (1973) confirm these findings in children and adolescents.

A more recent study, based on a computer analysis (Matsuura et al. 1985) reports on a population of 1416 normals of both sexes between 6 and 39 years. In this study, the percentage beta time turned out to show the greatest difference between males and females; there was more beta activity in the latter than in the former. In addition, these authors found that the percentage time of slower alpha was higher in males than in females, and that there was more faster alpha in females than in males after adolescence. In the delta band, no sex differences were found. Lateralization is not mentioned in any of these studies.

Studies on differences in evoked potentials between males and females are more numerous. Almost unanimously, EPs are reported to be larger and to have shorter latencies in females. This holds true for VEP (Rodin et al., 1965; Shagass & Schwartz, 1964; Straumanis et al., 1965) but also for AEP (Buchsbaum et al., 1974) and for somatosensory evoked potentials (Shagass, 1972). Ikuta and Furuta (1982) even showed, in a comparison between 100 male and 100 female students, that the group mean SEPs of each sex converge to given wave forms which significantly differ from each other.

Data from coherence studies with respect to sex differences are rare. Beaumont et al.

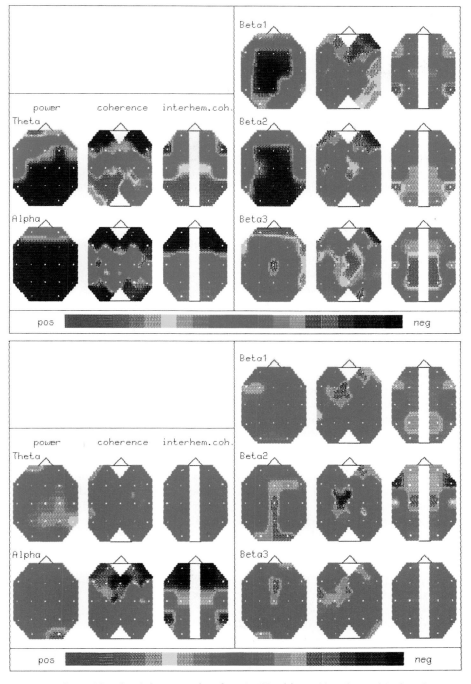

Figure 3. Same as Figure 2 but for doing *mental arithmetic* (64 subjects, 30 males and 34 females).

(1978) compared 8 male and 8 female right-handed healthy subjects and recorded between T3—P3 and between T4—P4; interhemispheric coherence was determined between the temporal and between the parietal electrodes. In this study, coherence between the parietal sites was greater than between temporal sites and females turned out to have higher coherence than males overall. This holds true for the alpha band and for different psychological tasks. As these data concern cognitive tasks different from ours and only the alpha band, a comparison with the present results is difficult. It has to be mentioned in this context that high coherence values may also be due to anatomical facts, such as an increased number of neuronal connections via the corpus callosum, but also to a smaller diameter of the head in females. This latter possibility may be rejected, as the higher interhemispheric coherence in females does not involve all frequency bands in the same way. However, the former possibility, a sex difference in the corpus callosum, may be worth considering. A larger corpus callosum in females is claimed by De-Lacoste-Utamsing and Holloway (1982); other investigators were unable to confirm these findings (Weber & Weis, 1986; Witelson, 1986). Sex-dependent differences must be considered between the two hemispheres (Galaburda, 1984; LeMay, 1984) that may involve neurochemical and neuroendocrinological asymmetries. These possibilities go beyond the scope of this paper. For review of sex differences see McGlone (1980).

The findings on sex differences in this study have to be considered under two aspects: one is the spontaneous EEG and the other mental tasks. Obviously the differences in the former are more likely to suggest sex dissimilarities of brain function whereas the latter could be taken as indices of a different form of information processing in males and females.

Regarding spontaneous activity, the larger beta content of the female EEG is accentuated over the posterior half of the skull, even in the eyes-closed situation, and even more so with eyes opened. A lateralization is seen in the coherence, which is, in both at rest conditions, lower to the left in females, and most distinct in the beta bands. There is also generally less interhemispheric coherence in women at rest with eyes closed, particularly in the alpha band over the frontal parts of the head. This might indicate that, in women, while resting with eyes closed, there is less information exchange between the two hemispheres than in men.

It must be remembered that the eyes-open-at-rest situation forces the brain to process a large amount of visual information. This information processing is accompanied by local and interhemispheric coherence decreases over the frontal areas and increases over the rear parts of the head. This could be interpreted by a need for a more specialized function of each of the two frontal lobes as soon as the flow of visual information into the brain begins, whereas the change of information between the two parietal and occipital lobes is increased.

This functional separation of the two hemispheres into their frontal parts seems to be still more pronounced in females than in males with eyes open, whereas the occipital information exchange seems to be greater, especially in beta1 and beta2. In beta3 it is lower than in males—the reason for this cannot yet be explained.

In this context it should be mentioned that the frequent absence of interhemispheric coherence changes between midtemporal regions can also be due to the fact that midtemporal (and also temporo-occipital) coherence values a priori are much lower than in any other area, so that hardly any significant differences during tasks can be found (Petsche et al., 1985).

All these findings taken together suggest that in the eyes-open condition, females are more engaged in scanning their visual environment than males.

References

Beaumont, JG, Mayes AR, Rugg MD (1978) Asymmetry in alpha coherence and power: effects of task and sex. *Electroenceph clin Neurophysiol, 45*, 393—401.

Buchsbaum MS, Henkin RI, Christiansen RL (1974) Age and sex differences in averaged evoked responses in a normal population, with observations on patients with gonadal dysgenesis. *Electroenceph clin Neurophysiol, 37,* 137–144.

De Lacoste-Utamsing C, Holloway RL (1982) Sexual dimorphism in the human corpus callosum. *Science, 216,* 1431–1432.

Edgington ES (1980) *Randomization tests.* Marcel Dekker Inc., New York and Basel.

Galaburda AM (1984) Anatomical asymmetries. In Geschwind N, Galaburda AM (Eds.) *Cerebral dominance.* Harvard University Press, Cambridge, 11–25.

Ikuta T, Furuta N (1982) Sex differences in the human group mean SEP. *Electroenceph clin Neurophysiol, 54,* 449–457.

Lebart L, Morineau A, Fenelon JP (1982) *Traitement des données statistiques: Methodes et programmes.* Dunod, Paris.

LeMay M (1984) Radiological development and fossil asymmetries. In Geschwind N, Galaburda AM (Eds.) *Cerebral dominance.* Harvard University Press, Cambridge, 26–44.

Matousek M, Petersen I (1973) Frequency analysis of the EEG in normal children and adolescents. In Kellaway P, Petersen I (Eds.) *Automation of clinical electroencephalography.* Raven Press, NY, 75–102.

Matsuura M, Yamamoto K, Fukuzawa H, Okubo Y, Uesugi H, Moriiwa M, Kojima T, Shimazono Y (1985) Age development and sex differences of various EEG elements in healthy children and adults—Quantification by a computerized wave form recognition method. *Electroenceph clin Neurophysiol, 60,* 394–406.

McGlone J (1980) Sex differences in human brain asymmetry: a critical survey. *Behav and Brain Sci, 3,* 215–264.

Mundy-Castle AC (1951) Theta and beta rhythm in the electroencephalogram of human adults. *Electroenceph clin Neurophysiol, 3,* 477–486.

Petersen I, Eeg-Olofsson O (1971) The development of the electroencephalogram in normal children from the age of 1 through 15 years. *Neuropäd, 2,* 277–304.

Petsche H, Pockberger H, Rappelsberger P (1985) EEG studies in musical perception and performance. In Spintge R, Droh R (Eds.) *Music and medicine.* Editiones Roche, 31–60.

Petsche H, Pockberger H, Rappelsberger P (1986) EEG topography and mental performance. In Duffy FH (Ed.) *Topographic mapping of the brain.* Butterworths, Boston, 63–98.

Petsche H, Rappelsberger P, Pockberger H (1987) EEG-Veränderungen beim Lesen. In Weinmann HG (Ed.) *Zugang zum Verständnis höherer Hirnfunktionen durch das EEG.* Zuckschwerdt, München, 59–74.

Rappelsberger P, Pockberger H, Petsche H (1986) Computer aided EEG analysis. *EDV in Med u Biol, 17,* 45–53.

Rappelsberger P, Krieglsteiner S, Mayerweg M, Petsche H, Pockberger H (1988, in press) Probability mapping of EEG changes: Application to spatial imagination studies. *J of Clinical Monitoring.*

Rodin EA, Grisell JL, Gudobba RD, Tachary G (1965) Relationship of EEG background rhythms to photic evoked responses. *Electroenceph clin Neurophysiol, 19,* 301–304.

Shagass C (1972) *Evoked brain potentials in psychiatry.* Plenum Press, New York.

Shagass C, Schwartz M (1964) Evoked potential studies in psychiatric patients. *Ann NY Acad Sci, 112,* 526–542.

Smith SM (1954) Discrimination between electroencephalograph recordings of normal females and normal males. *Ann Eugen (Lond), 18,* 344–350.

Straumanis JJ, Shagass C, Schwartz M (1965) Visually evoked cerebral response changes associated with chronic brain syndromes and aging. *J. Geront, 20,* 498–506.

Vogel F, Götze W (1962) Statistische Betrachtungen über die Betawellen im EEG des Menschen. *D Z Nervenheilk, 184,* 112–136.

Weber C, Weis S (1986) Morphometric analysis of the human corpus callosum fails to reveal sex-related differences. *J. Hirnforsch, 27,* 237–240.

Witelson SF (1986) Wires of the mind: anatomical variation in the corpus callosum in relation to hemispheric specialization and integration. In Lepore F, Ptito M, Jasper HH (Eds.) *Two hemispheres—one brain. Functions of the corpus callosum.* Liss, New York, 117–137.

A Pharmacological Model of "Local Cerebral Activation": EEG Cartography of Caffeine Effects in Normals

P. Etevenon*, P. Peron-Magnan**, S. Guillou**, M. Toussaint**,
B. Gueguen**, P. Deniker**, H. Loo**, E. Zarifian*

A control group of 10 volunteers, mean age 27.2 years, right-handed, was chosen for a randomized double-blind study of caffeine (400 mg p.o.) versus placebo. They were free of any medical treatment and in good health. Between placebo or caffeine administration there was a period of one week. During each of the two recorded sessions, each subject was recorded before the oral administration, for two baseline EEG cartographies: 2.5 minutes of resting EEG, eyes closed under diffuse attention, were followed by 2.5 minutes of active wakefulness, eyes opened. Spectral analysis was performed over 16 stimultaneously recorded EEG channels, using a common average reference. Three main spectral EEG parameters were computed: mean centroid frequencies, RMS absolute amplitudes, relative amplitude percentages for raw EEGs and EEGs filtered into five frequency bands (delta, theta, alpha, beta 1 and beta 2). Group EEG maps were computed, and averaged spectral parameters were tested between conditions by non-parametric permutation Fisher tests for descriptive data analyses.

The observed psychostimulant effects of caffeine are characterized by the following changes in the "differences of differences" in EEG spectral parameters (caffeine corrected from time zero, minus placebo corrected from time zero). Five main results were obtained for the eyes closed situation: (1) increase in mean alpha frequency; (2) decrease in mean alpha amplitude; (3) decrease in mean alpha %; (4) decrease in mean theta amplitude; (5) decrease in mean raw EEG amplitude. The left temporal area appears to be the most activated EEG location, followed by anterior right and left occipital areas. This cartographic EEG profile is in agreement with the previously published findings based on quantitative EEG analysis of fewer EEG channels. Descriptive and confirmatory data analyses confirm our concept.

Since the pioneering work in the fifties and after that the work of Pfeiffer et al. (1965), Fink (1969, 1974), Goldstein (1976), Goldstein et al. (1963), Itil (1968, 1974) in the United States, followed by Künkel (1972, 1976a, 1976b), Herrmann (1982a, 1982b), Herrmann and Schaerer (1986), Matejcek (1982), Matejcek et al. (1985), Saletu (1976), Sannita et al. (1983) and ourselves (Etevenon et al., 1982, 1986) in Europe, and many others, pharmaco-electroencephalography has developed a quantitative EEG strategy for psychotropic drug studies and profiles, based on a few quantified EEG channels. The EEG mapping that came into use about 10 years ago was based on quantification of 16 EEG channels or more, followed by computation and editing of EEG maps (Buchsbaum et al., 1982, 1985, 1986; Coppola, 1982; Coppola & Herrmann, 1987; Duffy, 1986; Etevenon, 1986; Etevenon et al., 1985a, 1985b). Buchsbaum et al. (1985) recently proposed EEG mapping for group studies of benzodiazepine effects. We have further developed this method in this present study and applied it to the effects of caffeine.

---

* Centre Esquirol, CHU Côte de Nacre, Caen, F-14033.
** Centre Hospitalier Sainte-Anne, Paris, F-75674. This research was supported by an INSERM grant (C.R.E. 84-8010), DRET (86-1155) and U.E.R. Cochin-Port-Royal (C.R. 85-86) grants and performed in Paris.

Moreover, the statistical treatment of data from mulitple EEG channels is still an unsolved problem despite corrected t-tests proposed by Abt (1986a). This author (Abt, 1986b) distinguished three kinds of statistical procedures: descriptive data analysis (DDA), exploratory data analysis (EDA) and confirmatory data analysis (CDA). We have proposed (Etevenon, 1986; Etevenon et al., 1985a, 1985b, 1986) applying a "non-parametric Fisher permutation test," which is more powerful than Mann-Whitney or Wilcoxon tests, not concerned with assumptions of normality of data implied in parametric statistics (t-tests, F-tests and ANOVAs, MANOVAs, z-scores) and easier to interpret when confronted with multivariate statistics (T of Hötelling, factor analysis, etc.). This statistical procedure is similar to the algorithm proposed by Streitberg and Roehmel (1986).

The purpose of the study is twofold: to assess the effects of a single large dose of caffeine on a group of young human volunteers, by computing group EEG maps and to apply to these averaged maps nonparametric Fisher tests for descriptive data analysis. From previous quantitative EEG studies on caffeine effects and psychostimulant compounds (Ammon & Künkel, 1976; Goldstein et al., 1963; Heinze & Künkel, 1979; Künkel, 1976a, 1976b; Pechadre et al., 1986; Pfeiffer et al., 1965) we expected that our concept of "EEG local activation cartography" (Etevenon, 1986; Etevenon et al., 1985a, 1985b, 1986) based on a simultaneous increase in alpha mean frequency and decrease in alpha amplitudes (over T3 and T5), would be confirmed. Therefore this study was also a "confirmatory data analysis study" (Abt, 1986b) in the sense that it would enable us to validate and further develop our concept of "EEG local activation cartography."

Methods and Protocol

A control group of 10 human volunteers (6 men, 4 women), mean age 27.2 years, academic background, right-handed, was chosen for a randomized double-blind study of caffeine (400 mg p.o.) versus placebo. All the subjects were habituated to the quantitative EEG laboratory conditions and were chosen after a standard EEG recording. They were free of any medical treatment and in good health. Between placebo or caffeine administration there was a period of one week. During each of the two sessions, each subject was recorded before the oral administration, for two baseline EEG cartographies: 2.5 minutes of resting EEG, eyes closed under diffuse attention, were followed by 2.5 minutes of active wakefulness, eyes opened. One hour after receiving either placebo or caffeine, the same two recordings were repeated. Thus, per subject 4 EEG recordings were carried out on each session involving, for all 10 subjects, 80 EEG recordings which had to be analysed. The day before each recording session, each subject was told not to take any tea, coffee, chocolate or cola drinks.

A bi-hemispheric symmetrical montage was choosen according to Giannitrapani's montage (1985). Spectral analysis was performed for each subject on 16 stimulaneously recorded EEG channels using a common average reference. Three main spectral EEG parameters were computed: mean centroid frequencies (for a frequency band, the centroid frequency is the center of gravity, computed by the sum of the spectral amplitudes multiplied by their respective frequencies, normalized after division by the sum of the spectral amplitudes, according to Lehmann and Koukkou, 1980), RMS root mean square absolute amplitudes, and relative amplitude percentages for raw EEGs and EEGs filtered into five frequency bands (delta, theta, alpha, beta 1 and beta 2). Each recording of the 16 EEG channels provided 17 different EEG maps. Group EEG maps were computed and averaged spectral parameters were tested between conditions by non parametric permutation Fisher tests (Lebart et al., 1982) for descriptive data analyses. In this present study of caffeine effects on topographic EEG changes we followed the Buchsbaum et al. (1985) procedure of testing topographic EEG differences.

All the multiple-channel EEG recordings were made on a Reega 16 polygraph (Alvar) under standardized conditions (Etevenon et al., 1985a, 1985b), using silver electrodes glued to the scalp with collodion. Details on spectral analysis have been described before

(Etevenon et al., 1985a, 1985b). After sampling the EEG at 200 Hz and passing the signals before sampling through anti-aliasing filters (48 dB octave, at 62.5 Hz), spectral estimates were calculated between 0 and 50 Hz using a frequency resolution of 0.39 Hz. Data from sample-and-hold 16-channel multiplexer linked with active filters (SOPEMEA) were then fed into a Hewlett-Packard Fourier analyzer (5451 C). The digitalized EEGs were stored on-line on a 800 bpi digital tape and spectral analyses were later made and stored on disc. Table 1 gives details of the 17 spectral parameters, the 5 frequency bands and the 7 series of experimental values obtained. Figure 1 shows the EEG montage according to Giannitrapani (1985), using a common average reference (Walter et al., 1984).

This was followed by a transfer into another minicomputer (21 MXF, HP 1000) after the spectral analyses, which permitted data reduction (Table 1) and storage of the 80 quantified multiple EEG recordings in a data base (IMAGE 1000 H.P.), and provided further computation of EEG maps from the numerical data as described by Etevenon (1986).

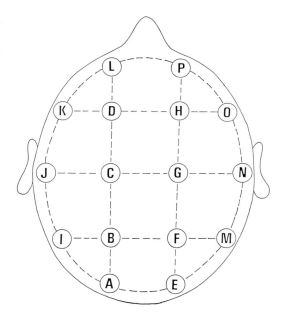

Figure 1. Multiple EEG channel montage: 16 derivations with common average electrode, according to Giannitrapani (1985).

Results

For each of the 17 spectral parameters averaged for the group of 10 subjects, tables were obtained. Table 2 gives an example for alpha mean RMS amplitude (eyes closed). Each column of Table 2 (P1, P0, PD, C1, C0, CD, DD) represents the 16 EEG channel mean values. The non-parametric Fisher permutation test was applied to the last column of "differences of differences" (CD−PD = DD), giving the exact probability for each EEG channel that caffeine difference (CD) differs (or not) from placebo difference (PD). To assess these probabilities two levels of confidence were chosen ($p < 0.05^*$ and $p < 0.01^{**}$) and represented by stars in Table 2 or dots in Figures 2 and 3. As regards the alpha mean RMS amplitudes, Table 2 shows that placebo differences (PD) after correction of time zero baselines presented 15 positive values and only 1 negative value. The caffeine differences (CD), however, after correction of time zero baselines, presented 16 negative values indicative of a general decrease in alpha amplitudes: All the values of the "differences of differences" (CD−PD) were also negative.

Table 1: Spectral parameters and sets of data.

17 Spectral Parameters:
- 6 centroid mean frequencies in Hz (on a, b, c, d, e, f)
- 6 mean RMS amplitudes in μV (on a, b, c, d, e, f)
- 5 mean relative amplitudes % (on b, c, d, e, f)

5 Spectral Frequency Bands:
- a. raw EEG: 1.56−49.61 Hz
- b. delta: 1.56−3.52 Hz
- c. theta: 3.91−7.42 Hz
- d. alpha: 7.81−14.06 Hz
- e. beta 1: 14.45−28.13 Hz
- f. beta 2: 28.52−49.61 Hz

7 Sets of Experimental Data:
- P1: time + 1 hour after placebo intake
- P0: time zero baseline before placebo intake
- P1−P0: placebo difference (PD)
- C1: time + 1 hour after caffeine intake
- C0: time zero baseline before caffeine intake
- C1−C0: caffeine difference (CD)
- CD−PD: differences of differences, caffeine minus placebo corrected from their time-zero baselines (DD)

Table 2: Mean spectral RMS alpha amplitudes (expressed in microvolts), eyes closed recordings, n = 10.

EEG channels	P1 after placebo	P0 before placebo	PD	C1 after caffeine	C0 before caffeine	CD	DD	p
A	62.78	66.16	−3.38	54.05	60.41	−6.36	−2.98	
B	40.14	35.08	5.06	30.24	35.37	−5.13	−10.19	**
C	25.81	23.64	2-17	21.70	26.26	−4.50	−6.73	**
D	36.32	33.31	3.01	26.80	32.00	−5.20	−8.21	**
E	70.29	65.30	4.99	57.10	65.25	−8.15	−13.14	
F	38.93	36.90	2.03	30.19	37.37	−7.18	−9.21	*
G	25.60	23.59	2.01	21.53	25.78	−4.25	−6.26	**
H	36.99	35.70	1.29	26,48	32.13	−5.65	−6.94	
I	47.74	45.11	2.63	35.48	43.66	−8.18	−10.81	*
J	31.53	28.95	2.58	22.70	28.87	−6.17	−8.75	**
K	35.37	34.43	0.94	26.05	31.48	−5.43	−6.37	
L	40.33	38.33	2.00	30.83	35.37	−4.54	−6.54	
M	47.44	44.41	3.03	35.80	42.18	−6.38	−9.41	*
N	28.87	26.97	1.90	21.34	26.50	−5.16	−7.06	**
O	40.38	38.96	1.42	30.13	35.09	−4.96	−6.38	*
P	35.71	34.28	1.43	26.23	31.04	−4.81	−6.24	*

Placebo differences corrected from time zero baselines: (P1−P0 = PD); caffeine differences corrected from time zero baselines (C1−C0 = CD); differences of differences: (CD−PD = DD); non-parametric Fisher tests on "difference of differences" values: descriptive data analysis: (p ≤ 0.05: *; P ≤ 0.01: **).

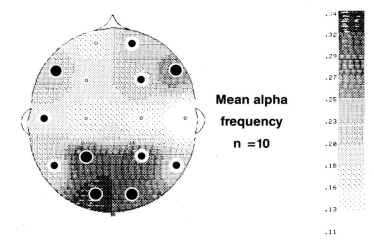

Mean alpha frequency n = 10

Figure 2. Mean alpha frequency in Hz for "differences of differences" (caffeine minus placebo, corrected from time zero baselines), n = 10, eyes closed condition, non-parametric Fischer tests (p ≤ 0.05 small dots, p ≤ 0.01 large dots). EEG map is made of 10 grey shades between a minimum of +0.11 Hz (white area) and a maximum of +0.34 Hz (black area).

Though all the EEG channels presented this trend of decreased alpha amplitudes, only 11 EEG channels among 16 reached statistical significance (B, C, D, G, J, N: **; F, I, M, O, P: *) for these descriptive data analyses. This is a confirmation of our hypothesis in terms of "confirmatory data analysis."

Table 3 summarizes the statistical results. Five main results were obtained:

1) increase in mean alpha frequency (up to 0.34 Hz, 11 EEG channels over 16)
2) decrease in mean alpha amplitude (Table 2): (down to −13 μV, 11 EEG channels over 16)
3) decrease in mean alpha % (down to 5%, 7 EEG channels over 16)
4) decrease in mean theta amplitude (down to −4 μV, 6 EEG channels over 16)

Table 3: Descriptive data analysis on "differences of differences": Caffeine minus placebo effects corrected from time zero baselines, sums of numbers of non-parametric Fisher tests (p ≤ 0.05: *; p ≤ 0.01: **); increased values: ↑; decreased values: ↓.

EEG channels	↑ alpha frequency	↓ alpha amplitude	↓ alpha %	↓ total RMS amplitude	↓ theta amplitude	SUMS
A	A**	—	—	—	—	1
B	B**	B**	—	B**	B**	4
C	—	C**	C**	C**	—	3
D	—	D**	—	D*	D*	3
E	E*	—	—	E*	E**	3
F	F*	F*	—	F*	F**	4
G	—	G**	G**	—	—	2
H	H*	—	—	—	—	1
I	I*	I*	I*	—	—	3
J	J*	J**	J**	J*	J*	5
K	K*	—	—	—	—	1
L	—	—	L*	—	—	1
M	M*	M*	M*	—	—	3
N	—	N**	N*	—	—	2
O	O**	O*	—	—	O*	3
P	P	P*	—	—	—	2
SUMS	11	11	7	6	6	41

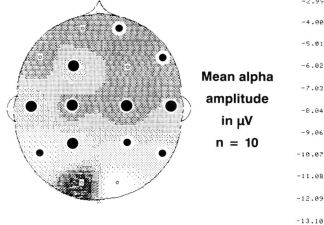
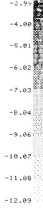

Mean alpha amplitude in µV n = 10

Figure 3. Mean alpha amplitude in microvolts for "differences of differences" caffeine minus placebo, corrected from time zero baselines. This EEG map is made of 10 grey shades between −3.0 µV (black area) and −12.1 µV (white area).

5) decrease in mean raw EEG amplitude (down to −22 µV, 6 EEG channels over 16).

For each of the 17 spectral parameters a similar analysis was done. This resulted in 272 Fisher tests, (17 × 16 EEG channels) for the 40 "eyes closed" quantified recordings. Only 41 of these tests reached statistical levels (Table 3). This corresponded to an increase in mean alpha frequency and decreases in mean amplitudes, namely in absolute and relative alpha values, total RMS amplitude and theta absolute amplitude values. This agrees with our hypothesis of "EEG local activation cartography" where we assumed that alpha frequency was increased and alpha RMS amplitude was decreased, but only for 7 EEG channels (B, F,

I, J, M, O, P) out of 16: anterior occipital areas, left temporal, right and left parietal and right frontal and pre-frontal areas. For these channels, we may consider that confirmatory data analyses were obtained, enabling us to determine the EEG cartographic profile of caffeine in normals. The other results, namely, the decreased amplitudes of alpha %, total RMS amplitudes and theta amplitudes, are in line with the preceding results and may be considered as descriptive data analyses.

The Concept of "EEG Local Activation Cartography"

Goldstein et al. (1963) and later Pfeiffer et al. (1965), reported that "definite EEG changes in the direction of stimulation were observed with the equivalent of two cups of coffee (250 mg total dose)." These changes observed in 15 normal volunteers and quantified over the left occipital area were "a rapid decrease in MEC (mean energy content, equivalent to total RMS amplitude) and a somewhat slower diminution of EEG variability." This last parameter reaches its lowest value 60 minutes following drug administration. Goldstein et al. (1963) then observed that "a stimulant effect is accompanied by a decrease in MEC: in other words the decrease in amplitude of brain waves is not compensated by their increase in frequency." They postulated "a refinement of the regulating properties of the brain with, as a result, an increased awareness of the environment. Not only caffeine but amphetamine and LSD-25 were producing these same quantified EEG changes."

Later on, Künkel (1972) simultaneously recorded 12 EEG channels which were quantified by spectral analysis and measured also for EEG variability. Künkel (1976a, 1976b) and Ammon and Künkel (1976) reported that "coffee and caffeine solution both produce a highly significant reduction of theta-amplitude, dominant theta frequency and theta-frequency-variation. The alterations within the alpha range are increase of dominant frequency and decrease of amplitude. These findings may be interpreted as signs of remarkable activation and elevation of vigil-

ance. It should be pointed out that the EEG effects of caffeine (at 200–250 mg), as well as those of other compounds with central effects, are characterized by topographically different effects. These are not only quantitative, but partially qualitative differences" (Künkel, 1976a).

In 12 human volunteers, Heinze and Künkel (1979) reported topographic differences of caffeine effects: The dominant alpha frequency was increased significantly, together with an increase of the dominant alpha frequency over frontal, antero-temporal, mid-temporal, temporo-basal areas, but not over postero-temporal and occipital areas. Simultaneously the mean absolute theta power was decreased significantly, together with absolute theta power values over mid-temporal, posterotemporal and temporobasal areas, but not over frontal, occipital and anterotemporal areas.

In agreement with these previous studies, we have observed that one hour after a high dose of caffeine (400 mg, p. o.), every subject (from tables of individual results) as well as the average group results (Figures 2 and 3, Tables 2 and 3) present an increase in alpha frequency and a decrease in alpha mean amplitudes mainly over temporal, parietal, anterior occipital, right pre-frontal and frontal areas, together with other decreased amplitudes (total RMS amplitudes, alpha relative percentages, theta amplitudes). This constellation of results may be considered as an "EEG local activation cartography" of specific areas produced by the psychostimulant effects of caffeine.

Obrist showed in 1963 that the slowing of EEG in old age was also accompanied by reduced cerebral metabolism. As early as 1933, Berger suggested that there could be a correlation between the EEG and the cerebral blood flow and metabolism (Ingvar et al., 1979). Following the studies of Sulg in animals (1969) and of Obrist (1963), Ingvar et al. (1976, 1979) have found that there is a positive correlation existing between mean EEG frequency from temporal and occipital areas and total hemispheric oxygen uptake. They have also found similar correlations between mean EEG frequency and regional blood flow in cortical grey matter (Ingvar et al., 1976).

It is likely that the "EEG local cortical activation," corresponding to increase of alpha frequency and decrease of alpha amplitude, may also be correlated with an increase in regional cerebral blood flow. This is further substantiated by PET-scan studies compared with EEG cartography (Buchsbaum et al., 1982, 1986; Coppola, 1982): The "EEG local cortical activation" pattern was also associated with increased glucose metabolism.

Discussion

The effects of psychotropic drugs inducing cortical activation can be described and quantified by changes in EEG parameters. However, these effects depend on many factors like the type of active administered compound, the dose, the time course, the route of administration, the choice of the group of subjects or patients. These changes appear to be specific for various EEG parameters: mean centroid frequency, absolute or relative spectral intensities (powers or root-mean-square amplitudes), spectral frequency bands, etc. Cortical activation produces visually desynchronized EEG tracings with increased frequencies and decreased amplitudes. Thus the alpha frequency is increased when the alpha intensity is decreased.

However, when the alpha band is split into a low alpha 1 (8.5–10.5 Hz) and high alpha 2 band (10.5–12.5 Hz), "vigilance stabilization" (Herrmann & Schaerer, 1986) may first increase the alpha 1 relative intensity, before decreasing it when the vigilance process is increased. Relative (power or amplitude) values provide less significant results than absolute values (Coppola & Herrmann, 1987) and are often in opposite directions (increased alpha 1 values) when compared with changes in absolute values.

In our previous study (Etevenon et al., 1982) of low doses of yohimbine (4 mg per os) given to human volunteers, we showed a theta frequency increase and alpha frequency increase over right and left central EEG channels (T4-C4, T3-C3), together with a beta spectral intensity increase over right and left parieto-occipital EEG channels (of +2% over P4-02 and 4,5% over P3-01), and a decrease of

slow waves (delta plus theta) over left parieto-occipital (−5% over P3-01), together with a slight but non-significant alpha intensity decrease over posterior areas. From this study, we suggested that yohimbine produced a possible "psychostimulant-like effect" over the left parieto-occipital area, considered as a part of the "dominant hemisphere." This effect was different from the "antidepressive-like effect" observed over the right parieto-occipital area that has recently been implied in depressive illness. This was in anticipation of the "EEG cartographic psychotropic profile," like the effects of a high dose of caffeine in normals that we have reported here.

The first findings of Goldstein et al. (1963) and Pfeiffer et al. (1965) of cortical activation (EEG) following oral administration of the equivalent of two cups of coffee were later confirmed and extented by Künkel et al. (1972), Künkel (1976a, 1976b) and Ammon and Künkel (1976), with a same range of doses (200–250 mg, p. o.). However, Herrman (1982) reported that after administration of 200 mg of caffeine to human volunteers and recording from right occipital region (O2-A2), the changes in relative power values could be misclassified into the placebo class (0.33 probability) instead of the psychostimulant class (0.26 probability) when compared to methylphenidate (30 mg), dextro-amphetamine (20 mg) or phenelzine (30 mg) administration. This may be related to the use of relative power values instead of absolute values.

Matejcek et al. (1985) also studied theophylline administration (600 mg), from the same chemical xanthine family to which caffeine belongs. They found an increase in EEG mean frequency, together with a significant increase in alpha 2 relative power values, over the right occipital area (O2-C7) recorded in 12 healthy male volunteers. Again, the results differ when relative power values instead of absolute values are studied. This result was also close to the previous findings of Matejcek (1982) in human volunteers receiving 5 or 10 mg of dextro-amphetamine. Pechadre et al. (1986) recently examined 5 volunteers for the effects of doses of 25, 50, 100 and 200 mg of caffeine on right and left rolandoparietal and parieto-occipital recordings, using our previous protocol for quantitative EEG study of psychotropic drugs. They found a decrease in mean frequency of the low alpha 1 band together with an increase in mean frequency of the high alpha 2 band, for the low doses (25,50 mg), which became an increase in mean frequency for alpha 1 and alpha 2 frequency bands for higher doses (100, 200 mg), similar to our findings after 400 mg. They also showed that alpha 1 power was unchanged and alpha 2 power was increased after 100 or 200 mg, but they have not tried a higher dose of 400 mg.

From the last table of results of this study, we have shown that topographic cortical activation (EEG) can differ statistically from place to place depending on the descriptive spectral EEG parameter used. Therefore we have proposed to find the electrode locations at which the first three parameters (alpha frequency, absolute and relative alpha RMS amplitudes) all show increased frequency together with decreased amplitude. This kind of "common denominator" between 3 main spectral EEG parameters appears to be a conservative strategy.

The most recent study of topographic brain mapping of caffeine effects has been published by Saletu et al. (1987). Two hours after oral administration of 250 mg of caffeine as compared with placebo, these authors found:

1) a significant increase of the alpha centroid frequency over the left and right occipital, parietal and occipito-temporal regions;
2) a significant attenuation of total power, specifically over the left occipital, occipito-temporal and parietal regions, together with the same decrease of slow alpha activity over parietal regions;
3) relative power values that did not change except for the slow alpha activity, which was decreased over left occipito-temporal and parietal areas and over right occipital area.

This study was carried out in 8 subjects. Group means of 36 EEG variables were computed and edited by the pharmaco-EEG imaging technique using our $1/d_3$ interpolation algorithm (Walter et al., 1984). Exploratory data analysis was made after computation of statistical probability maps based on t-values first described by Duffy et al. (1981).

These results are very close to our present findings on non-parametric Fisher tests. They are therefore in agreement with our proposed concept of local cerebral activation. From a technical point of view, the present study and the "caffeine model of local cerebral activation" should be verified and completed with complementary studies under the same protocol and statistical strategy. It is known that the common average reference may artificially introduce occipital alpha-like activity in frontal derivations and eye artifacts in occipital derivations. This would probably not be the case in our study, since we found decreased alpha EEG amplitudes after caffeine administration, especially over right frontal areas. Nevertheless, this study should be duplicated with the linked-ears reference and source derivation techniques.

As an elaboration of this study, we propose to apply this protocol of EEG cartography to a group of patients with high anxiety levels and compare their EEG cartography profile with the present results. This may lead to quantitative EEG cartography screening of anxious people versus a normal matched control group, and also to pharmaco-EEG trials of anti-anxiety compounds, based on their EEG cartography profile.

References

Abt K (1986a) Significance testing of many variables. *Neuropsychobiology, 9,* 47–51.

Abt K (1986b) *Experimental strategies and hypothesis testing.* Inferiential strategies, IPEG Training Course, IPEG Meeting Sta Margherita, 1–10.

Ammon HPT, Künkel H (1976) Welche Bedeutung kommt der Chlorogensäure bei der zentralstimulierenden Wirkung des Kaffeegetränkes zu? *Dtsch Med Wschr, 101,* 460–464.

Berger H (1933) Über das Elektroencephalogramm des Menschen. VIII *Mitt Arch Psychiat Nervenkr, 101,* 452–469.

Buchsbaum MS, Coppola R, Cappelletti J (1982) Positron emission tomography, EEG and evoked potential topography: New approaches to local function in pharmaco-electroencephalography. In Herrman WM (Ed.) *Electroencephalography in drug research.* G. Fischer, Stuttgart, 193–207.

Buchsbaum MS, Hazlett E, Sicotte N, Stein M, Wu J, Zetin M (1985) Topographic EEG changes with benzodiazepine administration in general anxiety disorder. *Biol Psychiatry, 20,* 832–842.

Buchsbaum MS, Hazlett E, Sicotte N, Ball R, Johnson S (1986) Geometric and scaling issues in topographic electroencephalography. In Duffy F (Ed.) *Topographic mapping of brain electrical activity.* Butterworths, Boston, 325–337.

Coppola R (1982) Topographic methods of functional cerebral analysis. In Potvin S, Potvin T (Eds.) *Frontiers of engineering in health care.* IEEE Press, New York.

Coppola R, Herrmann WM (1987, in press) Psychotropic drug profiles: Comparisons by topographic maps of absolute power. *Neuropsychobiology.*

Duffy FH (Ed.) (1986) *Topographic mapping of brain electrical activity.* Butterworths, Boston.

Duffy FH, Bartels PH, Burchfield JL (1981) Significance probability mapping: An aid in the topographic analysis of brain electrical activity. *Electroenceph clin Neurophysiol, 51,* 455–465.

Etevenon P (1986) Applications and perspectives of EEG cartography. In Duffy FH (Ed.) *Topographic mapping of brain electrical activity.* Butterworths, Boston, 113–141.

Etevenon P, Pidoux B, Peron-Magnan P, Lecrubier Y, Verdeaux G (1982) First computerized EEG effects of yohimbine in man. In Herrmann WM (Ed.) *Electroencephalography in drug research.* Gustav Fischer, Stuttgart, 539–553.

Etevenon P, Tortrat D, Benkelfat C (1985a) EEG cartography II-By-means of statistical group studies. Activations by visual attention. *Neuropsychobiology, 13,* 141–146.

Etevenon P, Tortrat D, Guillou S, Wendling B (1985b) Cartography EEG au cours d'une tâche visuo-spatiale. Cartes moyennes et statistiques de groupes. *Rev EEG Neurophysiol, 15,* 139–147.

Etevenon P, Peron-Magnan P, Boulenger JP, Tortrat D, Guillou S, Toussaint M, Gueguen B, Deniker P, Zarifian E (1986) EEG cartography profile of caffeine in normals. *Clin neuropharmacology, 9* (suppl 4), 538–540.

Fink M (1969) EEG and human psychopharmacology. *Ann Rev Pharmacology, 9,* 241–258.

Fink M (1974) EEG profiles and bioavailability measures of psychoactive drugs. In Ban TA, Freyhan FA, Poldinger W (Eds.) *Modern problems of pharmacopsychiatry, Vol. 8.* Karger, Basel, 76–98.

Giannitrapani D (1985) *The electrophysiology of intellectual functions.* Karger, Basel.

Goldstein L (1976) Quantitative EEG of "classical" psychoactive drugs. In Deniker P, Radouco-Thomas C, Villeneuve A (Eds.) *Neuropsychopharmacology, Vol 2.* Pergamon Press, Oxford, 1165–1171.

Goldstein L, Murphree HB, Pfeiffer CC (1963) Quantitative electroencephalography in man as a measure of CNS stimulation. *New York Acad Sci, 107,* 1045–1056.

Heinze HJ, Künkel H (1979) The significance of personnality traits in EEG evaluation of drug effects. *Pharmacopsychiat, 12,* 155–1.

Herrmann WM (Ed.) (1982a) *Electroencephalography in drug research.* Gustav Fischer, Stuttgart.

Herrmann WM (1982b) Development and critical evaluation of an objective procedure for the electroencephalographic classification of psychotropic drugs. In Herrman WD (Ed.) *Electro-encephalography in drug research.* Gustav Fischer, Stuttgart, 249–351.

Hermann WM, Schaerer E (1986) Pharmaco-EEG: Computer EEG analysis to describe the projection of drug effects on a functional cerebral level in humans. In Lopes da Silva FH, Storm van Leeuwen W, Remond A (Eds.) *Clinical applications of computer analysis of EEG and other neurophysiological signals.* (Handbook of Electroencephalography and Clinical Neurophysiology, revised series, Vol 2) Elsevier, Amsterdam, 385–445.

Ingvar DH, Sjölund B, Ardö A (1976) Correlation between dominant EEG frequency, cerebral oxygen uptake and blood flow. *Electroenceph clin Neurophysiol, 41,* 268–276.

Ingvar DH, Rosen I, Johanesson G (1979) EEG related to cerebral metabolism and blood flow. *Pharmakopsychiat, 12,* 200–209.

Itil TM (1968 Electroencephalography and pharmacopsychiatry. Clinical psychopharmacology. *Mod Probl Pharmacopsychiat, 1,* 163–194.

Itil TM (1974) Quantitative electroencephalography. In Ban TA, Freyhann FA, Poldinger W (Eds.) *Modern problems of pharmacopsychiatry, Vol. 8.* Karger, Basel, 43–75.

Künkel H (1972) Simultane Vielkanal-on-line EEG-Analyse in Echtzeit, *EEG-EMG, 3,* 30–38.

Künkel H (1976a) EEG-Spektral Analyse der Koffein-Wirkung. *Arzneim Forsch (Drug Res), 26,* 462–465.

Künkel H (1976b) Vielkanal-EEG-Spektralanalyse der Kaffein-Wirkung. *Z. Ernährungswiss, 15,* 71–79.

Lebart L, Morineau A, Fenelon JP (1982) *Traitement des données statistiques.* Dunod, Paris.

Lehmann D, Koukkou M (1980) Classes of spontaneous, private experience and ongoing human EEG activities. In Pfurtscheller G, Buser P, Lopes da Silva FH, Petsche H (Eds.) *Rhythmic EEG activities and cortical functioning.* Elsevier, Amsterdam, 289–297.

Matejcek M (1982) Vigilance and the EEG psychological, physiological and pharmacological aspects. In Herrmann WD (Ed.) *Electroencephalography in drug research.* Gustav Fischer, Stuttgart, 405–508.

Matejcek M, Irwin P, Neef G,. Abt K, Wehrli W
(1985) Determination of the central effects of the
asthma prophylactic ketotifen, the bronchodila-
tor theophylline, and both in combination: An
application of quantitative electroencephalography to the study of drug interactions. *Internl J
Clin Pharmacol, Therapy and Toxicology, 235,*
258—266.

Obrist WD (1963) Cerebral ischemia and the senes-
cent electroencephalogram. In Simonson E,
McCavack TH (Eds.) *Cerebral ischemia.* Thomas,
Springfield, 71—78.

Pechadre JC, Beudin P, Kantelip JP, Trolese F,
Mont-Chamont L (1986) A propos des effets
centraux de la caféine en EEG quantifiée. *Psy-
chiatrie, 27,* 690—692.

Pfeiffer CC, Goldstein L, Murphree HB, Sugerman
A (1965) Time-series, frequency analysis, and
electrogenesis of the EEGs of normals and
psychotics before and after drugs. *Am J Psychiatry, 121,* 1147—1155.

Saletu B (1976) *Psychopharmaka, Gehirntätigkeit
and Schlaf.* Karger, Basel.

Saletu B, Anderer P, Kinsperger K, Grünberger J
(1987) Topographic brain mapping of EEG in
neuropsychopharmacology. Part II. Clinical
applications (Pharmaco-EEG Imaging) *Meth
and find expl clin pharmacol, 9,* 385—408.

Sannita WG, Ottonello D, Perria B, Rosadini G,
Timitilli C (1983) Topographic approaches in
human quantitative pharmaco-EEG. *Neuropsychobiology, 9,* 66—72.

Sulg IA (1969) Manual EEG analysis. *Acta neurol
scand, 45,* 431—445.

Streitberg B, Roehmel J (1986) Exact distributions
for permutation and rank tests. An introduction
to some recently published algorithms. *Statistical
Software Newsletter,* 10—17.

Walter PO, Etevenon P, Pidoux B, Tortrat D, Guillou S (1984) Computerized topo-EEG spectral
maps: Difficulties and perspectives. *Neuropsychobiology, 11,* 264—272.

Topographical Mapping of Electrocortical Activity in Schizophrenia during Directed Nonfocussed Attention, Recognition Memory and Motor Programming

J. Gruzelier, D. Liddiard, L. Davis, L. Wilson

An approach is illustrated for testing the validity of EEG topographical mapping through monitoring EEG during neuropsychological testing in pathological groups. Here schizophrenic patients were found to be deficient in recognition memory for faces while recognition memory for words was normal. Deficits on faces recognition have been shown to occur after damage to right parietal and temporal regions. Probability maps of EEG power spectra revealed a right posterior abnormality in patients in beta II during the faces recognition tests. The potential for EEG topographical mapping in elucidating brain functional abnormalities is discussed.

In research on cerebral asymmetry and schizophrenia clinical syndromes have been shown to be important in delineating the direction of lateral imbalances in functional activation. Patients with a syndrome characterized by delusions and excitment (Active syndrome) show higher left than right hemispheric levels of activity, whereas patients characterized by withdrawal, slowness, poverty of speech and blunted affect (Withdrawn syndrome), show higher right than left hemispheric activity (Gruzelier & Manchanda, 1982; Gruzelier, 1983, 1984, 1987; Gaebel et al., 1986).

The neurophysiological basis of the syndromes has been elucidated with various methods including EEG topographic mapping. Investigation of schizophrenic patients with neuropsychological tests known to differentiate patients with unilateral temporal from those with temporofrontal lesions, indicated that unilateral losses of function corresponded to the hemisphere with the lower level of activation, except for a sub-group of Withdrawn patients who had severe bilateral deficits (Gruzelier et al., 1987). In the Withdrawn syndrome Andrews et al. (1986, 1987) have shown abnormal somatosensory evoked potentials to unimanual stimuli coupled with neuropsychological impairments, results which implicate left-sided deficits together with impaired interhemispheric transfer; patients with the Active syndrome were not differentiated from normal controls. The syndrome classification has also predicted the visual search performance of schizophrenic patients, such that the Active group displayed serial-type, left hemispheric processing, and the Withdrawn group gestalt or holistic, right hemispheric processing (Gaebel et al., 1986). Additional studies consistent with the syndrome classification were presented at the Third International Conference on Cerebral Dynamics, Laterality and Psychopathology (Takahashi et al., 1987), and confirm the association of positive versus negative symptoms with opposite imbalances in hemispheric levels of activation (Gruzelier, 1987).

The study with EEG topographical mapping involved examination of female schizophrenic patients, all with the Active syndrome, based on tests of recognition memory (War-

Department of Psychiatry, Charing Cross & Westminster Medical School, St Dunstan's Road, London, W6 8RP, England.

Assistance from the Wellcome Trust and Neuroscience Ltd. is gratefully acknowledged.

rington, 1984). This revealed a striking deficit in memory for faces whereas memory for words was normal (Gruzelier & Liddiard 1987). Concurrent monitoring of EEG with a 28 electrode array revealed abnormal elevations in fast beta in the posterior temporal-parieto-occipital region. This corresponded to the area in which neurological lesions have been found to impair memory for faces as distinct from memory for words. In controls there was a focal reduction in fast beta in this area. Abnormal elevations in beta occur in pathological conditions characterized by states of low functional arousal such as could be associated with poor recognition memory. Elevations also occur in states of anxiety and excitement which are both features of the Active syndrome. It is of importance to note that reductions in beta amplitude have been associated with information processing (Gibbs & Gibbs, 1961).

Topographical differences in patients were also found in alpha and slow beta during tests of recognition memory as well as during tests of motor sequencing devised by Luria. In the latter, effects were restricted to the left hand condition, again implicating disturbances of functional activation in the right hemisphere in patients with the Active syndrome. No differences were found in the eyes closed condition, endorsing the importance of functional activation of the brain in revealing differences between schizophrenic patients and controls. The present study set out to extend the sample by including male patients, also with the Active syndrome, and male controls. The Luria motor sequencing tests were also included along with an eyes closed and an eyes open directed, nonfocused attention condition to further explore the relevance for schizophrenia of the results of the previous study.

Subjects

Five female and five male DSM III hospitalised schizophrenic patients were compared with 10 age and gender matched normal controls. The patients all fulfilled criteria for the Active syndrome on the *Hemisphere Imbal-*

ance Syndrome Scale (Gruzelier & Wilson, in preparation). All patients had evidence of delusions and/or excitement, overactivity, cognitive acceleration, social involvement and emotional engagement. All subjects were dextral (Annett, 1970). The average age of patients was 34, range 23–55. All but two patients were medicated with antipsychotics prescribed in conventional doses.

Procedure

Apparatus

Brain electrical activity was monitored with a Brain Imager (Neuroscience Ltd.) from 28 scalp electrodes referenced to linked ears. Electrode placements were derived from the International 10–20 system. Electrodes were attached to a cap which was secured with elastic straps fastened to an elastic band placed around the chest. On average each test condition required two minutes of recording to obtain one minute of artefact-free EEG.

The two minute sections of trace were first examined for evidence of movement artefacts. After deletion of artefacts a Fast Fourier power spectrum analysis was carried out for delta 0.5–2 Hz, theta 3–9 Hz, alpha 10–12 Hz beta I 13–16 Hz, and beta II 17–30 Hz. For each 2.5 seconds a topographical map was made which was examined for evidence of raised bilateral frontal delta as a check on the adequacy of the artefact rejection procedure. Any further contaminated samples were removed. The remaining artefact free EEG was then averaged. Each task condition consisted of at least one minute of artefact free EEG. Topographical maps for both the mean square root of power and the standard deviation were then obtained for the five spectral bandwidths for all conditions for each group. In all cases the standard deviations for patients and controls were comparable. t-tests were then carried out on the standard deviations and none approached significance. With assumptions of homogeneity of variance, the groups were compared with t-tests for differences in power using two-tailed levels of significance.

Neuropsychological Tests

The first test condition included 2 minutes of eyes closed EEG. This was followed by 2 minutes with eyes open and attention directed to a square on the wall. This was done to minimise movements by the subjects and to structure the condition. It also provided a control for the directed attention component of the memory and motor tasks. The white square, 2 cm in diamter, was positioned on a dark grey background, 3.5' in front of the subject at eye level. The subject was instructed to look in the direction of the square without analysing it. The memory tasks involved recognizing words and unfamiliar faces, 50 items in each task with task order counterbalanced (Warrington, 1984). Each task was divided into an acquisition and a recognition phase. The acquisition phase involved showing one item at a time with the instruction to raise an index finger according to whether it was regarded as pleasant or unpleasant. In the recognition phase items were shown in pairs, only one of which was in the previous list. Subjects had to indicate which they had seen before by raising the index finger on the same side as the item. A forced-choice procedure was adopted. The final condition involved a programmed movement task of Luria which involved tapping one finger at a time in sequence with the thumb of the corresponding hand. Hand order was counterbalanced across subjects.

Results

Recognition Memory

In an analysis of variance with group and gender as between subject variables and memory for faces/words as a within subject variable there was a significant interaction between group, gender and memory (p < 0.009). Paired comparisons indicated that the schizophrenic women were distinguished by a poorer memory for faces p < 0.01). The means are shown in Table 1.

Topographical EEG

There were no differences between the groups in the frequency of delta, theta, alpha and

Table 1. Recognition memory scores for the various groups.

Warrington Recognition Memory		
	Words	Faces
Male schizophrenia	93.60	79.20
Male controls	83.60	71.60
Female schizophrenia	79.60	48.20
Female controls	76.80	63.60

Group x Sex x Memory (F = 8.74, df = 1,16, p < 0.009)

beta I. In beta II there were significant elevations in patients in (1) eyes open directed unfocused attention, (2) recall of faces, and (3) left hand programmed movement. The results are shown in Figure 1 maps a, b, c.

Inspection of group means (Figure 1 f—k) indicate that two factors appeared to account for the group differences. Firstly, in controls there was a focal reduction in activity in the region of maximum difference. Secondly, in patients there was a posterior rim of elevated activity which overlapped with the region of difference. Probability maps comparing eyes closed with the task-relevant condition confirmed that there was a dynamic decrease in beta II in controls and that the effect was absent in patients; probability maps are shown only for the directed attention condition comparisons (Figure 1 d, e.).

Discussion

The results, though preliminary, are consistent with the theoretical predictions based on our view of cerebral asymmetry of function in schizophrenia. They are also consistent with previous reports on elevations in fast frequency activity in schizophrenia. By coupling EEG topographical mapping with neuropsychological testing, the present results contribute to the validation of localisation and shed light on mechanisms responsible for information processing abnormalities in schizophrenia. They indicate that functional activation

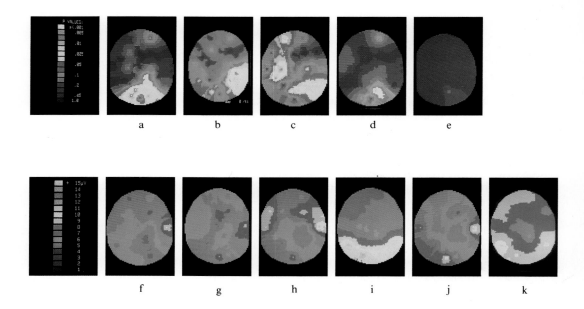

Figure 1. Maps depicting t-test probabilities — patients versus controls for (a) directed attention, (b) recall of faces, (c) left hand programmed movement; eyes closed versus eyes open directed attention controls (d) and patients (e); beta II spectral maps (controls left/patients right) for directed attention (f, g), recognition of faces (h, i) and left hand movements (j, k). The probability scale is one-tailed.

conditions are more sensitive than the resting state to the differentiation of schizophrenic patients from controls. These issues will be elaborated in turn.

In line with predictions based on the Hemisphere Imbalance Syndrome model the major effects were found in the face recognition task and the left hand programmed movement task, both tasks necessitating right hemispheric involvement, a requirement not necessary in the case of the right hand task or in word recognition. In this study, patients were all characterized by the Active Syndrome in which functional activation is greater in the left hemisphere than in the right, so that losses of function arise in tasks involving the right hemisphere or in tasks requiring interhemispheric coordination where right hemispheric participation is critical. A further test of the model will require examination of patients in the Withdrawn syndrome where left hemispheric losses of function would be predicted.

Previous authors have reported elevations in fast frequency activity in schizophrenia. Finley (1944) observed high amplitude activity above 20 Hz in the EEG tracings of 25—40% of undrugged schizophrenic patients. Lester and Edwards (1966) also observed this activity in more than 50% of schizophrenic patients withdrawn from drugs for three months or longer. It was present in the waking record and in REM sleep where muscle activity was inhibited and sometimes the amount of high amplitude beta in the awake record predicted the amount of activity in sleep. In studies including other psychiatric and neurological conditions they concluded that "the most clear cut association of the activity is with conditions associated with a psychotic disorder, a history of psychotic illness, and an immediate family history of mental illness." Furthermore "7 of the 8 alcoholic subjects with maximal activity had a history of alcoholic hallucinations or delusions of delirium tremens 1—8 months prior to the studies. However, none of these subjects were clearly psychotic at the time of the study." These observations indicate that the high amplitude beta phenomenon warrants study as a vulnerability trait for psychosis.

Flor-Henry (1983) also found excess 20—50 Hz activity in schizophrenia, in his case this was in the left temporal region. Coincidentally there was an excess of left sided activity from the masseter and temporalis muscles. In his review of evidence he concluded that only some of the excess beta could be attributed to muscle activity. This is also the implication of the sleep study of Lester and Edwards (1966) where the high amplitude beta activity persisted in the REM phase of sleep in which muscle activity is inhibited. Evidence from our study suggests that an explanation in terms of myogenic activity is also unlikely. As can be seen in Figure 1, the topography of beta II varies between tests even though postural and motor requirements of the tasks were identical, e. g., compare word association, word recall, face acquisition and face recall.

Another possible artefact is neuroleptic medication. In the literature both prior to computerized analysis of EEG (Gibbs & Gibbs, 1961) and subsequent to it (Fink, 1978) there is, however, complete agreement on the fact that neuroleptics, even when they induce drowsiness, which often accompanies high amplitude beta as is discussed below, do not produce increases in beta, on the contrary, beta activity is often reduced by neuroleptics.

Consideration of the significance and correlates of elevations in beta power may shed light on the nature and mechanisms responsible for the processing deficits in schizophrenia. Beta activity has been shown to reflect at least two factors. One factor is the EEG arousal response which occurs when attention is deployed to a stimulus or task. This is characterised by the blocking of the alpha rhythm which is replaced by low-amplitude fast-frequency desynchronised activity. In contrast, another factor is characterised by high amplitude fast frequency activity. This may accompany excitement and anxiety (Kennard et al., 1955; Lester & Edwards, 1966) or drowsiness (Gibbs & Gibbs, 1961), in which case it is indicative of depressed cognitive activity. Unfortunately the measurement of EEG power in this study, the magnitude of which is a function of both frequency of occurrence and amplitude, does not distinguish between these factors. Notwithstanding,

the issue is elucidated by inspection of the group means and the dynamic changes in beta that are seen when the eyes closed EEG is compared with the task related EEG. Here it can be seen that in schizophrenia there is no dynamic shift towards a reduction in beta power as may accompany the reduction in amplitude that occurs with the arousal response, a reduction that does occur in controls.

An extensive body of research has shown that it is the thalamo-cortical system which is responsible for the EEG arousal response especially when the cortical location corresponds to areas of neuropsychological relevance, such as the right posterior region for directed attention, face recognition and right hand movements, and the left anterior region for motor programming. If our interpretation is correct, it is the thalamo-cortical mechanism which appears deficient in schizophrenic patients with the Active syndrome when right hemispheric processing and the integration of right with left hemispheric processing is required. In view of the importance of dopaminergic function in the antipsychotic effects of neuroleptics, it is noteworthy that a clear influence of mesencephalic dopamine from the ventral tegmental area has been identified in the control of focused attention in the beta rhythms that accompany EEG arousal response (Bouyer et al., 1986).

Another factor that contributes to the topographical difference between the groups in beta II is seen in the distinctive topographical patterns of beta activity which extend beyond the regions in which the putative EEG arousal response occurs. These may well reflect the high amplitude beta phenomenon earlier documented in schizophrenia. It is noteworthy that one class of symptoms previously shown to be an accompaniment of high amplitude beta includes excitement and anxiety. These symptoms are both important components of the Active syndrome which characterised the patients (Gruzelier & Manchanda, 1982; Gaebel et al., 1986; Gruzelier & Wilson, in prep.).

The significance of beta activity for information processing and for psychopathology requires further investigation. The results presented here are preliminary and are part of an ongoing study comparing Active and Withdrawn syndrome patients subdivided further by chronicity, gender, handedness, medication and psychiatric status. The interesting gender differences in the face recognition task, in which female schizophrenic patients were significantly inferior to male patients, will await a larger number of subjects prior to detailed examination. In conclusion the study has shown the value of incorporating neuropsychological testing into studies of brain imaging with EEG neuropsychological testing. This provides a controlled procedure for the functional activation of the EEG and assists in the validation of the topographical abnormalities and elucidation of their functional significance. The EEG findings in turn hold promise of helping to understand the nature of the processing deficiencies.

References

Andrews HB, House AO, Cooper JE, Barber C (1986) The predicition of abnormal evoked potentials in schizophrenic patients by means of symptom pattern. *Brit Psychiat, 149,* 46–50.

Andrews HB, Cooper JE, Barber C, Raine A (1987) Early somatosensory evoked potentials in schizophrenia: Symptom pattern, clinical outcomes and interhemispheric functioning. In Takahashi R, Flor-Henry P, Gruzelier J, Niwa SI (Eds.) *Cerebral dynamics, laterality and psychopathology.* Elsevier, Amsterdam.

Annett M (1970) Classification of hand preference by association analysis. *Brit J Psychol, 61,* 303–321.

Bouyer JJ, Montaron MF, Fabre-Thorpe N, Rougeul A (1986) Compulsive attentive behaviour after lesions of the ventral striatum in the cat: A behavioural and electrophysiological study. *Exp. Neurol, 92,* 698–712.

Fink M (1978) EEG and psychopharmacology. In Cobb W A, Duijn V (Eds.) *Contemporary clinical neuropsychology (EEG), Suppl No. 34 L.* Seville Scientific Publishing Company, Amsterdam, 41–56.

Finley KH (1944) On occurrence of rapid frequency potential changes in human electroencephalogram. *Am J Psychiat, 101,* 194–200.

Flor-Henry P (1983) *Cerebral basis of psychopathology.* John Wright, London.

Gaebel W, Ulrich G, Frick K (1986) Eye-movement research with schizophrenic patients and normal controls using corneal reflection-pupil centre measurement. *Eur Arch Psych Neurol Sci, 235,* 243–254.

Gibbs FA, Gibbs EL (1961) Clinical and pharmacological correlates of fast activity in electroencephalography. *J Neuropsychiat, 3,* 573–578.

Gruzelier, JH (1983) A critical assesment and integration of lateral asymmetries in schizophrenia. In Myslobodsky M (Ed.) *Hemisyndromes, psychology, biology, neurology and psychiatry,* Academic Press, New York, 265–326.

Gruzelier JH (1984) Hemispheric imbalances in schizophrenia. *Int J Psychophysiol, 1,* 227–240.

Gruzelier JH (1987) Commentary on neuropsychological and information processing deficits in psychosis and neuro-psychophysiological syndrome relationship in schizophrenia. In Takahashi, R, Flor-Henry P, Gruzelier J, Niwa S (Eds.) *Cerebral dynamics, laterality and psychopathology.* Elsevier Science Publishers, Amsterdam, 23–54.

Gruzelier JH, Manchanda R (1982) The syndrome of schizophrenia: Relations between electrodermal response, lateral asymmetries and clinical ratings. *Brit J Psychiat, 141,* 488–495.

Gruzelier JH, Liddiard D (1988, in press) The neuropsychology of schizophrenia in the context of topographical mapping of electroencephalographic activity. In Maurer K (Ed.) *Topographic brain mapping of EEG and evoked potentials.* Springer-Verlag, Heidelberg, New York.

Gruzelier JH, Wilson L (in preparation) *The Hemisphere Imbalance Syndrome Rating Scale.*

Gruzelier JH, Seymour K, Wilson L, Jolley A, Hirsch S (1987) Neuropsychological evidence for hippocampal and frontal impairments in schizophrenia, mania and depression. In Takahashi R, Flor-Henry P, Gruzelier J, Niwa S-I (Eds.) *Cerebral dynamics, laterality and psychopathology.* Elsevier Science Publishers, Amsterdam 273–286.

Kennard MA, Ribanovitch MS, Fister WP (1955) The use of frequency analysis in the interpretation of the EEGs of patients with psychological disorders. *Electroenceph clin Neurophysiol, 7,* 29–38

Lester BK, Edwards RJ (1966) EEG fast activity in schizophrenic and control subjects. *J Neuropsychiat, 2,* 143–156.

Takahashi R, Flor-Henry P, Gruzelier J, Niwa SI (Eds.) (1987) *Cerebral dynamics, Laterality and Psychopathology.* Elsevier Science Publishers, Amsterdam.

Warrington EK (1984) *Recognition Memory Test Manual.* NFER-Nelson, Windsor.

Topographic Mapping of Auditory Evoked P300 in Psychiatric Disorders

K. Maurer, T. Dierks, R. Ihl

There is abundant evidence that, compared to normal controls, psychiatric patients suffering from psychosis and dementia demonstrate EP abnormalities. Of special interest in psychiatry is the late cognitive component P300 that is elicited by stimuli in any modality that are both relevant to the subject and surprising. In the present study normal persons and patients suffering from schizophrenia, depression and dementia fullfilling DSM-III and ICD-9 criteria were investigated. The EPs were recorded with a twenty channel brain mapping system (Brain Atlas III, Bio-logic Systems Corp.) For the group differences between normals and patients the t-test and two-way analysis of variance (ANOVA) were calculated. There were differences in P300 topography between schizophrenics, depressed and demented patients and controls. In schizophrenics localized P300 amplitude alterations have been found frontally and temporally, which supports the hypothesis that frontal and temporal lobe dysfunction may be one of various pathological processes relevant to our understanding of schizophrenia. In dementia the most prominent findings were increased bifrontal amplitudes and a decrease in parietotemporal areas. After ingestion of phosphatidylserine P300 amplitudes increased. Findings are discussed in order to delineate the advantage of the noninvasive P300 topography.

P300 is a well defined positive wave which appears in the late latency range between 200 and 400 ms. The wave is less dependent upon stimulus qualities such as intensity and frequency than upon psychophysiological conditions such as concentration, attention, ability to count and others. It can be elicited only if the person under investigation cooperates. In our stimulus context the person had to recognize and count the rare occurrences of a high-pitched tone (target stimulus).

It has been shown in animal studies, depth recordings in man and magnetencephalographic studies (Halgren et al., 1982; Okada et al., 1983) that the P300 originates probably not only in the cortex but also in subcortical structures, namely, in the hippocampus and nucleus amygdalae. Since hippocampal and parahippocampal structures play an important role in our understanding of memory function and pathogenesis of dementia and psychoses, our interest has been focused upon P300 topography in diseases where we suppose a hippocampal change of structure and function.

In the following study we investigated patients suffering from senile dementia of Alzheimer's type (SDAT) and patients with schizophrenia and depression. Another area of application of P300 topography is psychopharmacology. It will be shown by a study in volunteers that P300 can be augmented in amplitude by the nootropic substance phosphatidylserine.

Methods and Subjects

In order to delineate the auditory evoked P300 and topography we recorded auditory evoked potentials (AEP) due to frequent low-pitched (1000 Hz, 80 dB, non-target) and infrequent high-pitched (2000 Hz, 80 dB, tar-

Department of Psychiatry, University of Würzburg, 8700 Würzburg, F. R. G.

get) tones. The tones had a duration of 50 ms, rise and fall times of 10 ms and were presented in a random sequence with a probability of 20% of hearing the infrequent high pitched tone (target stimulus). The subjects had been carefully instructed at the beginning of each experiment. They were asked to pay attention to the target stimulus and to count its occurrences. At the end of the experiment the number of target stimuli counted by the subjects and those delivered by the computer were compared. In this study results will be described only from patients who were able to perform the P300-task properly. The electrical activity of the brain was recorded by 20 elec-

trodes applied to the scalp according to the 10-20 system. Two linked mastoid electrodes served as reference. The analog data obtained from the 20 electrodes were AD-converted and processed into topographical maps of electrical field distribution by means of linear interpolation. For baseline definition a pre-delay interval of 220 ms duration was used. Further analysis involved the construction of group averages and t-value maps (hybridic t-test procedure). The test allows the delineation of areas of differences between peak amplitude values of P300 obtained from controls and patients. Negative t-values (blue and green colors in Figure 1) indicate an area with

Figure 1. Topography of P300 amplitudes in normals and psychiatric patients. In the left column (a–e) head formats of topography of P300 amplitudes of controls are shown. The amplitude scale indicates values between -15 (blue) and $+15$ (red) µV. In the middle column head formats of topography of P300 amplitudes of the patient groups are shown (same amplitude scale), whereas the right column shows maps of t-values to delineate differences between normals and patients. Positive t-values are indicated by red and yellow and negative t-values by green and blue colors. The scale of t-values ranges from $+3.1$ to -3.1. The three head formats in part f of the figure represent the topographical display of P300 amplitudes.

First row (a)

a) *Left:* P300 amplitude topography in eight elderly controls (mean age: 74.2 years). At points P3, Pz, P4 amplitudes of 10 µV could be measured. *Middle:* P300 amplitude topography in 8 SDAT patients (mean age: 70.8 years). Frontally higher amplitudes and in temporal, parietal and occipital areas lower amplitudes were measured compared to controls. *Right:* t-value map exhibiting the difference between normals and SDAT patients. The higher frontal amplitudes could be varified by positive t- values (red color) and the lower parietal, temporal and occipital amplitudes by negative t-values (green and blue colors).

Second row (b, c and d)

Left single map: P300 topography in 10 adult controls (mean age 28.8 years)

b) *Middle:* P300 topography in 10 hebephrenic patients (mean age 25.5 years) with lower frontal amplitudes. *Right:* t-value map exhibiting the difference between normals and hebephrenic patients with signs of "hypofrontality." The lower frontal amplitudes could be verified by negative t-values (blue color).

c) *Middle:* P300 topography in ten paranoid patients (mean age 28.7 years) with lower parietotemporal amplitudes. *Right:* t-value map exhibiting the difference between normals and paranoid patients with signs of right temporoparietal hypofunction (blue color).

d) *Middle:* P300 topography in ten residual patients (mean age 41.2 years) with lower parietotemporal amplitudes. *Right:* t-value map exhibiting the difference between normals and residual patients with signs of temporoparietal hypofunction.

Third row (e)

e) *Left:* P300 topography in ten adult controls (mean age 43.8 years). *Middle:* P300 topography in ten patients suffering from major depression (mean age: 45.9 years) with lower parietal amplitudes. *Right:* t-value map exhibiting the difference between normals and depressed patients with signs of a slight parietal decrement (blue color).

Fourth row (f):

f) *Left:* P300 topography in 6 volunteers (mean age 26.3 years) after application of 60 mg phosphatidylserine. *Middle:* P300 topography 60 minutes after drug administration with an increase of P300 amplitude at Pz in the order of 5 µV. *Right:* P300 topography 120 minutes after drug administration; same pattern as in the left part of the figure.

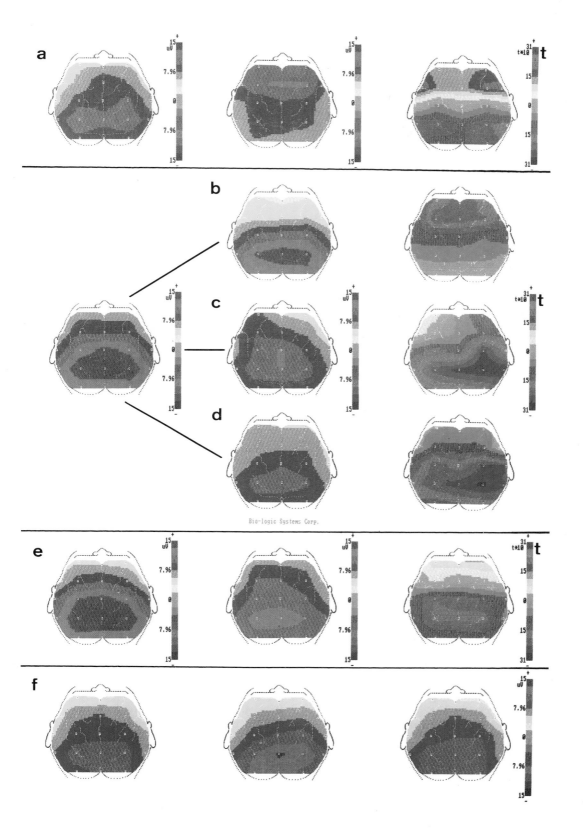

Bio-logic Systems Corp.

lower and positive t-values (red and yellow colors) an area with higher amplitudes. In elderly controls and SDAT-patients a two way analysis of variance (ANOVA) was calculated.

Ten adult control subjects (mean age 28.8 years) and ten elderly controls (mean age 74.2 years) with no history of neurologic or psychiatric illness were investigated. Patients were

a) 8 persons diagnosed as having SDAT,
b) 30 schizophrenic patients, ten clasified as being of the disorganized subtype (DSM-III, ICD-9: 295.1), ten of the paranoid subtype (DSM III, ICD-9: 295.3) and ten of the residual subtype (DSM III, ICD-9: 295.6).
c) 10 persons suffering form major depression (DSM III, ICD-9: 296.1, 296.3, 296.4 and 300.4).

All patients were right-handed. In 6 volunteers the P300 was recorded after parental administration of a single dose of 60 mg phosphatidylserine.

Results

The P300 topography of controls and patients is shown on Figure 1 a–e. The left side head formats exhibit group means of P300 of the age-matched controls. In the middle, group means of patients are shown, whereas the maps on the right side delineate the topography of t-values. Figure 1f shows P300 group means before and 60 and 120 minutes after phosphatidylserine administration.

SDAT-Patients

In elderly controls the topography of P300 was similar to that observed in younger normals. The amplitudes were lower in the range of about 5 μV in the parietal area (Figure 1a, left head format). The P300 fields in SDAT patients showed higher amplitude values bifrontally, no central change, and an amplitude loss over the temporal, parietal and occipital areas on both sides (Figure 1a, middle head format). The t-value maps were able to illustrate the regional differences topographically. Positive bifrontal t-values were found, whereas negative t-values were obtained in parietal, temporal and occipital areas. The bifrontal increase of P300 amplitude (red colors in the t-value map of Figure 1a) was significant as could be shown by ANOVA ($p < .01$).

Schizophrenic Patients

The single left head format in Figure 1b, c, and d shows P300 topography in an age-matched control group (28.8 years). The pattern was maximally positive at points P3, Pz and P4 with an amplitude decrement towards frontal and temporal structures. All schizophrenic subgroups had a generalized amplitude reduction. In the hebephrenic subgroup, however, a low frontal field with amplitude values around zero was measured (Figure 1b, middle head format). The t-value map (Figure 1b, right head format) confirmed the frontal decrement by its negative t-values (blue colors). The amplitudes were significantly lower at electrode sites F3, Fz, F4 ($.01 < p < .05$) The paranoid subgroup had a lateralized P300 pattern with lower amplitudes over the right temporoparietal lobes where negative t-values could be measured (Figure 1c, middle and right head format). The amplitudes were significantly lower at electrode sites P4 ($p < .01$) and Cz, C4, P3, Pz, T6 ($.01 < p < .05$). A similar pattern could be observed in the residual subgroup. The P300 distribution was less lateralized but also showed lower amplitudes mainly in the left temporo-parital area (Figure 1d, middle head format) with negative t-values (Figure 1d, right head format). The amplitudes were significantly lower at electrodes C3, Cz, C4, P3, Pz, P4, T4, T6 ($.01 < p < .05$).

Major Depressive Disorder

The left head format shows the P300 distribution in an age-matched control group (Figure 1e, left head format). In the middle row of P300 maps, a slight symmetrical decrease of P300 is evident over the parietal cortex; this was also confirmed by negative t-values (Figure 1e, right head format). The decrease of P300 amplitudes, however, was not significant.

Topographic Pharmaco-AEP 300

Decreased P300s have been found in psychiatric diseases monitored in this way to date. There are also pharmacologically induced conditions in normals where an increase of P300 at the cortex could be measured. This was the case at point Pz after administration of 60 mg of phosphatidylserine (Figure 1f, middle head format), where an amplitude increase of 5 µV could be observed ($.01 < p < .05$).

Discussion

If one takes into consideration the two assumed sources of P300, the hippocampus and the cortex, the P300 pattern in SDAT patients with a frontal increment and a parietotemporal decrement could be explained in two ways. According to measurements by Okada et al. (1983), a deep hippocampal dipole can be assumed to be responsible for the P300 fields. SDAT is known to involve a degeneration of nerve cells in hippocampal and parahippocampal structures (Ball et al., 1985). If, in SDAT patients, lesions occur in the posterior portion of the hippocampus, a shift and/or other changes of the dipole can be assumed to be responsible for the change in P300 observed and consecutive for the higher frontal amplitudes.

Considering the contribution of cortical neurons to P300 generation, the abnormal P300 pattern could be determined by lesions in temporal, parietal and occipital cortical areas. This would be in line with numerous studies where the same lesion pattern has been described by means of neuropathology, cerebral blood flow and glucose metabolism (Brun & Gustafson, 1976; Stigsby et al., 1981; Friedland et al., 1983). Brain imaging thus leads us to assume a pattern of posterior hippocampal and temporoparietal cortical involvement in dementia. In this context studies by Stigsby et al. (1981) are of interest, where the term "hyperfrontality" was used to describe the phenomenon of a selectively preserved frontal function in this disease.

In schizophrenia, P300 topography revealed a totally different pattern compared to that obtained in SDAT patients. There were signs of "hypofrontality" in the hebephrenic subgroup and signs of an underactivation on the right side and a relative overactivation on the left side in the paranoid subroup. The results in the residual subgroup showed less laterality. It is of interest that other functional imaging procedures such as rCBF and PET support the hypothesis of "hypofrontality." This may be interpreted as a further indication that frontal lobe dysfunction is an important factor in our understanding of schizophrenia (Ingvar & Franzen, 1974; Farkas et al., 1984). The reduction in P300 amplitude in the right posterior temporoparietal area of paranoid schizophrenics is consistent with research by Gruzelier et al. (1988), who found in paranoid schizophrenics evidence of reduced right temporal functioning by using neuropsychological tests of learning and long-term memory. The results in the residual subgroup cannot be interpreted at present in terms of over- and/or underactivation of one hemisphere. It may be of interest that Gruzelier et al. (1988) found that patients with negative symptoms in the learning and memory test showed either left sided or bilateral impairment. The findings in depressives need no further discussion since t-values did not indicate significant changes compared to those obtained in controls.

Results of an augmentation of P300 amplitude after administration of 60 mg phosphatidylserine suggest a reversible change in acetylcholine and/or dopamine turnover induced by the drug. There is no way of knowing at present whether the cholinergic or the dopaminergic system is more involved since we have to expect a P300 increase in both conditions. It is known, however, by the work of Bruni and Toffano (1982) that phosphatidylserine interferes with the dopamine uptake which undergoes an increase in limbic and paralimbic structures.

To summarize, P300 topography opens up a new field of electrodiagnosis in psychiatry and neuropsychology extending beyond conventional recordings with a limited number of electrodes. Our multichannel approach in combination with mapping augmented the specificity of findings and even allowed differentiation between dementia and psychoses. It is hoped that the reliability of the P300 test and its topography will remain so consistent that P300 can be regarded as a biological marker pointing to structural and/or functional lesions in psychiatric diseases.

References

Ball MJ, Hatchinski V, Fox A, Kirshe AJ, Fishman M, Blume W, Kral UA, Fox A (1985) A new definition of Alzheimer's disease: A hippocampal dementia. *Lancet,* Feb. 2, 14—16.

Brun A, Gustafson L (1976) Distribution of cerebral degeneration in Alzheimer's disease. *Arch Psychiatr Neur, 223,* 15—33.

Bruni A, Toffano G (1982) The principles of phospholipid pharmacology. In Antolini et al. (Eds.) *Transport in biomembranes: Model systems and reconstruction.* Raven Press, New York, 235—242.

Farkas T, Wolf AP, Jaeger J, Brodie JD, Christman DR, Fowler JS (1984) Regional brain glucose metabolism in chronic schizophrenia. *Arch Gen Psychiat, 41,* 293—300.

Friedland RP, Budinger TF, Ganz E, Yano Y, Mathis CA, Koss B, Ober BA, Huesman RH, De-renzo SE (1983) Regional cerebral metabolic alteration in dementia of the Alzheimer type: Positron emmission tomography with Fluorodeoxy-glucose. *J. Comp Assist Tomogr, 7,* 590—598.

Gruzelier J, Liddiard D (1988, in press) The neurophysiology of schizophrenia in the context of topographic mapping of electrocortical activity. In Maurer, K. (Ed.) *Topographic brain mapping of EEG and evoked potentials.* Springer-Verlag, Heidelberg, New York.

Halgren E, Squires NK, Wilson CL, Crandall PH (1982) Brain generators of evoked potential: The late (endogenous) components. *Bull Los Angeles Neurol Soc, 47,* 108—123.

Ingvar DH, Franzen G (1974) Abnormalities of cerebral blood flow distribution in patients with chronic schizophrenia. *Acta Psychiat Scand, 40,* 425—462.

Okada YC, Kaufman L, Williamson SJ (1983) The hippocampal formation as a source of the slow endogenous potentials. *Electroenceph clin Neurophysiol, 55,* 417—426.

Stigsby B, Johanneson G, Ingvar D (1981) Regional EEG anlysis and regional cerebral blood flow in Alzheimer's disease. *Electroenceph clin Neurophysiol, 51,* 537—547.

Pattern Differences in Two-Dimensional EEG Maps During Mental Calculation

J. Tatsuno

In order to evaluate objectively differences in EEG topographical distributions, the Mahalanobis' distance (Q value) was calculated using polynomial coefficient vectors. These were obtained by means of an unbiased polynomial interpolation procedure applied to the values of picture elements of individual EEG maps representing four-second epochs. The larger the Q value, the more distinct the differences between the topographical maps. The validity of this evaluation method was tested by comparing various isopotential maps obtained during mental calculation; the comparisons were made between maps of poor (or worst) and good (or best) calculators and maps of the distribution of different frequency bands were compared.

In order to assess two-dimensional EEG maps it is important to be able to compare them in an objective way. We have developed such a method (Ashida, 1986; Ashida et al., 1984) and applied it in a number of preliminary studies (Takao et al., 1988; Tatsuno, 1988; Tatsuno et al., 1988). It consists in the use of polynomial coefficients (PCs) obtained according to the unbiased polynomial interpolation procedure. This procedure is applied to calculate the values of the picture elements in the EEG maps. The PCs contain the information on both amplitude and location. A set of PCs corresponds to one pattern of the map. Therefore one group of PCs represents one group of individual maps. When two groups are to be compared, the Mahalanobis' distance in multidimensional space is calculated. In this way the degree of difference between two patterns is represented.

In this report various two-dimensional EEG maps obtained under different mental conditions were used and compared using this procedure. The aim of this study was to determine whether EEG maps recorded from normal subjects differed according to their ability to perform mental calculation.

Material and Method

Sixteen healthy medical students 20 to 22 years old were the subjects of this study. They were all male and right-handed. According to their performance in mental calculation, they were divided into two groups: poor calculators (9 subjects) and good calculators (7 subjects). The three worst calculators and the three best calculators were selected for comparison in this study.

Twelve electrodes were placed at Fp1, Fp2, F7, Fz, F8, C3, C4, T5, Pz, T6, O1, O2 according to 10–20 International System. The subjects were instructed to lie on a bed with their eyes closed. The EEGs were recorded using connected ear lobe electrodes as reference. Following a period of three minutes where a resting EEG recording was taken, the subjects were assigned the task, mentally subtracting 7 from a given number of 3 digits (e.g., 876) for two minutes. Then the subtraction was stopped and the subject reported the result.

The EEG was A/D converted with a sampling rate of 256 Hz. The signals of the twelve channels were checked by the computer;

Department of Physiology, National Defense Medical College, 3–2 Namiki, Tokorozawa, Saitama 359, Japan.

those 4 second long epochs which contained the amplitudes above 70 microvolts in any channel were discarded as artifactual. Human inspection was also employed to discard artifacts (e.g., EMG, etc.). Spectral analysis of each 4 second epoch was carried out using FFT. The square root of the power was calculated with 0.25 Hz resolution. The average values of the square root of power within the alpha, beta, theta and delta band were computed. Thus the average value within the alpha band corresponds to the average of square root of power at 7.75, 8.0, 8.25, ... 13.0, 13.25, and 13.5 Hz. Similar calculations were done for the other frequency bands. Since 12 derivations were used we obtained 12 amplitude data. Using the unbiased polynomial interpolation procedure, $10(a_1...a_{10})$ PCs were calculated. The relation between the value at a location x, y and PCs is shown in the equation (1).

$$f(x,y) = a_1 + a_2x + a_3y + a_4x^2 + a_5xy + a_6y^2 + a_7x^3 + a_8x^2y + a_9xy^2 + a_{10}y^3 \quad (1)$$

where a_1, a_2, ... a_{10} are the polynomial coefficients. In this way a map was constructed by interpolation. In the final form a map contained 4989 elements. The coordinates x and y are as follows: The x-axis is the line connecting the preauricular points of both sides; the y-axis is the median line connecting nasion and inion. The origin is Cz. X values are negative to the left of Cz and positive to the right of Cz. Y values are positive anterior to Cz and negative posterior to Cz.

For each comparison of a pair of maps the Mahalanobis' distance (Q value) in ten-dimensional space was calculated. The larger the distance (the larger the Q value), the greater the difference of the maps.

The statistical value of Q can be assessed by using the common test criterion F. The value of F is related to Q and indicated in equation (2). It has the degree of freedom of $(q, g_1 + g_2 - q - 1)$, where q is the number of PCs (= 10) and g_1 and g_2 are the numbers of vectors of group 1 and 2.

$$F = \frac{(g_1 + g_2 - q - 1) g_1 g_2}{(g_1 + g_2 - 2)(g_1 + g_2) q} Q$$

Results

Figure 1 shows the average amplitude maps for four frequency bands of the three worst and three best calculators. Q values, F values and p values are shown between the worst and best calculators's maps.

An important difference between the topographical patterns of the worst and best calculators' was seen in the alpha maps. In the former, the decrease in amplitude values down to, or under, 4.0 is seen over a wider area which spreads medially around F7, while in the latter the corresponding area of low amplitude values was a narrow strip in anteropost-

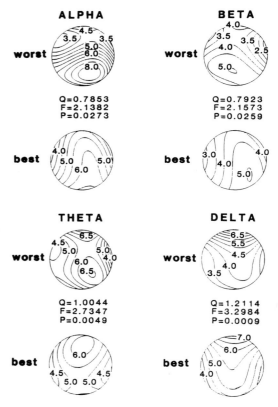

Figure 1. Average amplitude maps of the three worst and three best calculators for alpha, beta, theta and delta bands. In all maps, frontal is above and occipital is below; left is subject's left and right is subject's right. Numbers on isopotential lines in the maps indicate rms amplitudes in microvolts. Q, F and P values are shown in the spaces between two compared maps.

erior direction and laterally situated. We call here this area of decreased amplitude value the activation area. Another feature was that in the worst calculators an area of stronger activation was found also over the right hemisphere in an almost symmetrical position, though the area on the right was narrower than on the left. In the best calculators the activation area around F8 was negligible.

Concerning beta activity, the decrease in amplitude value was more conspicuous over the right temporal area in the worst calculators, while in the best calculators this was not observed. In the worst calculators the decrease in beta amplitude values was less pronounced over the left than over the right temporal area. In the best calculators such a decrease was only found over the left temporal area. Concerning theta activity in the worst calculators, amplitudes decreased in both anterior temporal areas on both sides, but in the best calculators the amplitude decreased down to the same level but over the more posterior temporal areas of both hemispheres. The area of the largest theta amplitude values was found at Fpz in the worst calculators, while in the best calculators it lay at Fz.

For both worst and best calculators, the area of the largest delta amplitude was located at Fpz, but in the best calculators the area over which large amplitudes were found spread in the occipital direction.

The Q value for the comparison between the worst and best calculators was the smallest in the alpha band, corresponding to p value of 0.0273. The Q and p values for the beta band were similar to those of the alpha band. The Q values of the theta and delta bands were larger than those of the alpha and beta bands.

Figure 2 shows the average maps of nine poor and seven good calculators for the four frequencies. The main features were quite similar to those in Figure 1, although the differences were less pronounced.

The Q value for the alpha band was the smallest, similar to that seen in the worst vs best comparison. The statistical significance of the difference was at the level of about 1.5%.

The Q values for the theta, beta and delta bands were almost equal, and were larger than

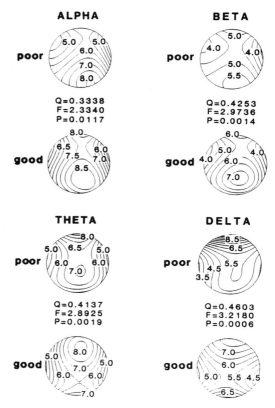

Figure 2. Average amplitude maps of nine poor and seven good calculators for alpha, beta, theta and delta bands.

that of the alpha band. The p values were much smaller that those of alpha band (p = 0.0019).

The large Q value of the beta band appeared to be mainly related to amplitude differences between the two maps. The large Q observed between the two maps of the theta band seemed to be mainly determined by different locations of the maximal amplitude area. The main difference between the maps for the delta band appeared to be the large amplitude in the frontopolar area in the poor calculators.

It must be noted that a direct comparison of Q values in Figure 1 and in Figure 2 is meaningless because of the difference in the size of the data and thus in number of degrees of freedom.

From formula (1) it can be understood that the first PC (a_1) is the term of the general level of amplitude. If this level is to be omitted, the Q value based on the other nine PCs (Q9: a_2 to a_{10}) should be considered. When laterality is considered, PCs related to the x-axis should be used (Qx: a_2, a_4, a_5, a_7, a_8, a_9). When an anteroposterior difference is discussed, such as delta dominance in the frontal area, PCs related to the y-axis should be used (Qy: a_3, a_5, a_6, a_8, a_9, a_{10}).

Table 1 shows these four Q values. The influence of a_1 which corresponds to the general level of amplitude can be examined by comparing Q10 and Q9. For the worst versus best calculators, the a_1, influence was smaller in the alpha and the beta band than in the theta and the delta band. This means that between the two groups of subjects there were less differences in the general level of amplitude for the higher (beta and alpha) than for the lower (theta and delta) frequency bands. As regards Qx, which can be considered a measure of the influence of laterality, the largest value was observed in the beta band. This corresponds to the fact that the maximal and minimal amplitude values of the beta band were found over in opposite locations (Figure 1). As regards Qy, which can be considered a measure of anteroposterior asymmetry, we may note that the higher frequency bands

(alpha and beta) show less anteroposterior differences than the lower bands (theta and delta).

The comparisons between poor and good calculators showed a similar general tendency as for the worst versus best groups. Here the a_1 influence was the smallest in the beta band. Concerning Qx, the low value in the theta band indicated a very small lateral difference, while the large values in the beta band corresponded to the fact that beta presented much larger amplitudes over the right than over the left hemisphere in the good calculators. Concerning Qy, the larger values were observed for the theta and the delta bands. These values may correspond to the fact that these activities presented frontal dominance in the poor calculators.

Table 2 shows Q values of the pattern differences of the maps for different frequency bands in the worst and best calculators. Here low Q values were found in the alpha-beta relationship, while large Q values were found in the alpha-delta and the beta-delta relationship.

Table 3 shows the results of the same analysis for poor and good calculators. Almost identical conclusions can be drawn as from Table 2.

Poor vs good calculators

d.f.	Q10 (10,283)	Q9 (9,284)	Qx (6,287)	Qy (6,287)
alpha	0.3338	0.2835	0.2352	0.1375
beta	0.4253	0.4249	0.3239	0.2632
theta	0.4137	0.3737	0.1070	0.3155
delta	0.4603	0.4222	0.2554	0.3679

Worst vs best calculators

d.f.	Q10 (10,108)	Q9 (9,109)	Qx (6,112)	Qy (6,112)
alpha	0.7853	0.7549	0.3330	0.5323
beta	0.7923	0.7308	4995	0.5276
theta	1.0044	0.6401	0.3023	0.6346
delta	1.2115	0.7749	0.2806	0.7260

Table 1. Q values from ten PCs (Q10), Q values from nine PCs (Q9), Q values x-related (Qx) and Q values y-related (Qy) for four bands of poor vs good calculators and worst vs best calculators. d.f. = degree of freedom.

worst calculators	alpha	beta	theta	delta
		degree of freedom (10,63)		
alpha	x x / x / x x	Q= 0.5645 / F= 0.9138 / p= 0.52633	Q= 1.6855 / F= 2.7285 / p= 0.00748	Q= 3.5250 / F= 5.7061 / p= 0.00000
beta	Q= 0.4822 / F= 1.6983 / p= 0.08678	x x / x / x x	O= 1.7394 / F= 2.8157 / p= 0.00597	Q= 3.8656 / F= 6.2575 / p= 0.00000
theta	Q= 0.6102 / F= 2.1491 / p= 0.02448	Q= 1.0129 / F= 3.5673 / p= 0.00031	x x / x / x x	Q= 0.9066 / F= 1.4676 / p= 0.17285
delta	Q= 1.5160 / F= 5.3392 / p= 0.00000	Q= 1.4510 / F= 5.1104 / p= 0.00000	Q= 0.5047 / F= 1.7776 / p= 0.07004	x x / x / x x
best calculators		degree of freedom (10,139)		

Table 2. Q values, F values, p values for the comparison of isopotential maps for two of four frequency bands of the three worst calculators (in upper diagonal) and the three best calculators (in lower diagonal). p = 0.00000 indicates p value is less than 0.100000E-05.

poor calculators	alpha	beta	theta	delta
		degree of freedom (10,283)		
alpha	x x / x / x x	Q= 0.2540 / F= 1.5555 / p= 0.12071	Q= 0.9465 / F= 5.7959 / p= 0.00000	Q= 1.9619 / F=12.0130 / p= 0.00000
beta	Q= 0.3906 / F= 3.1728 / p= 0.00067	x x / x / x x	Q= 0.7128 / F= 4.3645 / p= 0.00001	Q= 1.5082 / F= 9.2350 / p= 0.00000
theta	Q= 0.6480 / F= 5.2300 / p= 0.00000	p= 0.8205 / F= 6.6655 / p= 0.00000	x x / x / x x	Q= 0.6458 / F= 3.9542 / p= 0.00005
delta	Q= 1.5232 / F=12.3742 / p= 0.00000	Q= 1.3233 / F=10.7499 / p= 0.00000	Q= 0.2783 / F= 2.2605 / p= 0.01452	x x / x / x x
good calculators		degree of freedom (10,323)		

Table 3. Q values, F values, p values for the comparison of isopotential maps for two of four frequency bands of nine poor calculators (in upper diagonal) and of seven good calculators (in lower diagonal). p = 0.00000 indicates p value is less than 0.100000E-05.

Discussion

In order to generate two-dimensional maps, several researchers have employed large numbers of electrodes. For example, 37 electrodes were used by Lehmann (1977), 40 by Darcey et al. (1980), and 30 by Thickbroom et al. (1984). Maps may also be calculated even using a smaller number of electrodes with the help of interpolation methods. One of these is the unbiased polynomial interpolation (UPI) procedure. This has the advantage that the electrodes can be irregularly placed, while other methods require the electrodes to be placed in a rectangular grid (Ueno et al., 1975). Recently Perrin et al. (1987) published a surface spline interpolation (SSI), akin to our method. A difference between our method and Perrin's is that the latter uses some factors to terminate the operations in case abnormal oscillations take place. However, in our experience such factors are dispensable.

UPI and SSI procedures also provide the possibility of representing one topographical pattern by a set of factors, as shown in the text. One set of PCs corresponds to one pattern. Furthermore, some PCs have an obvious meaning in relation to the pattern; for example, a_1 is related to the general level of the map.

A very important fact is that the difference between two maps can be calculated using the Mahalanobis' distance. In this way two groups of PC vectors from the two groups can be compared. In this report the validity of the method was tested using EEG data recorded during mental calculation.

A detailed discussion about the physiological meaning of the EEG topographical patterns characteristic of mental calculation cannot be given here. However, two general points may be made. First, the topographical differences between worst and best calculators or poor and good calculators were confirmed and the differences were objectively evaluted. Second, we found that the main differences between EEG maps of poor versus good or worst versus best mental calculators involved particularly the beta, theta and delta activities. A further discussion will appear in a separate report.

References

Ashida H (1986) Further consideration on EEG topographical by unbiased polynomial interpolation. *BOEI IKA DAIGAKKO ZASSHI (J Natl Def Med Coll), 11*, 85–95.

Ashida H, Tatsuno J, Okamoto J, Maru E (1984) Field mapping of EEG by unbiased polynomial interpolation. *Comp Biomed Res, 17*, 267–276.

Darcey TM, Ary JP, Fender DH (1980) Spatio-temporal visually evoked scalp potentials in response to partial-field patterned stimulation. *Electroenceph clin Neurophysiol, 50*, 348–355.

Lehmann D (1977) The EEG as scalp field distribution. In Rémond A (Ed.) *EEG informatics. A didactic review of methods and applications of EEG data processing.* Elsevier, Amsterdam/Oxford/New York, 365–384.

Perrin F, Pernier J, Bertrand O, Giard MH, Echallier JF (1987) Mapping of scalp potentials by surface spline interpolation. *Electroenceph clin Neurophysiol, 66*, 75–81.

Takao A, Suzuki H, Ozaki M, Fujita M, Tatsuno J, Ashida H (1986) Statistical evalution of topographical difference between thiopental sodium and diazepam fast waves. *Electroenceph clin Neurophysiol, 64*, (4), 83.

Tatsuno J (1988, in press) EEG laterality during mental functions evaluted by Mahalanobis' distance using polynomial coefficents of hemispherical two dimensional maps. In *Proceedings of the 3rd Symposium on Two-Dimensional EEG Maps.* Nyuron-sha, Tokyo.

Tatsuno J, Ohiwa M, Ozawa K (1988, in press) Topographical studies on the EEg changes in hyperbaric heliox environment during saturated dive into 200 feet. In *Proceedings of the 9th International Symposium on Underwater and Hyperbaric Physiology.* Undersea Medical Society, Inc., Bethesda.

Thickbroom GW, Mastaglia FL, Carroll WM (1984) Spatiotemporal mapping of evoked cerebral activity. *Electroenceph clin Neurophysiol, 59*, 425–431.

Ueno S, Matsuoka S, Mizoguchi T, Nagashima M, Cheng CL (1975) Topographic computer display of abnormal EEG activities in patients with CNS deseases. *Memoirs of Face Engin Kyushu Univ, 34*, 195–209.

Section IV

PET and SPECT Imaging and Bioelectrical Activity

Positron Emission Tomographic Studies of Aging and Dementia

K.L. Leenders

Positron emission tomography (PET) makes it possible to determine in a three-dimentional way certain aspects of human cerebral tissue functions *in vivo*. So far this applies mainly to regional energy metabolism and the striatal dopaminergic neurotransmitter system. Here, a short review is given of the PET studies concerning the effect of age and dementia on cerebral tissue values. The functional changes in brain occurring during normal aging differ distinctly from those found in demented patients. In the latter group, apart from a moderate to market global decrease in neuronal functioning, a characteristic focal pattern of cerebral functions is seen.

Many attempts have been made to discover which changes occur in the brain during aging and in association with dementia.

Post-mortem studies can provide precise measurements of certain components of brain tissue structure and composition. However, these reflect only one point in time and, in the case of dementia, death usually occurs after a longstanding illness. Also, post-mortem changes may influence the measurements. Therefore, there is a need for reliable *in vivo* measurements of brain tissue functions to make possible the performance of longitudinal studies in selected patients.

The first *in vivo* measurements were performed by Kety and Schmidt (1948). They used the nitrous oxide technique to determine hemispheric brain blood flow, oxygen and glucose utilisation. These authors reported a decline of these functions with age (Kety, 1956). At a later stage, this was confirmed for cerebral blood flow by many groups using ^{133}Xe washout techniques which allowed a more focal type of measurement. After that, positron emission tomography (PET) developed slowly during the seventies and early eighties. PET makes possible a quantitative and really three-dimensional measurement of many functions (see below). Although PET scanning is expected to solve certain issues concerning the effect of age on brain tissue metabolism, some confusing data have already been produced.

This chapter will briefly review the published PET reports concerning age effect and dementia. In addition, new results in a group of healthy subjects obtained in our laboratory will be discussed.

Positron Emission Tomography

General Features

PET uses a special type of radio-labelled tracers. After administration, either by intravenous injection or via inhalation, the distribution of radioactivity derived from the administered tracer is measured in absolute units across a transaxial section of the body. The regional distribution of tracer in the brain can be followed during minutes to hours, depending on the type of tracer and radionuclide attached to it. Mathematical models can then be applied to convert the measured radioactivity

MRC Cyclotron Unit, Hammersmith Hospital, Du Cane Road, London W12, UK

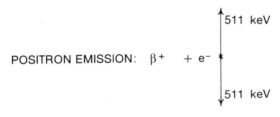

POSITRON EMISSION: β⁺ + e⁻

Figure 1. Diagram of positron emission resulting in two high energy gamma rays arising simultaneously and travelling in opposite directions.

into a specific tissue function, e.g., cerebral blood flow, oxygen or glucose utilisation, quantitation of blood-brain barrier transport, neurotransmitter precursor turnover, receptor densities. For general reference see Phelps et al. (1986).

A brief comment should be made about the radionuclides with which PET tracers are labelled. These radionuclides have a short life span and are usually isotopes of physiological atoms like oxygen-15 (physical half-life $(T_{1/2}) = \pm 2$ minutes) or carbon-11 $(T_{1/2} = \pm 20$ minutes). Fluorine-18 $(T_{1/2} = \pm 110$ minutes) is also a positron emitter and can often substitute hydrogen atoms. The short half-life makes it possible to administer a large signal while keeping the radiation dose low or acceptable. The fact that these radionuclides are physiological atoms makes it possible to incorporate them into chemicals without changing, or only slightly changing, the properties of these compounds. The third important feature of positron emitting nuclides is their characteristic mode of decay. This makes absolute quantitation possible. After emission of the positron (a positively charged particle with the mass of an electron) by the atom nucleus, it travels a short distance

and is then captured by an electron. The masses of the two particles are annihilated and converted into two high energy (511 keV) gamma rays, which arise simultaneously and travel in opposite directions (Figure 1). When two detectors are placed on opposite sides of the body (Figure 2), simultaneous stimulation of the detectors (coincidence event) indicates that a radionuclide decayed along the line between the two detectors. Multiple detectors placed around the body, as in Figure 3, constitute a system of precise electronic collimation of the signals emitted from the body. The distribution of radioactivity in the center of the field of view of a ring of detectors is especially clear.

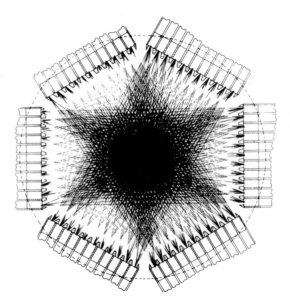

Figure 3. Diagram of a ring of detectors surrounding the body and defining a transaxial field of view. The numerous lines of coincidence allow accurate sampling of radioactivity.

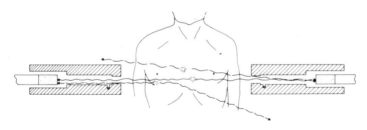

Figure 2. Diagram of two detectors placed on opposite sides of the body. Simultaneous stimulation of the two detectors is electronically recorded as a "coincidence event" and determines the line along which positron emission occurred.

Tracers for Measurement of Cerebral Energy Metabolism

Cerebral Glucose Utilization.

FDG (fluoro-deoxyglucose) is a glucose analogue (for review see Phelps et al., 1986), which is transported into the brain and enters the glycolytic pathway like glucose itself. However, after the first step, 6-phosporylation FDG cannot be metabolized further and is essentially trapped for the time of the PET scan. Several mathematical models can be applied to calculate from fluorine-18 (^{18}F) brain uptake the actual regional cerebral glucose consumption (CMR_{glu}) expressed as mg/100 g brain/min. For this, radioactivity in arterial blood after FDG administration has to be determined (arterial input curve). For a review of quantitation aspects, see Gjedde (1982).

Most PET studies on aging or dementia have used FDG. Although in principle glucose utilization can also be measured by carbon-11 labelled glucose, this tracer is still being explored and to my knowledge no systematic studies on aging or dementia have been reported so far.

Cerebral Blood Flow and Oxygen Utilization

Cerebral blood flow (CBF) and oxygen utilization ($CMRO_2$) are usually measured during the same procedure since oxygen-15 ($^{15}O_2$) labelled tracers can be used for both functions. After about 10 minutes continuous inhalation of $C^{15}O_2$, a steady state is reached of influx and outflow of $H_2^{15}O$ in brain which is directly related to tissue perfusion (Jones et al., 1976; Frackowiak et al., 1980a, 1980b). A simple mathematical model comparing regional tissue perfusion with arterial activity yields regional values of CBF.

Subsequent continuous inhalation of $^{15}O_2$ will equally result in steady state cerebral radioactivity distribution. Here, however, uptake of radioactivity is determined by oxygen extraction. Corrections need to be made for the signal from recirculating $H_2^{15}O$ and the non-extracted $^{15}O_2$ in the blood. The former can be established using the results of the $C^{15}O_2$ scan (Lammertsma et al., 1981, 1982) and the latter by using a third procedure, namely, a $C^{15}O$ or ^{11}CO scan (Lammertsma & Jones, 1983; Lammertsma et al., 1983; Pantano et al., 1985). The signal obtained from the last scan is derived from radio-labelled CO which adheres to hemoglobin. Regional cerebral blood volume values can be calculated from this (Phelps et al. 1979). The cerebral metabolic rate of oxygen ($CMRO_2$), which is also called oxygen utilisation, is calculated as: CBF × OER × arterial oxygen concentration (OER = oxygen extraction ratio). Figure 4 illustrates how the several functions can be displayed as quantitative images.

Dopaminergic Tracers

Radio-labelled ligands for the cerebral dopaminergic neurotransmitter system are available for both pre- and postsynaptic aspects of the transmitter system. L-^{18}F-fluorodopa (^{18}F-dopa) uptake can be used as an indicator of presynaptic dopamine turnover (Garnett et al., 1983; Leenders et al., 1985, 1986b), while

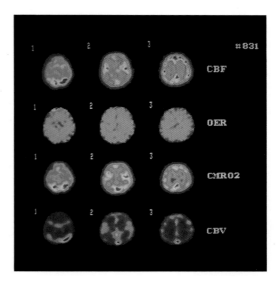

Figure 4. Quantitative images visualising the values of the functions CBF, OER, $CMRO_2$ and CBV measured in one healthy subject. See text. The left column (1) shows the images cutting through a lower level (cerebellum) of the brain. Columns 2 and 3 are two and four centimeters higher, respectively. The colour scale translates linearly the value of the displayed function, red indicating higher and blue lower values.

[11]C-N-methyl-spiperone (^{11}C-MSP) binds to dopamine D_2 receptors (in striatum mainly) and serotonin S_2 receptors (in cortex mainly) (Wagner et al., 1983; Fowler et al., 1986; Frost et al., 1987). See also Figure 5.

Recently, ^{11}C-raclopride was introduced as a specific ligand for D_2 receptors (Farde et al., 1985, 1986). Also, ^{11}C-nomifensine, which binds to presynaptic catecholamine re-uptake sites, was recently introduced (Aquilonius et al., 1987; Leenders et al., 1987). This tracer may prove useful as an indicator of striatal dopamine nerve terminal density and possibly thalamic noradrenergic nerve terminal density. Regional cerebral MAO-B enzyme concentrations may be assessed using the tracer ^{11}C-deprenyl (Fowler et al.,1987).

Most of these tracers need further validation—particularly the aspects of quantitation—before their usefulness for *in vivo* PET studies can be better defined. Since PET measures total radioactivity in a volume of brain tissue, the unravelling of the separate steps in the processing of the tracer compound in the tissue (Figure 6) needs to be performed by mathematical kinetic analysis. For this at least the time-activity curves of brain and arterial blood are required. Methods and problems of quantitation are discussed by Patlak et al. (1983) Patlak and Blasberg (1985), Wong et al. (1984), Farde et al. (1986), and Eckernäs et al. (1987).

The effect of age on the dopaminergic neurotransmitter system as measured by PET scanning has only been reported in one study using ^{11}C-MSP (Wong et al., 1984).

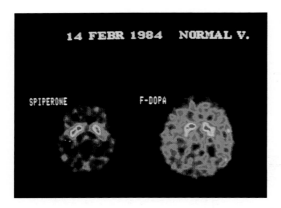

Figure 5a. Two images of the same healthy volunteer depicting (left) D_2 dopamine receptor binding and (right) ^{18}F-dopa uptake in a plane across the body of the striatum. Red in the colour scale indicates more radioactivity uptake.

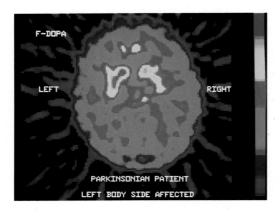

Figure 5b. ^{18}F-dopa uptake in patient with Parkinson's disease. The patient was more affected in his left body side. The right striatum shows less tracer uptake than the left.

Normal Values and Effect of Age

Cerebral Energy Metabolism

Under normal steady state conditions, CBF is proportional to the level of cerebral oxygen and glucose consumption (Sokoloff et al., 1977; LeBrun-Grandier et al., 1983). Glucose and oxygen consumption is determined by local brain tissue energy requirements, which are thought to be directly related to neuronal cell density and thus local synaptic density. Changes in focal neuronal (synaptic) activity or density (e.g., atrophy) are reflected by corresponding focal changes in $CMRO_2$ or CMR_{glu}. These two functions are stoichiometrically related to each other. How the coupling between $CMRO_2$ or CMR_{glu} and CBF is regulated is still unknown, although several theories have been advanced. For review, see Lou et al. (1987).

The studies which report cerebral energy metabolism *in vivo* in man have been partially conflicting. CBF, CMR_{glu}, and $CMRO_2$ are

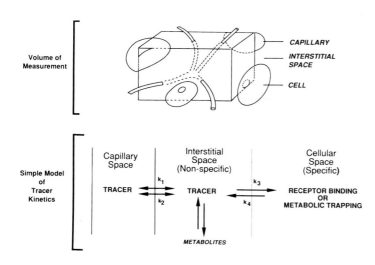

Figure 6. Diagram of theoretical and ideal tracer distribution over different compartments on the tissue. k_1 to k_4 denote the rate constants governing the transport of tracer or its metabolites over the several (here three) compartments.

the functions which have been measured either separately or in several combinations. The majority of studies using *in-vivo* techniques (like nitrous oxide or ^{133}Xe washout measurements or PET/SPECT) showed a decline of CBF with age. A notable exception is the study of Yamaguchi et al. (1986). The reason for this discrepancy is not clear.

However, the situation is less clear for oxygen or glucose utilization. Some studies reported a decline with age for $CMRO_2$ (Kety, 1956; Gottstein et al., 1971; Pantano et al., 1984; Yamaguchi et al., 1986) or CMR_{glu} (Kuhl et al., 1982), but others showed no such change for CMR_{glu} (Duara et al., 1983, 1984; DeLeon et al., 1984; Rapoport et al., 1985). Frackowiak and Lenzi (1982) and Lenzi et al. (1983) found only a non-significant decline of $CMRO_2$ with age. CBF, however, did significantly decrease with age, resulting in a non-significant increase of OER. Possibly, a real but small change with age may not be recognized as such statistically in view of the large interindividual variation (see also Figure 8) and the necessarily small number of subjects included in the studies. Moreover, most PET studies measuring $CMRO_2$ did not correct for intravascular nonextracted [15]O_2, thereby overestimating OER and thus $CMRO_2$.

Here, I will briefly report the results of CBF, OER, $CMRO_2$ and CBV PET studies in a new group of 34 healthy volunteers (age range 22–82 years; mean and median 45 years; 16 females and 18 males) recently performed in our laboratory. A more extensive report is in preparation. The improved steady-state [15]O inhalation method was used, applying OER correction (CBV scan) and multiple arterial sampling. Here, only the results of one region of interest (ROI) are given (Table 1, Figure 7 and Figure 8), namely, "insular grey matter," which is defined as the ROI around the peak value derived from temporal (insular) cortex and subcortical grey matter. It is thought that this region best reflects neuronal activity in the brain (lowest partial volume effect) since cortical and subcortical grey matter are in close proximity and densely folded there.

As is clear from the table and figures, the inter-individual variability of the values was large. The percentage standard deviation was ±13% for $CMRO_2$, ±20% for CBF, ±14% for OER and ±26% for CBV. Therefore, cohort comparisons between healthy subjects and patient groups will be unrewarding unless the

Table 1. Mean values (±SD) of grey matter ROI in "young" and "old" healthy subjects.
"Young" = average values of 17 subjects below 45 years (median). "Old" = average values of 17 subjects above 45 years of age. CBF and $CMRO_2$ are expressed as ml/100 ml brain/min; OER as percentage and CBV as ml blood/100 ml brain.

	CBF	CMRO$_2$	OER	CBV
young	57.3 ± 12.3	3.91 ± 0.43	36.9 ± 4.4	5.8 ± 1.4
old	53.1 ± 11.5	3.51 ± 0.50	39.6 ± 6.3	4.6 ± 1.0

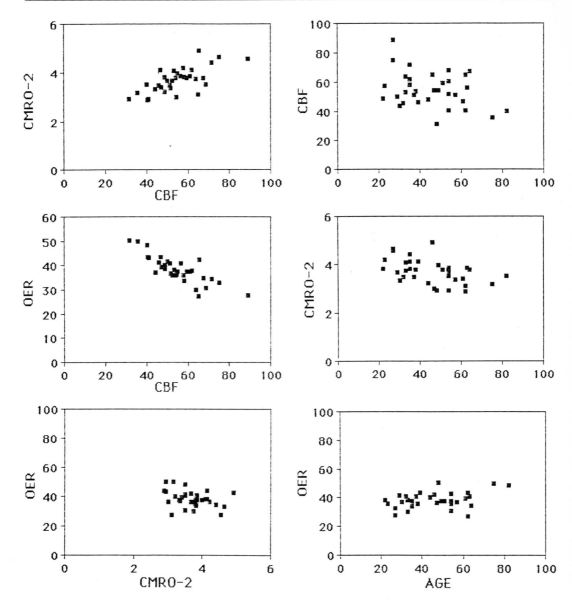

Figure 7. Scatter diagrams relating several functions in a group of 34 healthy subjects. The values are all from the grey matter region of interest (left and right side averaged). See text.

Figure 8. Scatter diagram of the same functions as in Figure 7 but now related to age. See text.

pathological changes are very large. But in that case a large control group is not needed. If brain disease results in small but real, focal or global changes of tissue function, it may remain undetectable in cohort comparisons unless large groups are studied. But that is not

very practical with the PET techniques available at present. To collect 34 subjects and analyse their scans is in itself a major undertaking.

As expected, CBF correlated positively with $CMRO_2$ (r = 0.72; p < 0.001) and negatively witn OER ($r = -0.84$; $p < 0.001$). This means that on the one hand a certain level of oxygen utilization dictates a range of CBF needed to comply with the tissue demands, while on the other hand the OER will adjust to the level of CBF which actually prevails. Therefore, OER does not directly depend on $CMRO_2$ (Figure 7). Notwithstanding the large interindividual variability, both CBF ($p < 0.05$) and $CMRO_2$ ($p < 0.01$) decreased significantly with age (Figure 8). The mean percentage decrease was -0.47% per year for $CMRO_2$ and -0.51% per year for CBF. OER did increase ($p < 0.05$) and CBV decrease ($p < 0.05$) with age. Table 1 shows the same trend if the studied population is arbitrarily divided in a "young" and "old" group. The majority of the other ROI's showed the same trend but less clearly and often not significantly. This is probably due to the large partial volume effects associated with the other, less well-defined ROI's. This is particularly evident for the scanner (a previous generation type) used here. The cerebellum values did not seem to be influenced by age at all. No differences between males and females were found for any of the measurements.

This data shows that with age in a seemingly healthy group of subjects there is a small but steady decline of oxygen utilization (neuronal cell loss ?) accompanied by a similar but slightly larger decline of CBF (decreased number of perfused capillaries?). It must be noted that the absolute changes during life are very small and it is quite unclear how these small differences translate in terms of numbers of functioning neurons. Even more unclear is how relevant the measured decreases are in relation to intellectual or daily life performances.

Dopaminergic Neurotransmitter Functions

Only one paper specifically adressing this topic has been published to date (Wong et al., 1984). The authors show a decline of D_2 dopamine receptor binding in striatum with age using the tracer ^{11}C-N-methylspiperone. The decline is steeper in the first decades of life, but after about age 30 a rather stable level appears to be maintained. This would be in line with

post-mortem findings (Seeman et al., 1987). Again, the interindividual variability is large.

The author's own results in healthy volunteers using ^{11}C-N-methylspiperone (Leenders et al., 1986c) are similar. In contrast, striatal ^{18}F-dopa uptake in a small ($n = 6$) group of healthy subjects (age range 24—65 yrs) did not change with age (Leenders, unpublished). However, only a relative measure for striatal dopamine turnover could be applied.

Dementia

Cerebral Energy Metabolism

Only one study has been published using [15]O techniques to measure CBF and oxygen utilization in dementing conditions (Frackowiak et al., 1981). In that study 13 patients with Alzheimer-type dementia (DAT) and 9 with multiple infarct dementia (MID) were reported. Average decrease of $CMRO_2$ was 20% in mildly to moderately affected patients and 40% in severely affected cases. The decline of metabolism appeared to relate to severity of disease, but not to type of dementia.

CBF was decreased to the same extent as $CMRO_2$. Thus the OER was found to be the same whether patients were moderately or severely affected and of degenerative or vascular type. This is taken as evidence that chronic ischaemic mechanisms are not the cause of cerebral decline. The regional patterns of decreased function varied, but temporal and parietal defects were commonly seen, accompanied by a profound frontal depression in the severely affected patients (Figure 9).

An early paper by Ferris et al. (1980) and later papers from the same group of workers (DeLeon et al., 1983) showed overall decreases of glucose utilization ranging from 17—24% relative to elderly healthy subjects. Foster et al. (1983) also found globally decreased glucose utilization, but in addition point to specific focal posterior parietal hypometabolism of 10% to 49% in 20 patients with probable Alzheimer's disease (Foster et al., 1984).

Kuhl et al. (1985) also performed FDG scans in 6 DAT, 6 MID, and 6 depressed patients. The latter group did not differ from

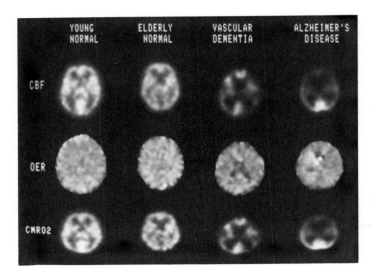

Figure 9. Images depicting quantitative cerebral functional values in four subjects: two healthy subjects (one young, one elderly) and two demented patients (one vascular, one Alzheimer type). See text.

normal, whereas the others showed changes comparable to those described above. The patients with DAT had a particularly profound decrease of metabolism (−47%) in parietal and dorsolateral occipital cortex.

Cutler et al. (1985) describe one case who was scanned several times over a period of 2.5 years. Although a progressive decline of global and focal glucose utilization was found, no straightforward relationship with clinical or cognitive performance was apparent.

Duara et al. (1986) studied a somewhat larger group of patients with DAT (n = 21) using FDG PET scans and compared these with healthy age-matched volunteers (n = 29). The results are essentially the same as obtained by the other authors.

Jagust et al. (1985) compared 17 patients with DAT and 3 patients with normal pressure hydrocephalus (NPH). Both groups showed lower cortical rates of glucose consumption, but the patterns were distinctly different: the patients with DAT showed bilateral temporal-parietal hypometabolism, whereas the NPH patients had only globally reduced values.

Several other reports have been published, demonstrating similar phenomena as already indicated. It is conspicuous that, although in most studies a crude relationship existed between degree of brain hypometabolism and severity of dementia, no clear quantitative relationship was found between measured impaired cognitive functions and the level of glo-

bal or focal cerebral energy requirements. Whether this is due to the limited technical performance of the early PET scanners remains to be seen.

Other conditions which are associated with one or other form of dementia may have a characteristic pattern of decreased energy metabolism. For instance Steele-Richardson-Olszewski syndrome is accompanied by severe frontal lobe hypometabolism (D'Antona et al., 1985; Leenders et al., 1987).

Dopaminergic Neurotransmitter Functions

To date no PET studies using dopaminergic tracers in patients with Alzheimer's disease have been performed to my knowledge, although one study is now in progress (Tyrrell, personal communication). It is conceivable that other types of tracers, e.g., for the cholinergic neurotransmitter system, might be more appropriate to study dementia; however, these are not yet available.

A combination of pre- and postsynaptic dopaminergic tracers can help to establish specific patterns of striatal functional deficits: a patient with Steele-Richardson-Olszewski syndrome will show decreased D_2 receptor binding and decreased dopamine turnover (Leenders et al., 1988); a patient with Huntington's disease will show normal dopamine turnover but decreased D_2 receptor binding (Leenders et al., 1986a); a patient with Parkinson's disease will show normal D_2 receptor binding but a marked decrease of dopamine turnover (Leenders et al., 1985).

References

Aquilonius SM, Bergström K, Eckernäs SA, Hartvig P, Leenders KL, Lundqvist H, Antoni G, Gee A., Rimland, A, Uhlin J, Långström B (1987) In vivo evaluation of striatal dopamine reuptake sites using 11C-nomifensine and positron emission tomography. *Acta Neurol Scand, 76*, 283–287.

Cutler N, Haxby J, Duara R, Grady C, Moore A, Parisi J, White J, Heton L, Margolin R, Rapoport S (1985) Brain metabolism as measured with positron emission tomography: serial assessment in a patient with familial Alzheimer's disease. *Neurology, 35*, 1556–1561.

D'Antona R, Baron J, Samson Y, Serdary M, Viader F, Agid Y, Cambier J (1985) Subcortical dementia: Frontal cortex hypometabolism detected by positron tomography in patients with progressive supranuclear palsy. *Brain, 108*, 785–800.

DeLeon M, Ferris S, George A, Reisberg B, Christman D, Kricheff I, Wolf A (1983) Computed tomography and positron emission transaxial tomography evaluations of normal aging and Alzheimer's disease. *J Cereb Blood Flow Metabol, 3*, 391–394.

DeLeon M, George AE, Ferris SH, Christman DR, Fowler JS, Gentes CI, Brodie J, Reisberg B, Wolf AP (1984) Positron emission tomography and computed tomography assessments of the aging human brain. *J Comp Assist Tomogr, 8*, 88–94.

Duara R, Margolin, RA, Robertson-Tchabo EA, London ED, Schwartz M, Renfrew JW, Koziarz BJ, Sundaram M, Grady C, Moore AM, Ingvar DH, Sokoloff L, Weingartner H, Kessler RM, Manning RG, Channing MA, Cutler NR, Rapoport SI (1983) Cerebral glucose utilization, as measured with positron emission tomography in 21 resting healthy men between the ages of 21 and 83 years. *Brain, 106*, 761–775.

Duara R, Grady C, Haxby J, Ingvar D, Sokoloff L, Margolin RA, Manning RG, Cutler NR, Rapoport SI (1984) Human brain glucose utilization and cognitive function in relation to age. *Ann Neurol, 16*, 702–713.

Duara R, Grady C, Haxby J, Sundaram M, Cutler N, Heston L, Moore A, Schlageter N, Larson S, Rapoport S (1986) Positron emission tomography in Alzheimer's disease. *Neurology, 36*, 879–887.

Eckernäs SA, Aquilonius SM, Hartvig P, Hägglund J, Jundqvist H, Någren K, Långström B (1987) Positron emission tomography (PET) in the study of dopamine receptors in the primate brain: evaluation of a kinetic model using ^{11}C-N-methyl-spiperone. *Acta Neurol Scand, 75*, 168–178.

Farde L, Ehrin E, Eriksson L, Greitz T, Hall H, Hedstrom CG, Litton JE, Sedvall G (1985) Substituted benzamides as ligands for visualisation of dopamine receptor binding in the human brain by positron emission tomography. *Proc Natl Acad Sci USA, 82*, 3863–3867.

Farde L, Hall H, Ehrin E, Sedvall G (1986) Quantitative analysis of D2 dopamine receptor binding in the living human brain by PET. *Science, 231*, 258–261.

Ferris SH, DeLeon MJ, Wolf AP, Farkas T, Christman DR, Reisberg B, Fowler JS, MacGregor R, Goldman A, George AE, Rampal S (1980) Positron emission tomography in the study of aging and senile dementia. *Neurobiol Aging, 1*, 127–131.

Foster N, Chase T, Fedio P, Patronas N, Brooks R, Di Chiro G (1983) Alzheimer's disease: Focal cortical changes shown by positron emission tomography. *Neurobiology, 33*, 961–965.

Foster N, Chase T, Mansi L, Brooks R, Fedio P, Patronas N, Di Chiro G (1984) Cortical abnormalities in Alzheimer's disease. *Ann Neurol, 16*, 649–654.

Fowler JS, Arnett CD, Wolf AP, Shiue CY, MacGregor RR, Halldin C, Långström B, Wagner Jr., HN (1986) A direct comparison of the brain uptake and plasma clearance of N-(^{11}C)methylspiroperidol and (^{18}F)N-methylspiroperidol in baboon using PET. *Nucl Med Biol, 13*, 281–284.

Fowler JS, MacGregor RR, Wold AP, Arnett CD, Dewey SL, Schlyer D, Christman D, Logan J, Smith M, Sachs H, Aquilonius SM, Bjurling P, Halldin C, Hartvig P, Leenders KL, Lundqvist H, Oreland L, Stålnacke CG, Långström B (1987) Mapping human brain monoamine oxidase A and B with 11C-suicide inactivators and positron emission tomography. *Science, 235*, 481–485.

Frackowiak RSJ, Lenzi GL (1982) Physiological measurement in the brain: From potential to practice. In Ell PJ, Holman BL (Eds.) *Computed emission tomography*. Oxford University Press, Oxford, 188–210.

Frackowiak RSJ, Jones T, Lenzi GL, Heather JD (1980a) Regional cerebral oxygen utilization and blood flow in normal man using oxygen-15 and positron emission tomography. *Acta Neurol Scandinav, 63*, 336–344.

Frackowiak RSJ, Lenzi GL, Jones T, Heather JD (1980b) Quantitative measurement of regional cerebral blood flow and oxygen metabolism in man using 15-O and positron emission tomography: Theory, procedure and normal values. *J Comp Assist Tomog, 4,* 727–736.

Frackowiak RSJ, Pozzilli C, Legg NJ, du Boulay GH, Marshall J, Lenzi GL, Jones T (1981) Regional cerebral oxygen supply and utilization in dementia. A clinical and physiological study with oxygen-15 and positron tomography. *Brain, 104* 753–778.

Frost JJ, Smith AC, Kuhar MJ, Dannals RF, Wagner Jr HN (1987) In vivo binding of 3H-N-methylspiperone to dopamine and serotonin receptors. *Life Sci., 40,* 987–995.

Garnett ES, Firnau G, Nahmias C (1983) Dopamine visualised in the basal ganglia of living man. *Nature, 305,* 137–138.

Gjedde A (1982) Calculation of glucose phosphorylation from brain uptake of glucose analogs in vivo: A re-examination. *Brain Res Rev, 4,* 237–274.

Gottstein U, Muller W, Berghoff W, Gartner H, Held K (1971) Zur Utilisation von nicht-veresterten Fettsäuren und Ketonkörpern im Gehirn des Menschen. *Klin Wschr, 49,* 406–411.

Jagust W, Friedland R, Budinger T (1985) Positron emission tomography with (18-F)fluorodeoxyglucose differentiates normal pressure hydrocephalus from Alzheimer-type dementia. *J Neurol Neurosurg Psychiatry, 48,* 1091–1096.

Jones T, Chesler DA, Ter-Poggossian MM (1976) The continuous inhalation of oxygen-15 for assessing regional oxygen extraction in the brain of man. *British J Radiol, 49,* 339–343.

Kety, S.S. (1956) Human cerebral blood flow and oxygen consumption as related to aging. *J Chronic Dis, 3,* 478–486.

Kety SS, Schmidt CF (1948) The nitrous oxygen method for the quantitative determination of cerebral blood flow in man: Theory, procedure and normal values. *J Clin Invest, 27,* 476–483.

Kuhl D, Metter EJ, Riege WH, Phelps ME (1982) Effects of human aging on patterns of local cerebral glucose utilization determined by the (¹⁸F)fluorodeoxyglucose method. *J Cereb Blood Flow and Metabol, 2,* 163–171.

Kuhl DE, Metter EJ, Riege WH, Hawkins RA (1985) Patterns of cerebral glucose utilization in dementia. In Greitz T, Ingvar DH, Widen L (Eds.) *The metabolism of the human brain studied with positron emission tomography.* Raven Press, New York, 419–431.

Lammertsma AA, Jones T (1983) The correction for the presence of intravascular oxygen-15 in steady state technique for measuring regional oxygen extraction in the brain, 1: Description of method. *J Cereb Blood Flow Metabol, 3,* 416–424.

Lammertsma AA, Jones T, Frackowiak RSJ, Lenzi GL (1981) A theoretical study of the steady state for measuring regional cerebral blood flow and oxygen utilisation using oxygen-15. *J Comput Assist Tomogr, 5,* 544–550.

Lammertsma AA, Heather JD, Jones T, Frackowiak RSJ, Lenzi GL (1982) A statistical study of the steady-state technique for measuring regional cerebral blood flow and oxygen utilization using 15-O. *J Comput Assist Tomogr, 6,* 566–573.

Lammertsma AA, Wise RJS, Heather JD, Gibbs JM, Leenders KL, Frackowiak RSJ, Rhodes CG, Jones T (1983) Correction for the presence of intravascular oxygen-15 in the steady-state technique for measuring regional oxygen extraction ratio in the brain, 2: Results in normal subjects and brain tumours and stroke patients. *J Cereb Blood Flow Metabol, 3,* 425–431.

Lebrun-Grandier P, Baron JC, Soussaline F, Loch'h C, Sassstre J, Bousser MG (1983) Coupling between regional blood flow and oxygen utilization in the normal human brain. A study with positron tomography and oxygen-15. *Arch Neurol, 40,* 230–236.

Leenders KL, Herold S, Palmer AJ, Turton D, Quinn N, Jones T, Frackowiak RSJ, Marsden CD (1985) Human cerebral dopamine system measured in vivo using PET. *J Cereb Blood Flow Metabol, 5* (suppl), 517–518.

Leenders KL, Frackowiak RJS, Quinn N, Marsden CD (1986a) Brain energy metabolism and dopaminergic function in Huntington's disease measured in vivo using positron emission tomography. *Movement Disorders, 1,* 69–77.

Leenders KL, Palmer AJ, Quinn N, Clark JC, Firnau G, Garnett ES, Nahmias C, Jones T, Marsden CD (1986b) Brain dopamine metabolism in patients with Parkinson's disease measured with positron emission tomography. *J Neurol Neurosurg Psychiat, 49,* 853–856.

Leenders KL, Palmer A, Turton D, Herold S, Frackowiak R, Jones T (1986c) In vivo measurements of the brain dopaminergic system in man using PET. In Valk, J. (Ed.) *Proceedings book, XIII Congress of the European Society of Neuroradiology.* Excerpta Medica, Amsterdam, 253–259.

Leenders KL, Aquilonius SM, Bergström, K, Bjurling P, Crossman AR, Eckernäs SA, Gee AG, Hartvig P, Lundqvist H, Långström B, Rimland A, Tedroff J (1987, in press) Unilateral MPTP lesion in a Rhesus monkey: Effects on the striatal dopaminergic system measured in vivo with PET using various novel tracers. *Brain Research.*

Leenders KL, Frackowiak RJS, Lees AJ (1988, in press) Steele-Richardson-Olszewski syndrome:

Brain energy metabolism, blood flow and fluorodopa uptake measured by positron emission tomography. *Brain.*

Lenzi GL, Gibbs JM, Frackowiak RSF, Jones T (1983) Measurements of Cerebral blood flow and oxygen metabolism by positron emission tomography and reproducibility and clinical application. In Magistretti PL (Ed.) *Functional radionuclide of the brain.* Raven Press, New York, 291—304.

Lou HC, Edvinsson L, MacKenzie E (1987) The concept of coupling blood flow to brain function: Revision required? *Ann Neurol, 22,* 289—297.

Pantano P, Baron JC, Lebrun-Grandie P, Duquesnoy N, Bousser MG, Comar D (1984) Regional cerebral blood flow and oxygen consumption in human aging. *Stroke, 15,* 635—641.

Pantano P, Baron JC, Crouzel C, Collard P, Sirou P, Samson Y (1985) The ^{15}O continuous-inhalation method: Correction for intravascular signal using C^{15}O. *Eur J Nucl Med, 10,* 387—391.

Patlak CS, Blasberg RG, Fenstermacher JD (1983) Graphical evaluation of blood-to-brain transfer constants from multiple-time uptake data. *J Cereb Blood Flow Metabol, 3,* 1—7.

Patlak CS, Blasberg RG (1985) Graphical evaluation of blood-to-brain transfer constants from multiple-time uptake data: Generalizations. *J Cereb Blood Flow Metabol, 5,* 584—590.

Phelps ME, Huang SC, Hoffman EJ, Kuhl DE (1979) Validation of tomographic measurement of cerebral blood volume with C-11 labeled carboxyhemoglobin. *J Nucl Med, 20,* 328—334.

Phelps ME, Mazziotta JC, Schelbert HR (Eds.) (1986) *Positron emission tomography and autoradiography. Principles and applications for the brain and heart.* Raven Press, New York.

Rapoport SI, Duara R, Grady CL, Cutler NR (1985) Cerebral glucose utilization in relation to age in man. In Greitz T, Ingvar DH, Widen L (Eds.) *The metabolism of the human brain studied with positron emission tomography.* Raven Press, New York, 339—350.

Seeman P, Bzowej NH, Guan HC, Bergeron C, Becker LE, Reynolds GP, Bird ED, Riederer P, Jellinger K, Watanabe S, Tourtelotte WW (1987) Human brain dopamine receptors in children and aging adults. *Synapse, 1,* 399—404.

Sokoloff L, Reivich M, Kennedy C et al (1977) The 14-C deoxyglucose method for the measurement of local cerebral glucose utilization: Theory, procedure and normal values in the conscious and anesthetized albino rat. *J Neurochem, 28,* 897—916.

Wagner HN, Burns HD, Dannals RF, Wong DF, Langstrom B, Duelfer T, Frost JJ, Ravert HT, Links JM, Rosenbloom SB, Lukas SE, Kramer AV, Kuhar MJ (1983) Imaging dopamine receptors in the human brain by positron tomography. *Science, 221,* 1264—1266.

Wong DF, Wagner Jr HN, Dannals RF, Links JM, Frost JJ , Ravert HT, Wilson AA, Rosenbaum AE, Gjedde A, Douglass KH, Petronis JD, Folstein MF, Toung JKT, Burns HD, Kuhar MJ (1984) Effects of age on dopamine and serotonin receptors measured by positron tomography in the living human brain. *Science, 226,* 1393—1396.

Yamaguchi T, Kanno I , Uemura K, Shishido F, Inugami A, Ogawa T, Murakami M, Suzuki K (1986) Reduction in regional cerebral metabolic rate of oxygen during human aging. *Stroke, 17,* 1220—1228.

Quantitative Measurements of Brain Metabolism During Physiological Stimulation

P. E. Roland and L. Widen

What progress in our understanding of brain functions has positron emission tomography (PET) provided? In all studies up to date designed for mapping of brain functions, changes in the regional metabolism or changes in regional cerebral blood flow (rCBF) were used as indicators of changes in neuronal function. The techniques for measurements of regional cerebral glucose consumption (rCMRgl) and regional cerebral oxidative metabolism (rCMRO$_2$) with PET are cumbersome. A certain amount of the studies in which quantitative changes in rCMR have been observed during physiological stimulation have been replications of already established physiological facts. However certain studies, among these many rCBF studies, have provided new insight in the function of the basal ganglia, cerebellum, supplementary motor area, supplementary sensory area, frontal eye fields and visual association cortices. A few new functionally delimited areas in the superior parietal lobule have been described. Hypotheses about organization of brain functions, among these the cortical field activation principle, have received support from PET studies. In other experiments PET investigators mapped the parts of the brain participating in production of language and complex cognitive functions. It has even been possible to map changes in rCMRO$_2$ due to pure mental activity and metabolic processes coupled to the learning phase. Examples of these new findings are given in this paper. The after all, quite limited progress, during ten years of active PET research is probably mainly due to the lack of a method that permits rapid regional measurements of neuronal acitivity which can be repeated several times during a day. So far only rCBF measurements with freely diffusible tracers fulfill these requirements.

With the advent of positron emission tomography it has become possible for the first time to perform direct, quantitative measurements of biochemical and physiological processes in the living human brain. The measurements can be performed regionally from all parts of the brain simultaneously with a spatial resolution that permits distinction of most of the anatomical subdivisions of the brain and a few major brainstem structures. Obviously this is a breakthrough in brain resarch.

Quantitative PET Measurements

Basic Requirements

A positron emission tomograph (PET) can measure concentrations of positron emitting isotopes (nCi/cc) simultaneously in all regions of the brain, brainstem and cerebellum. A series of PET-scans will show changes in tracer concentrations as a function of time. The tracer molecules usually enter the brain via the blood stream. Thus it is also necessary to measure the time-course of the tracer concentration in arterial blood in order to quantify changes of tracer concentrations in the brain. An appropriate kinetic tracer model that describes changes in concentrations of tracer and mother substance with time in the different compartments of the brain (e.g., vascular, interstitial, cytosol, subcellular) is also

Department of Clinical Neurophysiology, Karolinska Hospital, S-10401 Stockholm, Sweden.
We thank Monica Serrander, Göran Printz, Lars Eriksson and Sharon Stone-Elander for collaboration and assistance with the laboratory work reported here.

needed. The tissue compartments need not be anatomical. Often the compartments in tracer-kinetic models are identified as different biochemical states (e.g., precursor pool, metabolic compartment, metabolites).

In some circumstances the amount of tracer in the blood is so significant that it is necessary to measure the regional cerebral blood volume (rCBV). Additional measurements of the regional cerebral blood flow (rCBF) are needed if one wants to measure the transport of a tracer and mother substance across the blood brain barrier. Dynamic measurements of the regional cerebral metabolic rate for oxygen, for example, require measurements of both the rCBF and rCBV in addition to the measurements of the time course of oxygen in the brain tissue.

With the proper requirements fulfilled, PET in contrast to other imaging techniques, provides fully quantitative measurements of the dynamic biochemistry and rCBF in the entire human brain.

Synaptic Metabolism

There are, in principle, many ways of measuring biochemical correlates of changes in neuronal function. So far, all investigators have concentrated on measuring the changes in metabolism that accompany changes in neuronal activity. All regional energy-consuming processes in the brain tissue will raise the local metabolism. Autoradiographic studies of animals have shown that the highest metabolic rates (rCMR) are located in anatomical regions with the highest synaptic density (Hand et al, 1978; Kadareko et al., 1985). The synaptic activity: ionic transfers, transmitter synthesis, transmitter release, transmitter reuptake, formation of second and third messengers and protein phosphorylation are all energy-consuming processes that deplete energy-rich phosphates. However, it has been shown that the synaptic metabolic activity is dominated by the energy consumption of the sodium pump (Mata et al., 1980). The fast transient changes in neuronal metabolism are thus dominated by the ATP consumption of the sodium pump.

When an anatomical structure increases its metabolism the increase most likely originates from the active synaptic regions within the structure. This means that the increase in metabolism could originate from activity of the terminals of the afferent neurons (located elsewhere) and from activity of the intrinsic neurons, but under normal circumstances only to a negligible extent from the perikayra of the efferent neurons.

In the literature on PET imaging of brain functions, the metabolism of a structure is sometimes reported as a ratio between the mean metabolism of a brain slice and the structure or as right-left ratios. It should be stressed that the relation between neuronal activity and metabolism is valid only if the metabolism is measured in absolute values, that is, in mmol/100 g brain tissue/min or in ml/100 g brain tissue/min. Similarly, quantitative changes in rCMR accompanying physiological stimulation should be reported in the same units.

Methods Available for PET Measurements of Brain Activation

An increase in the regional cerebral metabolism is called an activation by convention. At present there are several methods of measuring the rCMR. All aim to measure either the regional cerebral metabolic rate for glucose (rCMRgl) or the regional cerebral oxidative metabolism (rCMRO$_2$).

For the measurement of rCMRgl, ^{11}C-deoxyglucose or ^{18}F-deoxyglucose are usually used. ^{11}C-glucose has also been employed, but at present this method is not quantitative because of the loss of tracer as [11]CO$_2$. The deoxyglucose methods require 40 min for a measurement. Since neuronal function is characterized by changes in the order of milliseconds, the rCMRgl measurements can only give the average rCMRgl for a given structure. One cannot ascertain whether a given structure shows increased rCMRgl because it was active throughout the 40 min or because it was strongly active only during certain phases. Even behavioral tasks having very complicated algorithms are usually solved in less than ten seconds. In consequence, special behavioral paradigms in which a given task is repeated over and over again have to be used. More problematic is the methodological requirement of a steady state of processing and metabolism during the 40 min: information processing cannot be repeated over and over again in the brain without habituation.

The deoxyglucose methods require that the so-called lumped constant is determined (Sokoloff et al., 1977). The lumped constant consists of several constants describing the Michaelis-Menten kinetics of tracer and mother substance, the distribution volumes of tracer and mother substance and the fraction of phosphorylated glucose that goes further down the glycolytic pathway. The lumped constant is difficult to determine in man and the rCMRglu values are inversely proportional to its value. This constitutes the Achilles heel of the deoxyglucose method. The advantage of the method is that only a single PET measurement is needed to determine the metabolic rate.

There are also two types of methods for $rCMRO_2$ measurements. Both require additional measurements of rCBF and rCBV. Thus, three separate PET measurements are needed to determine the $rCMRO_2$ of a single behavioral state. In the steady-state method (Jones et al. 1976) the subject continuously inhales $^{15}O_2$ for some 10–15 min until the brain tissue radioactivity reaches a steady state. The rCBF is usually measured after continuous inhalation of $C^{15}O_2$ which in the lungs is converted to $H_2^{15}O$ by carbonic anhydrase. The rCBV is measured after inhalation of $C^{15}O$ to label the erythrocytes. The problem with this method is the underestimation of rCBF in cerebral regions with a high rCBF.

In the dynamic method for $rCMRO_2$ determination the subject inhales the $^{15}O_2$ in a single breath (Mintun et al., 1984; Roland et al., 1987 a). The rCBF is usually determined after a single injection of $H_2^{15}O$ or after inhalation of an inert gas. The advantage of the method is that the $rCMRO_2$ can be determined from PET measurements lasting less than one minute. The drawback of the dynamic method is that the measurement of the regional oxygen extraction is dependent on the volume of distribution of the metabolically produced water. At present it is known that the volume of distribution changes with the state of activity of the local synapses, but it is not yet possible to quantify this dependency.

Since the deoxyglucose method requires a steady state of metabolism for 40 min, whereas the dynamic method for $rCMRO_2$ determination requires only 40 s the results obtained during activation with the two methods are not comparable. On the other hand, since $rCMRO_2$ measurements require three separate PET measurements one has to make sure that the specific behavioral state, the speed of information processing in the brain, the novelty of the task and the attention put into the task can be reproduced exactly during each measurement.

These problems could be solved if there were a method for measuring the rCMR after a single injection in less than a minute. Such a method is not yet available. However, it is possible to measure the rCBF in less than one minute with PET. It is usually assumed that the rCBF is adjusted to the local metabolic demands and that changes in rCBF in the normal brain are coupled to changes in rCMR. This view has recently been questioned (Fox & Raichle, 1986). At present, it is probably fair to say that the bulk of evidence speaks for a coupling, but that the issue is by no means resolved and that the postulated biochemical mechanism that couples the rCBF to the rCMR has not been identified. Despite these reservations, the rCBF has been widely used as a quantitative measure of neuronal activity. The tracer-kinetic model used in all studies of cerebral activation has so far been a single-compartment model in which it is assumed that the tracer instantaneously distributes uniformly in the brain tissue. The majority of PET experiments have been performed with $H_2^{15}O$ as the flow tracer. Because H_2O ist not a freely diffusible tracer, the results obtained with this method can only be considered semi-quantitative.

Localization of the Changes in Metabolism

All PETs have limited spatial resolution. In the available literature all data have been obtained with PETs for which the smallest volume of detection (voxel) ranged between 1 cm^3 and 8 cm^3. This means that many metabolically active and inactive cortial columns and nuclei are monitored within each detectable volume element. The rCMR that is mea-sured then is a weighted average of the meta-bolism within the volume element. The meta-bolic changes during physiological stimula-tion thus are only weighted averages of the changes in the bulk of tissue in each volume element of detection. In some measurements

the spatial resolution is so poor that a consid-erable amount of white matter is always pres-ent in each volume element. Since white mat-ter has a metabolism that is only 25% of that of gray matter the measured rCMR will be lower than the true rCMR due to such partial volume effects.

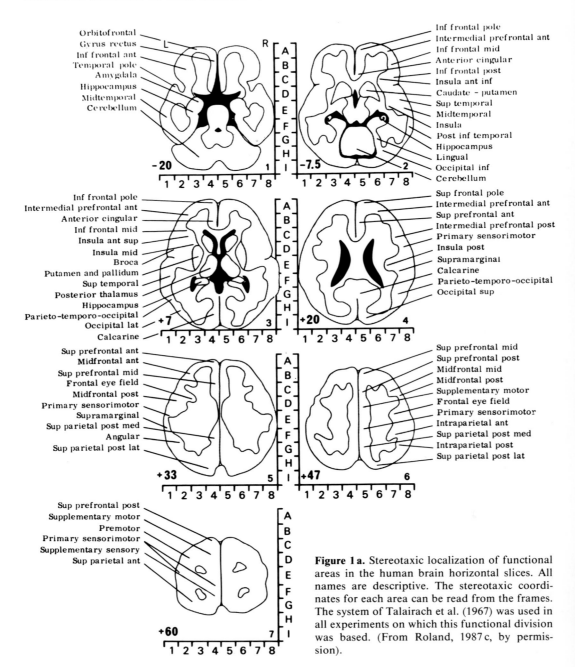

Figure 1a. Stereotaxic localization of functional areas in the human brain horizontal slices. All names are descriptive. The stereotaxic coordi-nates for each area can be read from the frames. The system of Talairach et al. (1967) was used in all experiments on which this functional division was based. (From Roland, 1987c, by permis-sion).

The spatial resolution of the PETs does not permit a direct visualization of many anatomical structures in the brain. It is therefore desirable to know from which anatomical structure a change in metabolism originated. Since the rCMR (or rCBF) must be measured in at least two separate behavioral states in order to detect changes in neuronal metabolism, it is mandatory that the head is fixed in exactly the same position during the measurements. This in turn requires a reliable fixation method and a stereotaxical system. Because individual brains are of different sizes and of different shapes one also needs a common system of reference. This is usually referred to

as a stereotaxic brain atlas. Not all investigators have made use of this tool, which is a pity because it is then not possible to compare functional mapping studies from different PET centers. Fixation devices, and stereotaxic brain atlases also vary. The most advanced atlas at present is that of Bohm et al. (1985).

Figure 1 displays an example of a stereotaxic brain atlas with a number of functional subdivisions of the human cortex determined in stereotaxic coordinates. These subdivisions are still the result of a limited number of functional mapping experiments and it is to be expected that new functional territories will appear as more experimental data become

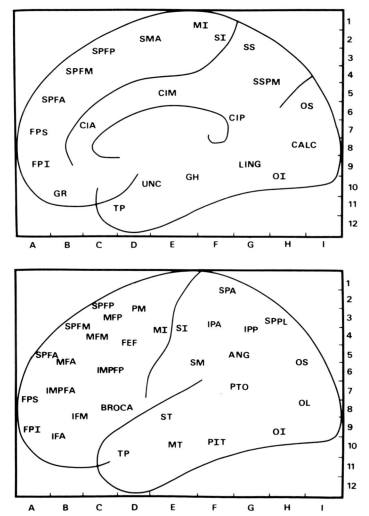

Figure 1 b. Stereotaxic localization of functional areas in the human cerebral cortex, lateral and medial view. The abbreviations refer to the names listed in Figure 1a. Frames according to the Talairach system.

available. The basic principle behind the construction of such a functional brain atlas is that regions activated in one class of experiments which are not activated in other classes of experiments are treated as separate entities.

Behavioral Control

Research prior to the PET era showed that movements, unwanted stimuli, anxiety, arousal and irrelevant thought influence the metabolic pattern of the brain. It is consequently necessary to maintain strict behavioral control if one wants to study metabolic changes associated with a particular task. Video-monitoring, EEG, measurements of blood pressure and heart rate are a minimum.

In all types of behavioral neurophysiology task-related changes in neuronal activity have to be judged against a non-task state or a control state without any specific stimulation. The control state in PET experiments is usually called "rest." Thus magnitude of metabolic changes between rest and test are depend also on the rCMR during rest. Traditionally, subjects have both eyes closed and ears plugged ("ears covered") during rest. Mazziotta et al. (1982b) showed that subjects demonstrated a progressive decrease of rCMRgl while going from the eyes-closed state to the ears-covered state and from the ears-covered state to the state where both eyes and ears were closed. Thus the resting state in which eyes and ears are closed is a state associated with a kind of baseline metabolism against which increases due to task-specific neural activity are easy to detect. Table 1 gives the rCMRO$_2$ in all the functional divisions of the brain shown in Figure 1 in resting (eyes closed, ears covered) healthy young volunteers aged from 20 to 35 years old.

A special problem arises in behavioral neurophysiology with PET because the processing in the brain has to be repeated over and over again: if the task that the subjects performs leaves time over between the trials of specific brain processing, this time will be occupied with other irrelevant kinds of brain work and the rCMR would change accordingly. Therefore the processing in the brain must be paced in such a way that no time is left over for other mental activity. This is not always done.

Contributions of PET to our Understanding of Brain Functions

It is only natural, after nine years of functional mapping studies with PET, to try to answer the question of whether PET has provided any new data, not known from earlier animal experiments or from studies using other techniques in man, on the normal physiology of the brain and its information processing.

When the first functional mapping experiment with PET was published (Reivich et al., 1979) the intracarotid method for rCBF measurements (Lassen & Ingvar, 1961) was already established. This method provided a wealth of new information about the functional anatomy of the brain (for reviews see Roland, 1984, 1985a; Raichle, 1986—among others). With the Lassen-Ingvar method it was, however, only possible to obtain information about the superficial parts of the cerebral cortex supplied by the branches of the carotid artery. One of the achievements of PET is that regions of the central nervous system inaccessible with the Lassen-Ingvar method now have been functionally mapped.

Many of the early studies were replications of experiments done on animals, carried out with the primary purpose of validating the PET technique. Also, many experimentors did not provide quantitative results. This leaves rather few studies in which new data on functions of the brain are reported.

Relation Between Stimulus Parameters and Metabolism in Sensory Cortices

Phelps et al. (1981) showed that, compared to rest state in which the subjects had their eyes closed, white light stimulation increased the rCMRgl in the primary visual cortex by 11.5%. Checkerboard stimulation of one eye increased the rCMRgl by 17.4% whereas checkerboard stimulation of both eyes increased the rCMRgl by 27.6%. The largest increase, 45.1%, was obtained when the subjects watched a scene in a park (university campus). The corresponding increases for the lateral temporo-occipital visual association cortex were 6.1%, 21.9%, 26.7% and 58.9%.

Region	Code	Left hemi-sphere	Right hemi-sphere
Inferor frontal ant	IFA	3.86 ± 0.66	4.16 ± 0.90
Inferor frontal mid	IFM	3.94 ± 0.68	4.19 ± 0.47
Broca		4.76 ± 0.89	5.09 ± 0.66
Inferor frontal pole	FPI	4.38 ± 0.84	4.21 ± 0.84
Superor frontal pole	FPS	3.94 ± 0.80	4.52 ± 0.95
Intermedial prefrontal ant	IMPFA	4.68 ± 0.95	4.64 ± 0.76
Intermedial prefrontal post	IMPFP	5.49 ± 0.83	5.47 ± 1.00
Midfrontal ant	MFA	5.39 ± 1.12	5.17 ± 0.79
Midfrontal mid	MFM	5.31 ± 0.94	5.58 ± 0.56
Midfrontal post	MFP	5.60 ± 0.91	5.77 ± 0.94
Frontal eye field	FEF	5.59 ± 0.85	6.17 ± 0.79
Superior prefrontal ant	SPFA	5.21 ± 0.91	5.46 ± 1.02
Superior prefrontal mid	SPFM	5.47 ± 1.20	6.04 ± 1.03
Superior prefrontal post	SPFP	6.54 ± 1.14	6.00 ± 1.36
Premotor	PM	5.35 ± 1.06	5.75 ± 1.05
Supplementary motor	SMA	5.82 ± 1.15	6.08 ± 1.08
MI hand area	MI	5.64 ± 1.03	5.39 ± 1.11
MI remaining parts	MI	5.03 ± 0.82	5.15 ± 1.14
SI hand area	SI	5.19 ± 1.27	5.33 ± 0.92
SI remaining parts	SI	5.14 ± 1.22	4.88 ± 1.01
Supplementary sensory	SS	5.78 ± 1.49	5.78 ± 1.42
Superior parietal ant	SPA	4.68 ± 0.91	4.72 ± 0.75
Intraparietal ant	IPA	5.49 ± 1.21	5.76 ± 1.44
Intraparietal post	IPP	5.34 ± 1.24	5.39 ± 1.15
Supramarginal	SM	5.27 ± 0.97	5.47 ± 0.67
Angular	ANG	4.91 ± 0.88	5.06 ± 1.07
Superior parietal post med	SSPM	6.28 ± 1.25	6.19 ± 1.36
Superior parietal post lat	SSPL	5.24 ± 1.02	4.71 ± 1.06
Occipital sup	OS	4.12 ± 0.79	4.19 ± 0.72
Occipital lat	OL	3.56 ± 0.41	3.53 ± 0.60
Occipital inf	OI	3.95 ± 0.60	3.53 ± 0.47
Calcarine	CALC	5.56 ± 0.55	5.23 ± 0.90
Posterior inf temporal	PIT	3.79 ± 0.64	3.70 ± 0.53
Parieto-temporo-occipital	PTO	4.41 ± 0.64	4.52 ± 0.70
Midtemporal	MT	4.19 ± 0.72	4.25 ± 0.66
Superior temporal	ST	4.81 ± 0.74	4.66 ± 0.83
Temporal pole	TP	3.68 ± 0.78	3.68 ± 0.94
Insula ant inf		5.31 ± 0.90	5.88 ± 1.33
Insula ant sup		5.56 ± 0.93	4.97 ± 1.16
Insula mid		5.75 ± 1.31	5.40 ± 0.95
Insula post		5.49 ± 1.38	5.26 ± 1.05
Orbitofrontal post		4.01 ± 0.83	4.07 ± 0.87
Orbitofrontal ant		3.63 ± 0.54	3.70 ± 0.92
Gyrus rectus	GR	5.35 ± 0.65	4.84 ± 0.95
Anterior cingular	CIA	6.03 ± 1.04	6.03 ± 1.04
Cingular mid	CIM	5.07 ± 0.94	5.07 ± 0.94
Gyrus lingualis	LING	4.67 ± 0.76	4.37 ± 0.65
Hippocampus	GH	3.46 ± 0.80	3.29 ± 0.70
Caput n caudatus		4.13 ± 0.81	3.81 ± 1.03
Caudate–putamen		4.72 ± 0.67	4.69 ± 0.52
Putamen–pallidum		5.55 ± 1.19	4.91 ± 1.12
Thalamus		5.03 ± 1.14	5.17 ± 1.29
Parasagittal cerebellum		4.18 ± 0.80	4.07 ± 0.82
Lat cerebellum lob post		4.60 ± 0.81	4.09 ± 0.66
Vermis		4.07 ± 1.01	4.07 ± 1.01
White matter		1.40 ± 0.23	1.41 ± 0.20

Table 1. Regional oxidative metabolism ($rCMRO_2$) during rest in functional subdivisions of the human brain. All values are mean ± SD in ml/100 g/min (n = 11).

Fox and Raichle (1984) exposed their subjects to flicker stimulation and demonstrated that the rCBF increase in the primary visual cortex was a non-monotonic function of the stimulation frequency (Figure 2 a). We changed the illumination time of a colored stimulus from 92% of the PET measurement time to 4% of the PET measurement time (Figure 5); from these experiments it was concluded that the decrease in rCBF in the primary visual cortex was not proportional to the decrease in exposure time. In an experiment in which the stimulus energies were measured, we demonstrated that the rCMRO$_2$ in the primary somatosensory area only increased slightly with stimulus power (Figure 2 b). These experiments demonstrated that the metabolic increase in a primary receptive cortical area is only moderately dependent on the physical stimulus parameters (stimulus power, exposure time and frequency). Far stronger determinants are the selective attention and interest the subjects put into the afferent signals they receive.

Organization of Voluntary Movements

The cortical motor areas (premotor PM, supplementary motor area SMA, primary motor area MI and the frontal eye field FEF) were functionally characterized in ^{133}Xe intracarotid studies. With the emergence of PET, the basal ganglia, the cerebellum and the cortex buried in the longitudinal fissure and the sylvian fissure became available for study. With the exception of the primar motor area MI, the cortical motor areas are bilaterally activated although the voluntary movements are strictly unilateral (Roland et al., 1982). Subcortical areas, namely the caudate, putamen, globus pallidus, the ventral thalamus and anterior lobe of the cerebellum are bilaterally activated (Figures 3 and 5) (Roland et al., 1982; Mazziotta & Phelps, 1984; Fox et al., 1985 a). The reason for this bilateral elabora-

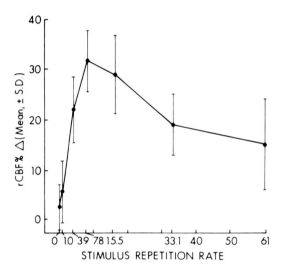

Figure 2 a. Changes of the rCBF in the striate cortex as a function of the frequency of a patterned visual stimulus to both eyes. Mean change of rCBF in % and SD shown for eight subjects. (From Fox & Raichle, 1984, by permission).

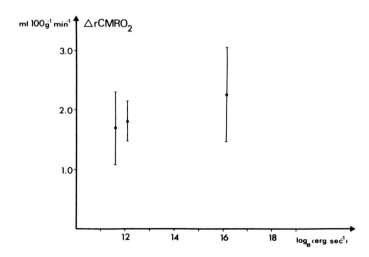

Figure 2 b. Changes in rCMRO$_2$ (mean ± SD) in ml/100 g/min in the contralateral primary somatosensory cortex in response to somatosensory stimulation of different energy (From Roland et al., in prep.).

tion of motor programs and motor control of unilateral movements is not known.

The anterior lobe of the cerebellum is now being functionally mapped. Fox et al. (1985a) and Roland et al. (1987b) showed that the parasagittal part is bilaterally activated during strictly unilateral finger movements. Vibration applied to the fingers produced an ipsilateral increase of rCBF that was coexistent with the increase produced by the finger movements

(Fox et al., 1985b). Saccadic eye movements produced rCBF increases in vermis, presumably located near lobus VI (Fox et al., 1985a, b).

Although the basal ganglia and cerebellum certainly participate in elaboration of motor programs and motor control, it would be wrong to assume that the function of these structures is entirely motor. The posterior lobe of the cerebellum and the caudate-putamen

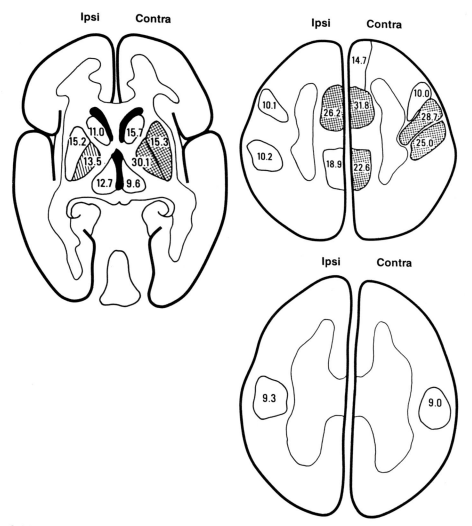

Figure 3. Mean percentage increase in rCBF and mean extents of increases while a complicated sequence of right hand finger movements was performed by ten normal volunteers. Crosshatched areas p < 0.001, hatched areas p < 0.01, other areas p < 0.05 (From Roland et al. 1982, by permission of the American Physiological Society).

are also activated in non-motor acitivities (Figures 4 and 5) (Roland et al., 1987 a, b).

Motor activities and sensori-motor activities also frequently activate somatosensory association areas. Figure 3 shows that unilateral finger movement sequences activate the fronto-parietal operculum (secondary somatosensory area, SII) and the supplementary sensory area (SS). Tactile exploration of unknown objects in addition activates the anterior part of the lobulus parietalis superior (SPA) and the parietal operculum-retroinsular cortex (RI-PO) (Figure 5).

Functional Organization of Language

Although many aspects of the cortical organization of language were revealed by studies performed with the Lassen-Ingvar method, recent PET studies have now given a more comprehensible view. Heiss et al. (1987) asked their subjects to speak spontaneously on a topic chosen by themselves. The language production increased rCMRgl bilaterally in the somatosensory cortex, the primary motor area for the mouth, the posterior superior temporal area (Wernicke), the inferior prefrontal cortex (Broca), the thalami and the cerebellum. In addition, a unilateral left prefrontal rCMRgl increase appeared. Mazziotta et al. (1982a) had their subjects listen to a Sherlock Holmes story during the PET measurement of rCMRgl. Afterward the subjects were questioned about details of the story. This language apprehension increased rCMRgl bilaterally in the auditory cortex, the posterior superior temporal cortex (Wernicke) and the thalami. An additional increase was seen in the Broca area. When subjects were requested to explain the use of an object whose name was shown to them on a screen, Fox et al. (1987a) found increases of rCBF in the primary motor area of the mouth, the SMA, head of caudate, cerebellum, superior and inferior prefrontal cortex (Broca), angular cortex, cingulate cortex plus visual areas. With a careful series of control experiments, Fox et al. (1987a) were able to dissect out the mouth area and SMA as participating in motor organization of language and the visual areas as participating in the visual analysis without being involved in the language production.

The picture that emerges from these studies is that the Broca area, Wernicke area, left prefrontal cortex and possibly the thalamus and angular cortex participe both in language comprehension and language production.

Mental Activity

From an operational point of view, mental activity is intrinsic activity initiated by the brain in the absence of immediate prior stimulation and in the absence of voluntary motor activity. In a study with the Lassen-Ingvar method, Roland and Friberg (1985) showed that specific mental activity increased rCBF in segregated cortical fields of $2-9$ cm^2 located outside the primary sensory and motor cortices. It was also shown that different types of mental activity gave rise to rCBF field increases with different localizations (Roland & Friberg, 1985). One major problem had to be solved: it was still debated whether mental activity increased the rCMR in some parts of the brain whereas other (inactive) regions showed a decrease in rCMR such that mental activity would not be associated with any net increase in brain metabolism. This question could only be solved by a measurement of the rCMR with PET.

Roland et al. (1987a) performed an experiment in which the $rCMRO_2$ was measured during rest and during purely mental activity. The subjects imagined that they walked out their front door and then turned to the left. When the first opportunity came they imagined turning down the street to the right, and then alternatively to the right and left each time they reached a corner. When the PET measurement was finished their final position was looked up on a map. The main results were (1) that no structure or region of the brain showed any decreases in $rCMRO_2$; (2) that $rCMRO_2$ increased in segregated cortical fields in the prefrontal cortex, parietal cortex and temporo-occipital cortex, but not in the primary visual cortex (Figure 4); (3) that $rCMRO_2$ increased in the neostriatum, posterior thalamus and posterior lobe of the cerebellum despite the absence of sensory stimuli and motor activity (Figure 4). The largest $rCMRO_2$ increases appeared in the posterior

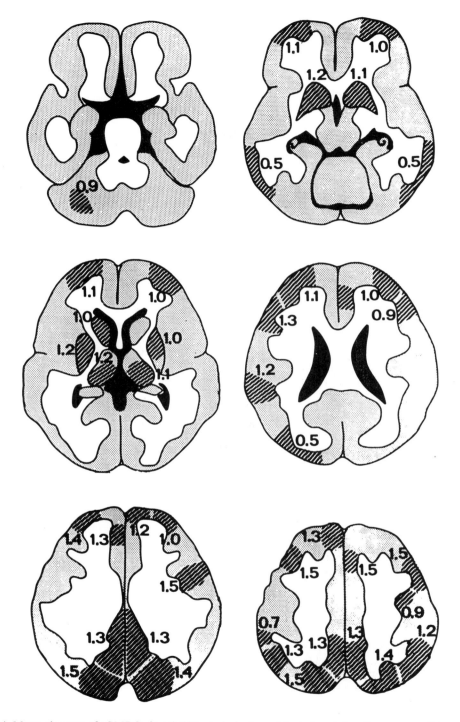

Figure 4. Mean changes of rCMRO$_2$ in ml/100 g/min in ten subjects imagining they were walking alternatively to the left and right in familiar surroundings (see text). Their eyes were closed and their ears plugged. The semi-diagrammatic slices of the brain were taken −20 mm, −7 mm, +20 mm, +34 mm, +47 mm above the commissural plane.

superior parietal cortex (regions SPPM and SPPL). Activations here were not seen if the material to be recalled was auditory or non-visual (Roland & Friberg, 1985). Similarly, the pattern of rCMRO$_2$ increases in the prefrontal cortex was different if auditory and other material was retrieved. This led Roland et al.

(1987a) to propose that the SPPM and SPPL were visual association areas, and that part of the memories for the visually spatially famil-iar sceneries were retrieved from these areas and that some of the prefrontal fields partic-ipated in the retrieval, which might occur via the pulvinar.

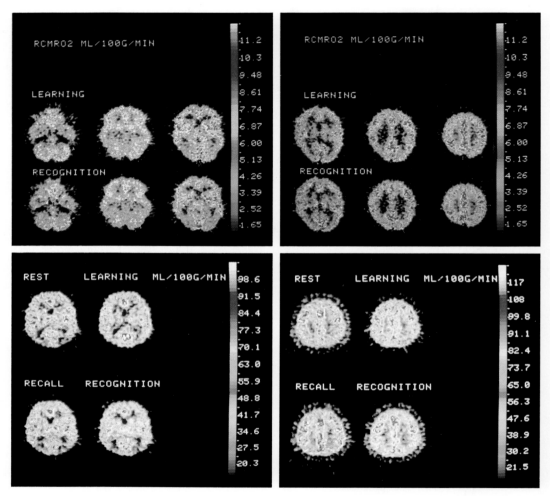

Figure 5. *Top:* rCMRO$_2$ in ml/100 g/min in the same subject during tactile learning and tactile recognition with the right hand. The main difference in metabolism occurred in the posterior lobe of cerebellum where rCMRO$_2$ was higher by 0.6 ml/100 g/min during learning. This difference was significant (p < 0.01; n = 8). Smaller, but still significant differences occurred in the left SMA and left sensorimotor region where the rCMRO$_2$ was higher during tactile recognition by 0.3–0.4 ml/100 g/min due to the higher frequency of exploratory movements with the right hand. *Lower left:* section of brain taken 15 mm above commissural plane showing rCBF in ml/100 g/min during (1) rest (eyes closed), (2) visual learning of colored geomet-rical patterns (eyes open, visual stimulation 92% of PET measurement time), (3) mental recall of the same patterns (eyes closed) and (4) visual recognition (eyes open, visual stimulation 4% of PET measurement time). Note the increase of rCBF in the thalamus during recall and the differences in primary visual cortex. *Lower right:* same subject, section 42 mm above commissural plane. Note the rCBF increase in the posterior mesial parietal cortex (SSPM) during recall.

The studies of mental acitivity constitute a radical change in behavioral neurophysiology. Hitherto, neuronal activity in the brain has been related to sensory input or motor output. The mental activity studies and the studies reported above emphasize that changes of metabolism in any cortical area or subcortical structure could be the result mainly of intrinsic brain processing.

Learning and Memory

There are three important questions with regard to how the brain stores and retrieves memorized information about the outside world: (1) Are the anatomical structures that participate in the storage the same as those participating in the analysis of the sensory information? (2) Are the anatomical structures that store the information the same as those participating in the retrieval of the stored information? (3) Is it possible to measure biochemical effects due to learning in the mammalian brain?

Duara et al. (1987) had their subjects read passages of the Wechsler intelligence test. After each reading the subjects recalled the contents. The rCMRgl was measured during 15 such learning and recall episodes. These procedures increased the rCMRgl in "all regions of the brain and even the cerebellum." Roland et al. (1987b) measured $rCMRO_2$ in normal healthy volunteers in three different stages: rest, tactile learning and tactile recognition. During tactile learning, blindfolded subjects had to learn 10 complicated geometrical objects they manipulated in their right hand. In tactile recognition these objects were mixed with similar, but previously unknown objects. The task was then to recognize the known objects. The frequency of manipulatory movements during tactile recognition was twice that of tactile learning.

Tactile learning with the right hand increased $rCMRO_2$ in six prefrontal cortical areas (lt FPS, r MFA, r MFM, r MFP, r + lt IMPFP, lt SPFP), bilaterally in the supplementary motor areas (SMA), the premotor areas (PM) and the left primary motor (MI) area. In addition, $rCMRO_2$ increased in supplementary sensory areas (SS), the left primary sensory area (SI), in the left anterior superior parietal lobule (SPA), bilaterally in the secondary somatosensory area (SII), the anterior insula, lingual gyri, hippocampus, basal ganglia, anterior parasagittal cerebellum, and lobus posterior cerebelli (Figure 5). Except for the anterior insular cortex, the posterior intermediate prefrontal cortex and the posterior lobe and lateral parts of cerebellum—all these structures had previously been found to participate in manipulatory movements and analysis of somatosensory information (Roland, 1987b,c).

Tactile recognition increased $rCMRO_2$ in the same structures as did tactile learning (Figure 5). The storage of tactile information thus engaged the same structures as did the retrieval of tactile information. Although identical structures were activated, there were important quantitative differences in the $rCMRO_2$ in a few structures between tactile learning and tactile recognition. The $rCMRO_2$ increases in the left premotor cortex, supplementary motor area and left somatosensory hand area were larger during tactile recognition in accordance with the higher frequency of manipulatory movements and higher flux of somatosensory information from the periphery during recognition. More important, despite the greater motor activity during tactile recognition the $rCMRO_2$ was significantly higher in the neocerebellar cortex during tactile learning (Figure 5).

In the records of the subjects it was not possible to find any effects of learning on the way the subjects manipulated the objects. So the extra metabolic activity in the lateral cerebellum was attributed to energy-demanding processes necessary for the storage of somatosensory information. Since the climbing fiber activity is higher during learning (Gilbert & Thach, 1977) and since climbing fiber activity is very energy demanding (Eccles et al., 1967) the extra metabolic activity in the posterior lobe of the neocerebellum during learning was probably due to climbing fiber activity. To our knowledge, this is the first demonstration of biochemical effects due to learning in the living human brain.

In a very recent experiment (Roland et al., in prep.), we studied learning, recall and recognition of colored geometrical patterns. In the learning session the subjects learned ten colored geometrical patterns. The expo-sure time for each pattern was 10 s. According to a preliminary evaluation of these data the rCBF increased in several prefrontal areas, the neostriatum, anterior insula, hippocampus, thalamus, and the visual association areas in the lateral temporo-occipital cortex and the visual association areas in the superior parie-tal lobule (SSPM). During the learning session the eyes were open and this resulted in an additional strong rCBF increase in the primary visual cortex (Figure 5). During the recall the subjects, with their eyes closed, recalled the appearance of each colored pat-tern in the same order as it was originally shown to them. This purely intrinsic retrieval of the stored images increased the rCBF in the prefrontal cortex, neostriatum, anterior insula, and in particular in thalamus and the post-erior parietal visual association cortex (Figure 5). This supports the hypothesis that the pre-frontal cortex via the thalamus (pulvinar?) participates in the retrieval of visual informa-tion stored in the visual association cortex. In the visual recognition experiment the learned geometrical patterns were mixed with other very similar patterns and the subjects's task was then to indicate by a subtle extension of the thumb each known pattern that he saw. During the recognition the rCBF, still accord-ing to a very preliminary analysis, increased in roughly the same regions as visual learning did. The exposure time of each stimulus was

only 100 ms. For this reason the rCBF increase in the primary visual cortex was quite modest (Figure 5). The rCBF in the cerebel-lum did not change during visual learning.

These experiments show that limbic and paralimbic structures plus the relevant sensory association areas are activated in learning and recognition. A special selection of prefrontal areas is also activated, the selection being dependent on the type of information to be stored or retrieved. The cerebellar involve-ment in learning is probably confined to sen-sori-motor activities. If any conclusion can be drawn from the recall experiments about the storage site for the sensory information that is learned, it is that the information is stored out-side the primary receptive area and its imme-diate surroundings.

Cortical Field Activation

One of the main findings from the intracarotid ^{133}Xe-studies was that cortical neurons always seem to be activated in a large ensemble that covers an area of some 3–9 cm^2 (Figure 6). This is the basis of the cortical field activation hypothesis (Roland, 1985b). But single pho-ton imaging techniques are inadequate in detecting the exact origin of rCBF changes and are incapable of measuring rCMR changes. Therefore it was necessary to ascer-tain whether the rCBF increases found during

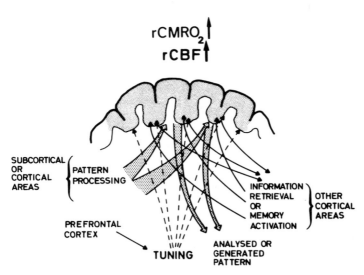

Figure 6. The physiological mecha-nisms that can increase metabo-lism and blood flow in a cortical field outside a primary sensory and motor area. Lesion studies have shown that the information processing is spread over the entire field. Direction of attention towards the field results in a tun-ing of selected neuron ensembles in the field. The prefrontal cortex is assumed to participate in the direction of attention. The pre-frontal cortex might also partic-ipate in retrieval of patterns from memory. (From Roland, 1984, by permission of The Australian Academy of Sciences).

earlier experiments corresponded to local rCMR increases. This was verified in a PET experiment in which the rCBF and rCMRO$_2$ was measured in the same individuals (Roland et al., 1987a).

In the primary motor area and primary somatosensory area the active fields are organized somatotopically. In the primary visual cortex the active fields are organized retinotopically (Fox et al., 1987b). In the auditory cortex the fields are organized tonotopically (Lauter et al., 1985). No clear topical organization has been seen outside these areas. The active fields do not seem coextensive with cytoarchitectural areas. In the somatosensory cortex this is probably because it is impossible to activate area 3b without activating areas 1 and 2 as well. From Figure 1 it is apparent that the space that is usually allocated to area 9 of Brodmann seems to consist of several functional subdivisions.

This principle of field organization has several implications. Two of the more important are that the information processing in the non-primary areas is spread out over a larger field (for a more detailed discussion see Roland, 1985b) and that the non-metabolic biochemical changes occurring when neurons are working also are spread out over a cortical field.

References

Bohm C, Greitz T, Kingsley D, Berggren BM, Olsson L (1985) A Computerized Individually Variable stereotaxic brain atlas. In Greitz T, Ingvar DH, Widén L (Eds.) *The metabolism of the human brain studied with positron emission tomography.* Raven Press, New York, 85—91.

Duara F, Yoshii F, Chang J, Barker W, Apicella A, Parks R, Emran A (1987) Complex reading memory task during PET in normal and memory-impaired subjects. *J Cereb Blood Flow and Metab, 7* (suppl 1), 312.

Eccles JC, Ito M, Szentagothai J (1967) *The cerebellum as a neuronal machine.* Springer, Heidelberg.

Fox PT, Raichle ME (1984) Stimulus rate dependence of regional cerebral blood flow in human striate cortex, demonstrated by positron emission tomography. *J Neurophysiol, 51,* 1109—1121.

Fox PT, Raichle ME (1986) Focal physiological uncoupling of cerebral blood flow and oxidative metabolism during somatosensory stimulation in

human subjects. *Proc Natl Acad Sci USA, 83,* 1140—1144.

Fox PT, Fox JM, Raichle ME, Burde RM (1985a) The role of cerebral cortex in the generation of voluntary saccades: A positron emission tomographic study. *J Neurophysiol, 54,* 348—369.

Fox PT, Raichle ME, Tach WT (1985b) Functional mapping of the human cerebellum with positron emission tomography. *Proc Natl Acad Sci USA, 82,* 7462—7466.

Fox PT, Petersen SE, Posner MI, Raichle ME (1987a) Language-related brain activation measured with PET: Comparison of auditory and visual word presentations. *J Cereb Blood Flow and Metab, 7* (suppl 1), 294.

Fox PT, Miezin FM, Allman JM, Van Essen DC, Raichle ME (1987b) Retinotopic organization of human visual cortex mapped with positron-emission tomography. *J Neurosci, 7* (3), 913—922.

Gilbert PFC, Thach WT (1977) Purkinje cell activity during motor learning. *Brain Research, 128,* 309—328.

Hand P, Greenberg JH, Miselis RR, Weller WK, Reivich M (1978) A normal and altered cortical column. *Neurosci Abstr, 4,* 553.

Heiss WD, Pawlik G, Hebold I, Herholz K, Wagner R, Wienhard K (1987) Metabolic pattern of speech activation in healthy volunteers, aphasics and focal epileptics. *J Cereb Blood Flow and Metab, 7* (suppl 1), 299.

Jones T, Chester DA, Ter-Pogossian MM (1976) The continuous inhalation of oxygen-15 for assessing regional oxygen extraction in the brain of man. *Br J Radiol, 49,* 339—343.

Kadareko M, Crane AM, Sokoloff L (1985) Differential effects of electrical stimulation of sciatic nerve on metabolic activity in spinal cord and dorsal root ganglion in the rat. *Proc Natl Acad Sci USA, 82,* 6010—6013.

Lassen NA, Ingvar DH (1961) The blood of the cerebral cortex determined by radioactive krypton-85. *Experientia, 17,* 42—43.

Lauter LL, Herscovitch P, Formby C, Raichle ME (1985) Tonotopic organization in human auditory cortex revealed by positron emission tomography. *Hearing Research, 20,* 199—205.

Mata M, Fink DJ, Gainer H, Smith CB, Davidsen L, Savaki H, Schwartz WH, Sokoloff L (1980) Activity-dependent energy metabolism in rat posterior pituitary primarily reflects sodium pump activity. *J Neurochem, 34,* 213—215.

Mazziotta JC, Phelps ME (1984) Positron computed tomographic studies of cerebral metabolic responses to complex motor tasks. *Neurology, 34,* 116.

Mazziotta JC, Phelps ME, Carson RE, Kuhl DE (1982a) Tomographic mapping of human cerebral metabolism: Auditory stimulation. *Neurology, 32,* 921—937.

Mazziotta JC, Phelps ME, Carson RE, Kuhl DE (1982b) Tomographic mapping of human cerebral metabolism: Sensory deprivation. *Ann Neurol, 12,* 435—444.

Mintun MA, Raichle ME, Martin WRW, Herscowitch P (1984) Brain oxygen utilization measured with [15]O radiotracers and positron emission tomography. *J Nucl Med, 25,* 177—187.

Phelps ME, Mazziotta JC, Kuhl DE, Nuwer M, Packwood J, Metler J, Engel J Jr (1981) Tomographic mapping of human cerebral metabolism: visual stimulation and deprivation. *Neurology, 31,* 517—529.

Raichle ME (1986) The circulatory and metabolic correlates of brain function in normal human subjects. Research strategies and problems of interpretation. In Plum F (Ed.) *Handbook of physiology, Section Neurophysiology, Vol. 3.* Am Physiol Soc., Bethesda.

Reivich M, Kuhl D, Wolf A, Greenberg J, Phelps M, Ido T, Casella V, Fowler J, Hoffman E, Alavi A, Sam P, Sokoloff L (1979) The ^{18}F-fluordeoxyglucose method for the measurement of local cerebral glucose utilization in man. *Circ Res, 44,* 127—137.

Roland PE (1984) Intensity and localization of cortical activations in man during sensory discrimination, directed attention and thinking. In Garlick ED, Korner PI (Eds.) *Frontiers in physiological research.* The Australian Academy of Science, Canberra, 306—324.

Roland PE (1985a) Cortical organization of voluntary behavior in man. *Hum Neurobiol, 4,* 155—167.

Roland PE (1985b) Application of imaging of brain blood flow to behavioral neurophysiology: The cortical field activation hypothesis. In Sokoloff L (Ed.) *Brain imaging and brain function.* Raven Press, New York, 87—104.

Roland PE (1987a) Changes in brain blood flow and oxidative metabolism during mental activity. *News in Physiological Sciences, 2,* 120—123.

Roland PE (1987b) Somatosensory detection of microgeometry, macrogeometry and kinesthesia after localized lesions of the cerebral hemispheres in man. *Brain Res Rev, 12,* 43—44.

Roland PE (1987c, in press) Metabolic mapping of sensori-motor integration in the human brain. In Porter R (Ed.) *Motor areas of the cerebral cortex.* Wiley, Chichester.

Roland PE, Friberg L (1985) Localization of cortical areas activated by thinking. *J Neurophysiol, 53,* 1219—1243.

Roland PE, Meyer E, Shibasaki T, Yamamoto YL, Thompson CJ (1982) Regional cerebral blood flow changes in cortex and basal ganglia during voluntary movements in normal human volunteers. *J Neurophysiol, 48,* 467—480.

Roland PE, Eriksson L, Stone-Elander S, Widén L (1987a) Does mental activity change the oxidative metabolism of the brain? *J Neurosci, 7,* 2373—2389.

Roland PE, Eriksson L, Widén L, Stone-Elander S (1987b, in press) Changes in regional oxidative metabolism induced by tactile learning and tactile recognition in man. *Soc Neurosci Abstr, 13.*

Sokoloff L, Reivich M, Kennedy C, DesRosiers M, Patlak CS, Pettigrew KD, Sakurada O, Shinohara M (1977) The (^{14}C)-deoxyglucose method for the measurement of local cerebral glucose utilization: Theory, procedure and normal values in the conscious and anaesthesized albino rat. *J Neurochem, 28,* 897—916.

Talairach J, Szikla G, Tournoux P, Prossalentis A, Bordas-Ferrer M, Covello L, Iacob M, Memple E (1967) *Atlas d'anatomic stéréotaxique du telencéphale.* Masson, Paris.

Comparison of Positron Emission Tomography and Electroencephalography as Measures of Cerebral Function in Epilepsy

J. Engel, Jr.

Positron Emission Tomography (PET) with 18F-fluorodeoxyglucose (FDG) and 15-oxygen has been used to examine patterns of cerebral metabolism and blood flow during the interictal state in patients with partial epilepsy, petit mal epilepsy, and some forms of secondary generalized epilepsy. Epileptogenic tissue is commonly characterized by decreased metabolism and perfusion in the partial and secondary generalized epilepsies, but no interictal PET disturbance has been identified in the primary generalized epilepsies. When present, the zone of hypometabolism or hypoperfusion is more extensive than any structural pathology, suggesting that it reflects functional reorganization associated with epileptogenesis. 2-deoxyglucose (2DG) autoradiographic studies of a variety of animal models of partial epilepsy have failed to demonstrate decreased glucose utilization beyond areas of obvious cellular destruction. Consequently, hypotheses concerning the neuronal mechanisms of interictal hypometabolism are based on additional data from epileptic patients. Electrophysiological studies have shown decreased unit firing rates and attenuated evoked potentials interictally in and around the site of seizure generation suggesting that neurons are hypoactive and have fewer connections. The hypometabolism, therefore, appears to reflect a reduction in synaptic activity within the epileptogenic zone and its projection fields. This can not be accounted for by selectively suppressed GABA mediated synaptic inhibition since paired pulse depression is enhanced in the epileptogenic zone interictally, and GAD terminals on remaining principal neurons in this area are normal or even increased.
PET studies with FDG during partial and generalized convulsive seizures indicate that the ictal event is associated with increased metabolism while the postictal period is associated with decreased metabolism. Petit mal seizures are associated with the highest rates of glucose metabolism, presumably because there is no postictal hypometabolism to influence the final weighted average. Ictal hypermetabolism during partial seizures occurs within the region of interictal hypometabolism, further supporting a conclusion that the latter involves a reversible functional component. Patterns of propagation during partial seizures are also revealed by PET with FDG, and have been studied by 2DG autoradiography in a variety of experimental animal models. As experience with kindling would suggest, the anatomical distribution of propagation from an experimental epileptic focus is greater than that produced by electrical stimulation of the same site, indicating that the epileptiform discharge has properties which facilitate transmission across certain synapses beyond what would normally occur.

Previous studies from our laboratory (Engel et al., 1982 a, b, c, d; 1983 a, b; 1984 a, b; 1985 a, b; Kuhl et al., 1980; Chugani & Engel, 1986; Chugani et al., 1987; Ackermann et al., 1986) and others (Theodore et al., 1984, 1985, 1987; Yamamoto et al., 1983; Bernardi et al., 1983; Ochs et al., 1987), using positron emission tomography (PET) with ^{18}F-fluorodeoxyglucose (FDG) to measure local cerebral meta-

Departments of Neurology and Anatomy, Laboratory of Nuclear Medicine, Brain Research Institute, UCLA School of Medicine, Los Angeles, CA 90024, USA.
Studies from UCLA reported here were supported in part by Grants NS-02808 and NS-15654 from the National Institutes of Health, Contract DE-AC03-76-SF00012 from the Department of Energy, and a grant from the David H. Murdock Foundation for Advanced Brain Studies.

bolic rate for glucose (LCMRGlc) as well as ^{13}N and $^{15}O_2$ to measure local cerebral blood flow, have demonstrated characteristic patterns of cerebral metabolism and perfusion in various forms of epilepsy. These patterns correlate poorly with certain aspects of epileptiform electrical activity recorded with scalp EEG and depth electrodes. It has been concluded that PET and EEG are complementary techniques which measure different aspects of cerebral function (Engel, 1983; 1984, 1985). This paper is concerned with characterizing these differences and attempting to define their pathophysiological bases.

The PET data examined here were derived from studies with FDG, although similar results have been obtained in some cases using tracers which indicate cerebral flood flow (Phelps et al. 1986). The FDG technique requires steady-state conditions and cannot be quantitatively applied to transient events such as epileptic seizures. FDG-PET is also unable to dissect out specific metabolic contributions of brief transients such as EEG spikes from ongoing background cerebral activity (Engel et al., 1985a). Data on cerebral metabolism obtained by this technique represents a weighted average over 40—60 minutes of FDG uptake and incorporation, with events occurring in the first few minutes after injection contributing most heavily to the final value obtained. Temporal resolution, therefore, is poor, but spatial resolution is excellent. Available FDG-PET equipment can create three-dimensional images of the entire brain with a resolution approaching 4 mm.

Electrophysiologic measurements, on the other hand, have excellent temporal resolution and can easily display brief epileptiform transients. EEG cleanly separates ictal from postictal and interictal phenomena. Spatial resolution, however, is poor since activity in deeper structures cannot be accurately inferred from scalp and sphenoidal activity, and stereotaxically implanted depth electrodes sample only from selected cerebral structures (Engel et al., 1983a; Wieser, 1983; Talairach et al., 1974). Scalp recordings were obtained routinely during all FDG-PET scan studies discussed here. In some cases, this also included sphenoidal and/or depth electrodes. In addition, most epileptic patients who par-

ticipated in these studies underwent long-term inpatient EEG telemetry and video monitoring using scalp and sphenoidal electrodes, and often depth electrodes as well (Engel et al., 1983a). Further confirmation of the location and nature of the epileptogenic region was obtained for many patients who underwent resective surgical therapy since pathological substrates and postoperative outcome are known (Engel et al., 1981b; 1982b, c, 1984b; Engel, 1987a).

Interictal Abnormalities

Local Metabolism

Interictal FDG-PET studies of partial epilepsy have consistently revealed one or more zones of hypometabolism in approximately 70% of patients (Engel et al., 1982a; Theodore et al., 1984; Yamamoto et al., 1983). Similar zones of hypoperfusion have also been demonstrated with ^{13}N and $^{15}O_2$ (Kuhl et al., 1980; Bernardi et al., 1983). The region of decreased LCMRGlc usually includes the demonstrated site of ictal onset (Engel et al., 1982a, c) and any observed pathological lesion (Engel et al., 1982b). However, the zone extends well beyond brain tissue which is electrophysiologically and structurally abnormal.

Typically, hypometabolism will involve an entire temporal lobe. In many cases, the contralateral temporal lobe also appears to be somewhat hypometabolic (Engel et al., 1982a; Bernardi et al., 1983). Depth electrode recordings, however, usually demonstrate that seizures originate in one hippocampus, and hippocampal sclerosis is often the only abnormality found on histological examination of resected tissue (Babb & Brown, 1987). This suggests that at least part of the decrease in LCMRGlc reflects functional disturbances of the brain. Such a conclusion is further supported by the fact that metabolism in the same area can be increased during seizures (Engel et al., 1983b; Theodore et al., 1984).

Diffuse, unilateral, and focal areas of hypometabolism are seen on interictal FDG-PET scans of children with secondary generalized epilepsies who are known to have diffuse and multifocal cerebral pathology (Chugani & Engel, 1986; Chugani et al., 1987; Theodore et al., 1987). Interictal FDG-PET scans are normal, however, in children with petit mal epilepsy, which has no known structural substrates (Engel et al., 1985b).

Electrophysiology

Cerebral areas generating the predominant interictal EEG spikes, as well as the site of ictal onset, are usually included within the interictal FDG-PET demonstrated hypometabolic zone. However, there is relatively poor correlation between the extent of the metabolic defect and the spatial distribution of interictal epileptiform EEG abnormalities, and no correlation between the degree of hypometabolism and any parameter of interictal EEG spike activity (Engel et al., 1982a) (Figure 1).

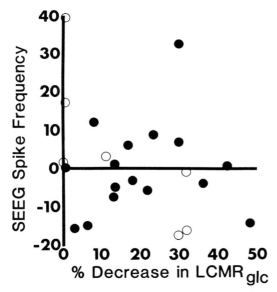

Figure 1. Graph to show the lack of correlation between interictal mesial temporal SEEG recorded spike frequency and percent relative hypometabolism within the less metabolically active temporal lobe. Each filled circle indicates a separate patient who had PCT with FDG and concurrent SEEG recordings. Open circles indicate repeat studies on seven patients during thiopental activation. Note that negative spike frequencies were obtained in 11 studies, indicating that interictal spike activity during these studies was greater contralateral to the zone of hypometabolism.

In temporal lobe epilepsy, interictal EEG spikes are usually most prominently recorded from sphenoidal derivations (Sperling et al., 1986), are commonly bilateral and independent (Engel et al., 1975, 1981b), and may be recorded independently over the lateral temporal cortex as well. Depth electrode recordings indicate that these sphenoidal spikes represent propagation from mesial temporal structures to some unknown cortical region, perhaps the uncus (Engel & Crandall, 1987). Multiple interictal spike foci are characteristically encountered in hippocampus, hippocampal gyrus and amygdala bilaterally, and the most active spike focus is not necessarily the site of ictal onset (Engel et al., 1981a, b; Lieb et al., 1981). This indicates that chronic human partial epilepsy is not due to a discrete epileptic focus, as suggested by experimental animal models, but rather to extensive, and perhaps multifocal, regions of epileptiform dysfunction (Engel, 1987b). Widespread, chronically epileptogenic regions of brain tissue may be necessary before clinical seizures are manifested (Engel, 1987b; Soper et al., 1978).

Basic Mechanism

There is no animal model of interictal focal hypometabolism beyond the area of cell loss induced by the epileptogenic lesion. 2-deoxyglucose autoradiography (2DG) reveals normal interictal cerebral metabolism in amygdala kindled rats with no identifiable structural pathology (Engel et al., 1978). Interictal 2DG studies of penicillin-induced epileptic foci in rats, however, demonstrate increased LCMRGlc at the site of interictal EEG spike discharges (Collins et al., 1976).

The neuronal membrane events underlying focal interictal EEG spike-and-wave discharges produced by topical penicillin, and a number of other epileptogenic agents, are known to be the synchronous occurrence of paroxysmal depolarization shifts, followed by prolonged afterhyperpolarization (Matsumoto & Ajmone-Marsan, 1964a). Unit recordings from human epileptogenic hippocampus demonstrate burst firing, followed by cessation of action potentials, during the interictal EEG spike-and-wave (Babb & Crandall, 1976). This suggests that similar membrane events underlie epileptiform transients in human chronic epilepsy. However, burst firing is encountered much less frequently in human epileptic brain than in experimental focal epilepsy, and synchronization is much less prominent (Babb & Crandall, 1976). Whereas 95% of recorded neurons in the penicillin focus may fire at the time of the interictal EEG spike (Matsumoto & Ajmone-Marsan, 1964a), less than 5% of neurons demonstrate burst firing during this time in the epileptic human hippocampus (Babb & Crandall, 1976). This might explain why interictal glucose metabolism is increased in the penicillin focus, but not in human epileptic brain regions.

Evidence from the amygdala kindling model (Engel & Ackermann, 1980), and from hippocampal slice (Swartzwelder et al., 1987), suggests that some interictal spikes reflect a state of seizure refractoriness. Since the wave of the spike-and-wave presumably represents membrane hyperpolarization, this interictal phenomenon may indicate that the "brakes are on." There is other evidence that chronic epileptogenic tissue is hypoexcitable during the interictal state. In both animals (Tuff et al., 1983) and humans (Engel & Wilson, 1986), the epileptic hippocampus can demonstrate paired pulse suppression rather than the normal paired pulse facilitation. This prolonged poststimulus refractory period may be analogous to the afterhyperpolarization which follows spontaneous paroxysmal depolarization shifts (Engel & Wilson, 1986). The human epileptic hippocampus also has elevated thresholds for electrical stimulation-induced afterdischarges (Cherlow et al., 1977). The interictal hypometabolic zone, therefore, appears to correspond to a region of neuronal suppression, perhaps reflecting endogenous mechanisms that act to contain epileptiform events, or to prevent transition to ictal state.

Ictal Abnormalities

Local Metabolism

Ictal FDG-PET studies carried out during partial seizures usually demonstrate regions of hypermetabolism which correspond to the site

of ictal onset and propagation of ictal discharge (Engel et al., 1983b; Theodore et al., 1984). Ictal FDG-PET studies of generalized convulsions induced by electroconvulsive shock (Engel et al., 1982d; Ackermann et al., 1986), and petit mal absences induced by hyperventilation (Engel et al., 1982d, 1985b), demonstrate diffusely increased cerebral metabolism. Some ictal scans during partial and generalized convulsive seizures, however, demonstrate little or no metabolic changes in regions clearly involved in ictal EEG discharges (Engel et al., 1982d, 1983b; Ackermann et al., 1986). Atypical absences also may not be associated with increased metabolism (Theodore et al., 1985; Ochs et al., 1987). Ictal hypermetabolism in these latter situations may be cancelled out by the contribution of postictal hypometabolism to the final weighted average, whereas postictal depression is not seen with typical absences (Engel et al., 1985b).

Electrophysiology

In ictal FDG-PET scans of partial epilepsy, there is good correlation between the location of EEG ictal onset and spread and the region of increased LCMRGlc. Nonetheless, it is not possible to differentiate sites of onset from sites of spread with PET (Engel et al., 1983b).

In all seizure types observed so far, there is no correlation between the duration of ictal discharges or the number of ictal events occurring during a FDG-PET study and the degree of hypermetabolism (Figures 2 and 3) (Engel et al., 1983b, 1985b). The increase in metabolic rate is uniformly greater during typical absences, which consist of 3/s spike-and-wave EEG patterns, than with other seizure disorders associated with low voltage fast, or polyspike ictal EEG patterns. This correlation is not true for all spike-and-wave phenomena, since atypical absences are not necessarily associated with increased metabolism (Theodore et al., 1985; Ochs et al., 1987).

Basic Mechanisms

2DG autoradiographic studies of rats with various types of experimental focal seizures have demonstrated a pattern of hypermetabo

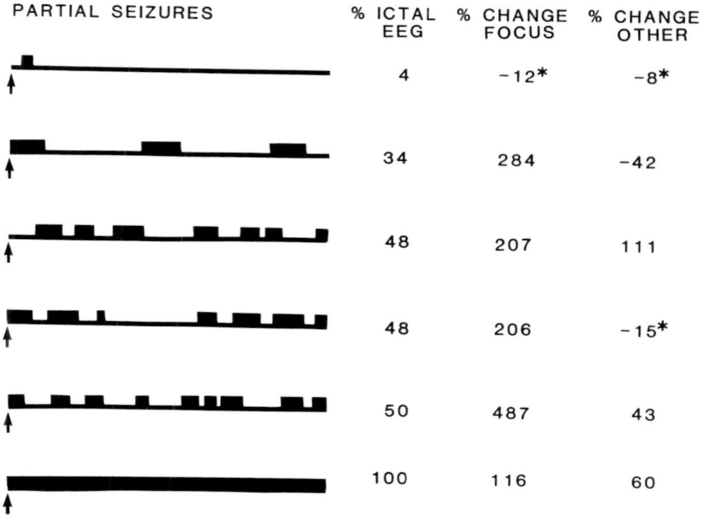

PARTIAL SEIZURES

	% ICTAL EEG	% CHANGE FOCUS	% CHANGE OTHER
	4	−12*	−8*
	34	284	−42
	48	207	111
	48	206	−15*
	50	487	43
	100	116	60

Figure 2. Demonstration of the temporal pattern and duration of partial seizures that occurred during the first 30 minutes after FDG injection, and metabolic data for six ictal scans. Arrows indicate time of FDG injection. Total time represented is 30 minutes. Patients are shown in order of increasing duration of ictal activity; numbers in text appear at left. % ICTAL EEG refers to the percentage of time during the first 30 minutes occupied by ictal EEG discharge; % CHANGE FOCUS indicated the relative change in LCMRGlc in the area of primary epileptiform discharge, compared with the same area interictally; and % CHANGE OTHER represents the same measurement for the remainder of the brain not directly involved in the epileptic discharge. Asterisks indicate three values that are not significantly different from paired studies in normal volunteers (Adapted from Engel et al., 1982a).

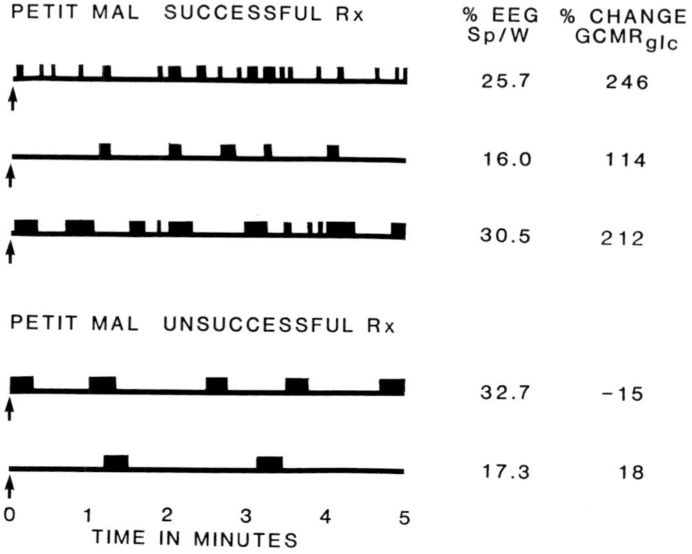

PETIT MAL SUCCESSFUL Rx

	% EEG Sp/W	% CHANGE GCMRglc
	25.7	246
	16.0	114
	30.5	212

PETIT MAL UNSUCCESSFUL Rx

	% EEG Sp/W	% CHANGE GCMRglc
	32.7	−15
	17.3	18

0   1   2   3   4   5
TIME IN MINUTES

Figure 3. The time lines on the left represent the first 5 minutes of hyperventilation following [18F]fluorodeoxyglucose (FDG) injection (arrow) for one FDG study in 3 patients and two FDG studies in a fourth with childhood absence epilepsy. The time of occurrence and duration of electroencephalographic (EEG) spike-and-wave (Sp/W) discharges are indicated as bars. Also indicated for each patient is the percentage of time during the first 5 minutes following FDG injection occupied by spike-and-wave discharges, and the percentage of change in the global cerebral metabolic rate for glucose (GCMRGlc) of the ictal scan, compared with the hyperventilation control scan. The percentage of change in GCMRGlc indicated for each of the two scans of Patient 4 refers to change with respect to the other scan. Note that there is no quantitative relationship between the increases in metabolic rate and aspects of the EEG-recorded absences. (Adapted from Engel et al., 1983b).

lism in regions of ictal onset and spread similar to that seen in human epilepsy (Collins, 1978; Collins & Caston, 1979; Collins et al., 1976; Engel et al., 1978). Patterns of ictal 2DG uptake with amygda kindling in rats are more stereotyped than those found with temporal lobe seizures in humans (Engel & Cahan, 1986). When amygdala kindled seizures remain partial, increased 2DG is seen in limbic structures receiving amygdalar projections, but when seizures are generalized, hypermetabolism appears more diffusely in cortex, thalamus, and substantia nigra (Engel et al., 1978). With these generalized seizures, amygdala and entorhinal cortex no longer show increased 2DG uptake even though ictal discharges can be recorded from these areas after stimulation (Engel et al., 1978). This animal model therefore demonstrates dissociation between ictal electrophysiological and metabolic measures of cerebral function similar to that seen in some epileptic patients.

Depth electrode recordings from human epileptogenic temporal lobe reveal that seizures originate in the cell-sparse areas of sclerotic hippocampus, not in the more normal appearing surrounding tissue (Babb et al., 1984). Presumably these areas of cell loss undergo synaptic reorganization conducive to the generation of epileptiform activity, while progagation may require projection areas to be abnormally receptive to these discharges (Engel, 1987b, 1988). Mechanisms of ictal onset therefore may be different from those that underlie subsequent recruitment.

At least two types of ictal discharge patterns exist clinically and often both can be seen at different stages of the same seizure. In any given ictus, one pattern may occur on ictal onset while the other may appear at sites of propagation. The pattern typically seen with most partial seizures and generalized convulsions consists of low voltage fast activity that builds up to a polyspike recruiting rhythm. The other pattern of rhythmic high amplitude spike-and-wave discharges is characteristic of absences, but a focal form can also occur with partial seizures (Engel & Wilson, 1986; Engel, 1988). The mechanism of the former is believed to be a breakdown of afterhyperpolarization leading to prolonged membrane depolarization and continuous

burst discharges (Matsumoto & Ajmone-Marsan, 1964b). The mechanism of the latter appears to be excessive synchronization of depolarization-hyperpolarization complexes, perhaps provoked by synchronizing afferent input (Gloor, 1979; Gloor et al., 1977; Quesney, et al., 1977). This form of ictal discharge would seem to require powerful inhibitory mechanisms (Engel & Wilson, 1986).

2DG autoradiographic studies carried out during continuous synaptic inhibition of hippocampus revealed hypermetabolism which may have been even greater than that seen with some forms of synaptic excitation of hippocampus (Ackermann et al., 1984). The inhibition in this study was mediated by rapidly firing GABA-containing interneurons, and it is not surprising that this activity requires energy. Ictal hypermetabolism seen on 2DG autoradiographs, as well as FDG-PET scans in patients therefore could be accounted for by excitatory or inhibitory synaptic events, or both. Failure to show increased metabolism with EEG ictal discharge, on the other hand, might reflect averaging of postictal hypometabolism, or increased efficiency of neuronal interactions at the region of ictal onset (Engel et al., 1978).

Postictal Abnormalities

Local Metabolism

Ictal FDG-PET scans during some partial seizures have demonstrated diffuse hypometabolism outside the areas of increased LCMRGlc (Engel et al., 1982d, 1983b). To date, this finding has been seen only in patients who have had complex partial seizures, and is presumed to reflect the more diffuse postictal changes following ictal events associated with impaired consciousness. One patient who had an FDG-PET scan during a single complex partial seizure induced by hippocampal stimulation showed only lateral temporal hypometabolism (Engel et al., 1983b). This was presumed to be due to postictal changes limited to that temporal lobe. These influences may have reduced the ictally hypermetabolic hippocampus to normal values, and the less activated lateral temporal cortex to subnormal values in the final weighted average.

The association of postictal depression with hypometabolism has been clearly demonstrated with electroconvulsive shock-induced generalized seizures (Engel et al., 1982d; Ackermann et al., 1986). Diffuse hypometabolic PET images are obtained when FDG is injected at the time the ictal EEG discharge terminates and postictal depression begins.

Electrophysiology

Complex partial and generalized convulsive seizures are usually followed by EEG depression which can persist for many minutes while postictal clinical symptoms remain. The EEG may be initially flat or contain polymorphic slow waves with marked attenuation or absence of normal activity. Localized EEG depression can also occur after simple partial seizures.

Impaired consciousness during complex partial seizures is usually an indication of bilateral hippocampal involvement in the ictal EEG discharge (Wieser, 1983). This bilateral seizure activity results in more diffuse postictal EEG and behavioral depression. No studies have been carried out to determine if the degree or duration of postictal EEG depression is correlated with the degree of focal or diffuse hypometabolism seen on ictal FDG-PET scans. Studies that have reported no change in global metabolism during atypical absences (Theodore et al., 1985; Ochs et al., 1987) did not note whether postictal EEG changes occurred.

Basic Mechanisms

Postictal 2DG autoradiographic studies of rats, following kindling-induced generalized convulsions, have revealed diffuse cerebral hypometabolism with relative hypermetabolism of hippocampus and substantia nigra (Ackermann et al., 1986). The duration of postictal behavior change appears to correlate with the persistence of hippocampal and substantia nigra metabolic abnormalities (Caldecott-Hazard & Engel, 1987). The role of these structures in mediating postictal depression

and other aspects of postictal behavior is unknown.

Endogenous opioids have been implicated in some postictal phenomena (Caldecott-Hazard & Engel, 1987; Engel et al., 1984a). These peptides are known to be released during epileptic seizures in animals (Hong et al., 1979). Pretreatment of kindled rats with morphine exacerbates postictal depression (Frenk et al., 1979), while pretreatment with naloxone shortens postictal depression (Frenk et al., 1979) and reduces certain other postictal behavioral disturbances (Caldecott-Hazard & Engel, 1987).

Epileptic seizures are terminated by active inhibitory mechanisms and not neuronal exhaustion (Caspers & Speckman, 1972). The inhibition involved would seem not to be GABA-mediated, at least outside of hippocampus and substantia nigra, since the brain is generally hypometabolic during this time. If opioid inhibition were not energy requiring, this might explain the postictal 2DG pattern obtained in rats. Endogenous opioids are generally inhibitory in the central nervous system, but excitatory in the hippocampus (Dingledine, 1981). Indeed, the 2DG metabolic pattern induced in rats by intracerebroventricular injection of opioids resembles the postictal pattern after amygdala kindling (Chugani et al., 1984).

Synthesis

FDG-PET and EEG appear to measure different aspects of cerebral function. The metabolic images revealed by PET reflect weighted averages over 40—60 minutes of FDG incorporation, and are influenced by the number of cells activated, and the degree of their activation during this time. These metabolic measurements are not affected by the types of cells activated, their particular function, or their orientation within the brain. Electrical signals measured by the EEG reflect the degree of synchrony of graded membrane potentials generated immediately beneath the recording electrodes. These signals are influenced by the functional relationships of neuronal elements and their dipolar orientations. Electrophysiological measures do not indicate the number of neuronal elements involved in producing the recorded signals. Hypersynchrony of a few cells can produce large EEG transients with no change in metabolic rate, while active GABA-mediated inhibition of neurons may be associated with hypermetabolism. Neuronal areas that are hypoactive due to inhibitory or suppressive mechanisms that require little energy would be hypometabolic. Such mechanisms could include intrinsic calcium-dependent potassium currents, or effects of neuromodulators released into the intercellular space without specific synaptic activation.

Ictal onset and spread of electrographic discharges undoubtedly reflect several mechanisms. Disinhibition leading to increased excitability utilizes energy. Hypersynchronous ictal patterns most likely involve GABA-mediated inhibitory mechanisms which would also be associated with increased energy requirements. There is no evidence that any ictal epileptic phenomena are associated with decreased metabolism.

Termination of ictal events is due to active inhibition which does not appear to be GABA-mediated since postictal depression is associated with hypometabolism. Generalized electrical and behavioral postictal depression may, in part, be due to opioid mechanisms since postictal 2DG metabolic patterns resemble those induced by intracerebroventricular opioid injections.

Interictal hypometabolism at the site of ictal onset may, in part, reflect neuronal loss. This region is also hypoactive and the hypoactivity is apparently not due to active GABA-mediated inhibition since this would increase LCMRGlc. Inhibitory mechanisms are prominent in the chronic epileptogenic zone, however, and presumably contribute to the development of hypersynchronization.

Hypometabolism extending beyond the structural epileptogenic lesion could reflect decreased input from the cell-sparse hypoactive region, or these areas might also be hypoexcitable. Recent PET studies with ^{11}C-carfentanil in patients with complex partial seizures have demonstrated increased mu receptor binding in the lateral cortex of the hypometabolic temporal lobe (Frost et al, 1987). The increase in mu receptor binding correlates directly with the decrease in LCMRGlc measured with FDG-PET. Just as postictal hypometabolism may in part reflect suppression of neuronal activity by endogenous opioids, these peptides may also contribute to more localized hypoactivity in the region of the epileptogenic lesion, perhaps developing as a natural mechanism to maintain the interictal state. This same opioid effect might also account for the appearance of the hypometabolic zone.

References

Ackermann RF, Finch DM, Babb TL, Engel J Jr (1984) Increased glucose metabolism during long-duration recurrent inhibition of hippocampal pyramidal cells. *J Neurosci, 4,* 251—264.

Ackermann RF, Engel J Jr, Baxter L (1986) PET and autoradiographic studies of glucose utilization following electroconvulsive seizures in humans and rats. *Ann NY Acad Sci, 462,* 263—269.

Babb TL, Brown WJ (1987) Pathological findings in epilepsy. In Engel J Jr (Ed.) *Surgical treatment of the epilepsies.* Raven Press, New York, 511—540.

Babb TL, Crandall PH (1976) Epileptogenesis of human limbic neurons in psychomotor epileptics. *Electroenceph clin Neurophysiol, 40,* 225—243.

Babb TL, Lieb JP, Brown WJ, Pretorius J, Crandall PH (1984) Distribution of pyramidal cell density and hyperexcitability in the epileptic human hippocampal formation. *Epilepsia, 25,* 721—728.

Bernardi S, Trimble MR, Frackowiak RSJ, Wise RJS, Jones T (1983) An interictal study of partial epilepsy using positron emission tomography and the oxygen-15 inhalation technique. *J Neurol Neurosurg Psychiat, 46,* 473—477.

Caldecott-Hazard S, Engel J Jr (1987, in press) Limbic postictal events: anatomical substrates and opioid receptor involvement. *Prog Neuro-Psychopharmacol and Biol Psychiat.*

Caspers H, Speckmann EJ (1972) Cerebral pO_2, pCO_2 and pH: changes during convulsive activity and their significance for spontaneous arrest of seizures. *Epilepsia, 13,* 699—725.

Cherlow DG, Dymond AM, Crandall PH, Walter RD, Serafetinides EA (1977) Evoked response and after-discharge thresholds to electrical stimulation in temporal lobe epileptics. *Arch Neurol, 34,* 527—531.

Chugani HT, Engel J Jr (1986) PET in intractable epilepsy. In Morselli PL, Schmidt D (Eds.) *Workshop on intractable epilepsy: Experimental and clinical aspects.* Raven Press, New York, 119—128.

Chugani HT, Ackermann RF, Chugani DC, Engel J Jr (1984) Opioid-induced epileptogenic phenomena: Anatomical, behavioral, and electroencephalographic features. *Ann Neurol, 15,* 361—368.

Chugani HT, Mazziotta JC, Engel J Jr, Phelps ME (1987) The Lennox-Gastaut syndrome: Metabolic subtypes determined by 2-deoxy-2[^{18}F]fluoro-D-glucose positron emission tomography. *Ann Neurol, 21,* 4—13.

Collins RC (1978) Use of cortical circuits during focal penicillin seizures: an autoradiographic study with ^{14}C deoxyglucose. *Brain Res, 150,* 487—501.

Collins RC, Caston TV (1979) Functional anatomy of occipital lobe seizures: an experimental study in rats. *Neurol, 29,* 705—716.

Collins RC, Kennedy C, Sokoloff L, Plum F (1976) Metabolic anatomy of focal motor seizures. *Arch Neurol, 33,* 536—542.

Dingledine R (1981) Possible mechanisms of enkephalin action on hippocampal CA1 pyramidal neurons. *J Neurosci, 1,* 1022—1035.

Engel J Jr (1983) Metabolic patterns of human epilepsy: Clinical observations and possible physiological correlates. In Baldy-Moulinier M, Ingvar DH, Meldrum BS (Eds.) *Current problems in epilepsy: 1, Cerebral blood flow, metabolism and epilepsy.* John Libbey Eurotext Ltd, London 6—18.

Engel J Jr (1984) The use of Positron Emission Tomographic scanning in epilepsy. *Ann Neurol, 115* (Suppl. 1), 180—191.

Engel J Jr (1985) Positron emission tomography (PET) in the diagnosis of epilepsy. In Porter RJ, Morselli PL (Eds.) *The epilepsies.* Butterworths, London, 242—266.

Engel J Jr (1987a) Outcome with respect to epileptic seizures. In Engel J Jr (Ed.) *Surgical treatment of the epilepsies.* Raven Press, New York, 553—572.

Engel J Jr (1987b) New concepts of the epileptic focus. In Weiser HG, Speckmann EG, Engel J Jr (Eds.) *The epileptic focus.* John Libbey Eurotext Ltd, London, 83—94.

Engel J Jr (1988, in press) Pathophysiology of human brain metabolism in epilepsy. In Dichter, M (Ed.) *Mechanisms of epileptogenesis.* Plenum Press, New York.

Engel J Jr, Ackermann RF (1980) Interictal EEG spikes correlate with decreased, rather than increased epileptogenicity in amygdaloid kindled rats. *Brain Res, 190,* 543—548.

Engel J Jr, Cahan L (1986) Potential relevance of kindling to human partial epilepsy. In Wada J (Ed.) *Kindling 3.* Raven Press, New York, 37—51.

Engel J Jr, Wilson CL (1986) Evidence for enhanced synaptic inhibition in epilepsy. In Nistico G, Morselli PL, Lloyd KG, Fariello RG,

Engel J Jr (Eds.) *Neurotransmitters, seizures and epilepsy, III.* Raven Press, New York, 1—13.

Engel J Jr, Crandall PH (1987) Intensive electrodiagnostic monitoring with intracranial electrodes. In Gumnit R (Ed.) *Advances in neurology, Vol 46: Intensive neurodiagnostic monitoring.* Raven Press, New York, 85—106.

Engel J Jr, Driver MV, Falconer MA (1975) Electrophysiological correlates of pathology and surgical results in temporal lobe epilepsy. *Brain, 98,* 129—156.

Engel J Jr, Wolfson L, Brown L (1978) Anatomical correlates of electrical and behavioral events related to amygdaloid kindling. *Ann Neurol, 3,* 538—544.

Engel J Jr, Ackermann RF, Caldecott-Hazard S, Kuhl DE (1981a) Epileptic activation of antagonistic systems may explain paradoxical features of experimental and human epilepsy: A review and hypothesis. In Wada JA (Ed.) *Kindling 2.* Raven Press, New York, 193—211.

Engel J Jr, Rausch R, Lieb JP, Kuhl DE, Crandall PH (1981b) Correlation of criteria used for localizing epileptic foci in patients considered for surgical therapy of epilepsy. *Ann Neurol, 9,* 215—224.

Engel J Jr, Kuhl DE, Phelps ME, Mazziotta JC (1982a) Interictal cerebral glucose metabolism in partial epilepsy and its relation to EEG changes. *Ann Neurol, 12,* 510—517.

Engel J Jr, Brown WJ, Kuhl DE, Phelps ME, Mazziotta JC, Crandall PH (1982b) Pathological findings underlying focal temporal lobe hypometabolism in partial epilepsy. *Ann Neurol, 12,* 518—528.

Engel J Jr, Kuhl DE, Phelps ME, Crandall PH (1982c) Comparative localization of epileptic foci in partial epilepsy by PCT and EEG. *Ann Neurol, 12,* 529—537.

Engel J Jr, Kuhl DE, Phelps ME (1982d) Patterns of human local cerebral glucose metabolism during epileptic seizures. *Science, 218,* 64—66.

Engel J Jr, Crandall PH, Rausch R (1983a) The partial epilepsies. In Rosenberg RN (Ed.) *The clinical neurosciences, Vol. 2.* Churchill Livingstone, New York, 1349—1380.

Engel J Jr, Kuhl DE, Phelps ME, Rausch R, Nuwer M (1983b) Local cerebral metabolism during partial seizures. *Neurology, 33,* 400—413.

Engel J Jr, Ackermann RF, Caldecott-Hazard S, Chugani HT (1984a) Do altered opioid mechanisms play a role in human epilepsy? In Fariello RG, Morselli PL, Lloyd K, Quesney LF, Engel J Jr (Eds.) *Neurotransmitters, seizures, and epilepsy II.* Raven Press, New York, 263—274.

Engel J Jr, Sutherling WW, Cahan L, Crandall PH, Kuhl DE, Phelps ME (1984b) The role of positron emission tomography in the surgical therapy of epilepsy. In Porter RJ, Mattson RH,

Ward AA Jr, Dam M (Eds.) *Advances in epileptology: XV Epilepsy International Symposium.* Raven Press, New York, 427–432.

Engel J Jr, Ackermann RF, Kuhl DE, Phelps ME (1985a) Brain imaging of glucose utilization in convulsive disorders. In Sokoloff L (Ed.) *Brain imaging and brain function* (Association for Research in Nervous and Mental Disease, Research Publication, Vol. 63). Raven Press, New York, 163–184.

Engel J Jr, Lubens P, Kuhl DE, Phelps M (1985b) Local cerebral metabolic rate for glucose during petit mal absences. *Ann Neurol, 17,* 121–128.

Frenk H, Engel J Jr, Ackermann RF, Shavit Y, Liebeskind JC (1979) Endogenous opioids may mediate post-ictal behavioral depression in amygdaloid-kindled rats. *Brain Res, 167,* 435–440.

Frost JJ, Mayberg HS, Fisher RS, Douglass KH, Dannals RF, Links JM, Wilson AA, Ravert HT, Rosenbaum AE, Snyder SH, Wagner HN (1987, in press) Mu-opiate receptors measured by positron emission tomography are increased in temporal lobe epilepsy. *Ann Neurol.*

Gloor P (1979) Generalized epilepsy with spike-and-wave discharge: A reinterpretation of its electrographic and clinical manifestations. *Epilepsia, 20,* 571–588.

Gloor P, Quesney LF, Zumstein H (1977) Pathophysiology of generalized penicillin epilepsy in the cat: The role of cortical and subcortical structures. II. Topical applications of penicillin to the cerebral cortex and to subcortical structures. *Electroenceph clin Neurophysiol, 43,* 79–94.

Hong JS, Gillin JC, Yang HY, Costa E (1979) Repeated electroconvulsive shocks and the brain content of endorphins. *Brain Res, 177,* 273–278.

Kuhl DE, Engel J Jr, Phelps ME, Selin C (1980) Epileptic patterns of local cerebral metabolism and perfusion in humans determined by emission computed tomography of ^{18}FDG and ^{13}NH3. *Ann Neurol, 8,* 348–360

Lieb JP, Engel J Jr, Gevins AS, Crandall PH (1981) Surface and deep EEG correlates of surgical outcome in temporal lobe epilepsy. *Epilepsia, 22,* 515–538

Matsumoto H, Ajmone-Marsan C (1964a) Cortical cellular phenomena in experimental epilepsy: Interictal manifestations. *Exp Neurol, 9,* 286–304.

Matsumoto H, Ajmone-Marsan C (1964b) Cortical cellular phenomena in experimental epilepsy: Ictal manifestations. *Exp Neurol, 9,* 305–326.

Ochs RF, Gloor P, Tyler JL, Wolfson T, Worsley K, Andermann F, Diksic M, Meyer E, Evans A (1987) Effect of generalized spike-and-wave discharge on glucose metabolism measured by positron emission tomography. *Ann Neurol, 21,* 458–464

Phelps ME, Mazziotta JC, Schelbert HR (1986) *Positron emission tomography and autoradiography. Principles and applications for the brain and heart.* Raven Press, New York.

Quesney LF, Gloor P, Kratzenberg E, Zumstein H (1977) Pathophysiology of generalized penicillin epilepsy in the cat: The role of cortical and subcortical structures. I. Systemic application of penicillin. *Electroenceph clin Neurophysiol, 42,* 640–655.

Soper HV, Strain GM, Babb TL, Lieb JP, Crandall PH (1978) Chronic alumina temporal lobe seizures in monkeys. *Exp Neurol, 62,* 99–121.

Sperling MR, Mendius JR, Engel J Jr (1986) Mesial temporal spikes: A simultaneous comparison of sphenoidal, nasopharyngeal, and ear electrodes. *Epilepsia, 27,* 81–86.

Swartzwelder HS, Lewis DV, Anderson WW, Wilson WA (1987, in press) Seizure-like events in brain slices: Suppression by interictal activity. *Brain Research.*

Talairach J, Bancaud J, Szikla G, Bonis A, Geier S, Vedrenne C(1974) Approche nouvelle de la neurochirurgie de l'epilepsie. Methodologie stereotaxique et resultats therapeutiques. I. Introduction et historique. *Neurochir, 20* (Supp 1), 240.

Theodore WH, Newmark ME, Sato S, De LaPaz R, Di Chiro G, Brooks R, Patronas N, Kessler RM, Manning R, Margolin R, Channing M, Porter RJ (1984) ^{18}F-fluorodeoxyglucose positron emission tomography in refractory complex partial seizures. *Ann Neurol 14,* 429–437

Theodore H, Brooks R, Margolin R, Patronas N, Sato S, Porter RJ, Mansi L, Bairamian D, DiChiro G (1985) Positron emission tomography in generalized seizures. *Neurol, 35,* 684–690.

Theodore WH, Rose D, Patronas N, Sato S, Holmes M, Bairamian D, Porter RJ, DiChiro G, Larson S, Fishbein D (1987) Cerebral glucose metabolism in the Lennox-Gastaut syndrome. *Ann Neurol 21,* 14–21.

Tuff LP, Racine RJ, Adamec R (1983) The effects of kindling on GABA-mediated inhibition in the dentate gyrus of the rat. I. Pairedpulse depression. *Brain Res 277,* 79–90.

Wieser HG (1983) *Electroclinical features of psychomotor seizure. A stereoelectroencephalographic study of ictal symptoms and chromatographical seizure patterns including clinical effects of intracerebral stimulation.* Butterworths, London.

Yamamoto YL, Ochs R, Gloor P, Ammann W, Meyer E, Evans AC, Cooke B, Sako K, Gotman J, Feindel WH, Diksic M, Thompson CJ, Robitaille Y (1983) Patterns of rCBF and focal energy metabolic changes in relation to electroencephalographic abnormality in the inter-ictal phase of partial epilepsy. In Baldy-Moulinier M, Ingvar D-H, Meldrum BS (Eds.) *Current problems in epilepsy: 1. Cerebral blood flow, metabolism and epilepsy.* John Libbey, London 51–62.

Quantitative EEG and Positron Emission Tomography in Brain Ischemia

K. Nagata*, K. Tagawa*, S. Hiroi*,
M. Nara**, F. Shishido***, K. Uemura***

Quantitative EEG data were analyzed with respect to CBF and $CMRO_2$ measured at cortical regions corresponding to the location of EEG electrodes in 43 patients with unilateral cerebral infarction. Percentage power fraction (PPF) was defined as a relative value of the square root of average power within each frequency band. Power ratio index (PRI) was calculated by dividing the combined delta-PPF and theta-PPF by the combined alpha-PPF and beta-PPF. Delta-PPF correlated negatively with CBF and $CMRO_2$ at all regions except for the frontopolar region. Theta-PPF and PRI correlated negatively with CBF and $CMRO_2$ at all regions, whereas alpha-PPF correlated positively at all regions. Their correlation coefficients were largest at the parietal and posterior temporal regions. Beta-PPF correlated significantly with CBF and $CMRO_2$ only at the frontal, central and parietal regions. In the acute stage of cerebral infarction, the EEG parameters correlated more closely with CBF than with $CMRO_2$, but this tendency was reversed in the subacute stage. All parameters but beta-PPF correlated significantly with both CBF and $CMRO_2$ in the chronic stage.

With respect to the reduction of cerebral blood flow (CBF) and oxygen uptake, the EEG data have been analyzed in patients with cerebral ischemia. Obrist and associates (1963) found that the slow-wave activity correlated negatively with CBF and oxygen uptake in patients with arteriosclerotic dementia. In regional CBF studies with ^{133}Xe intra-arterial method, Ingvar and Sulg (1969) concluded that the quantitative EEG data correlated not only with the hemispheric mean CBF values but also with the regional CBF values in pa-

tients with cerebral ischemia. Topographic multichannel EEG data were used in the correlation study with two-dimensional regional CBF measurements in patients with cerebral infarction (Nagata et al., 1982; Nagata et al., 1984). The topographic focus of the slow-wave activity corresponded to the ischemic lesion provided by the two-dimensional CBF measurements. Although the relationship between EEG and CBF or oxygen metabolism might vary according to the methodological difference and the timing of examination, the slowing of the background EEG activity seems to correlate in general with the reduction of CBF and oxygen metabolism in patients with cerebral ischemia. However, because of the individual variability of the EEG data and the technical limitation in the measurement of circulatory and metabolic variables, the study of the correlation between EEG and CBF or cerebral metabolism in patients with cerebral ischemia was rather limited.

Positron emission tomography (PET) has made it possible to visualize the quantitative data of the cerebral circulation and metabolism. Our preliminary report suggested that there was a close correlation between slowing of the background EEG activity and reduction of cortical blood flow and oxygen metabolism that were measured by PET in patients with

Department of Neurology*, EEG Laboratory**, Department of Radiology and Nuclear Medicine***, Research Institute for Brain and Blood Vessels, Akita, Japan

neuropsychological syndromes due to cerebral infarction (Nagata et al. 1986a,b). The purpose of the present study is to elucidate the relationship between quantitative EEG data, cortical blood flow and oxygen metabolism in patients with cerebral infarction utilizing the topographic EEG and PET studies.

Subjects and Methods

Subjects

The present study was based on 43 patients with a unilateral cerebral infarction. The patients' mean age was 62.9 years. Fifty-two series of CT, EEG and PET studies were performed on these 43 patients. Multichannel EEG recording was carried out within 24 hours of the PET studies. Thirty-two patients had a left hemisphere lesion and 11 patients had a right hemisphere lesion. The present study included 34 patients with an infarct in the territory of the middle cerebral artery (MCA), 7 patients with an infarction in the territory of the posterior cerebral artery (PCA) and 2 patients with an occlusion of the anterior choroidal artery. Seventeen examinations were done within 14 days of onset (acute stage), and 16 examinations were performed between 15 days and 30 days after onset (subacute stage). Nineteen examinations were performed more than 31 days after onset (chronic stage). The mean timings of the examinations were at 8th, 21st and 134th day after onset, for the acute, subacute and chronic stages, respectively. The mean ages of the patient groups were 62.8, 62.6 and 63.2 years for the acute, subacute and chronic stages, respectively.

Quantitative EEG Analysis

Using the international 10-20 system, electrical activity was recorded from the 16 scalp electrodes using the 17-channel EEG polygraph (1A88, NEC-San'ei): Fp1, Fp2, F3, F4, C3, C4, P3, P4, O1, O2, F7, F8, T5, T6, Fz and Pz. Referential derivations were used with both earlobes serving as reference. Using the Fast Fourier transformation, power spectral analysis was carried out between 2.0 and

29.8 Hz by an on-line data processor (7T17, NEC-San'ei; CME-100, Japan System). This data acquisition system provided a good reproducibility as shown in a previous report (Nagata et al., 1982). The square root of the average power was calculated for the particular frequency ranges: delta (2.0–3.8 Hz), theta (4.0–7.8 Hz), alpha (8.0–12.8 Hz), and beta (13.0–29.8 Hz). Percentage power fraction (PPF) was defined as the relative value of the square root of the average power within each frequency band to that of the whole frequency spectrum (Nagata et al., 1986b; Tagawa et al., 1986). As indicated below, four PPFs, delta-PPF, theta-PPF, alpha-PPF and beta-PPF, were calculated for each derivation. The hemispheric mean value of PPF was calculated by averaging the values from the 7 derivations over each hemisphere; Fz and Pz derivations were not included.

$$\text{delta-PPF} = \frac{\text{square root of average power (2.0-3.8 Hz)} \times 100}{\text{square root of average power (2.0-29.8 Hz)}}$$

$$\text{theta-PPF} = \frac{\text{square root of average power (4.0-7.8 Hz)} \times 100}{\text{square root of average power (2.0-29.8 Hz)}}$$

$$\text{alpha-PPF} = \frac{\text{square root of average power (8.0-12.8 Hz)} \times 100}{\text{square root of average power (2.0-29.8 Hz)}}$$

$$\text{beta-PPF} = \frac{\text{square root of average power (13.0-29.8 Hz)} \times 100}{\text{square root of average power (2.0-29.8 Hz)}}$$

As a single parameter is reflecting the degree of the slowing of the background EEG activity, a power ratio index (PRI) was defined as a ratio of the slow-wave components to the fast-wave components (Nagata et al., 1985; Nagata et al., 1986b).

$$\text{PRI} = \frac{(\text{delta-PPF} + \text{theta-PPF}) \times 100}{\text{alpha-PPF} + \text{beta-PPF}}$$

$$= \frac{\text{square root of average power (2.0-7.8 Hz)} \times 100}{\text{square root of average power (8.0-29.8 Hz)}}$$

The PRI was calculated for each derivation. The hemispheric mean value of PRI was calculated by averaging the values from the 7 derivations over each hemisphere.

Positron Emission Tomography

The PET study was carried out using HEAD-TOME III (Kanno et al., 1983; Uemura et al., 1985) during continuous inhalation of three kinds of oxygen-15-labeled compounds. According to the oxygen-15 steady state method

(Lammertsma & Jones, 1983), four kinds of circulatory variables were obtained by the PET studies: cerebral blood flow (CBF), cerebral metabolic rate of oxygen (CMRO$_2$), cerebral blood volume (CBV) and oxygen extraction fraction (OEF), which is defined as a ratio of CMRO$_2$ value relative to CBF value. Regional values of CBF and CMRO$_2$, rCBF and rCMRO$_2$, were calculated at 14 cortical sites corresponding to the location of the EEG electrodes over the scalp. In the calculation of the rCBF and rCMRO$_2$, the regions of interest, consisting of 81 pixels (18 × 18 mm), that correspond to the location of the scalp EEG electrodes were determined on the print-out PET images (Tagawa et al., 1986). The mean of the 7 regional values over each hemisphere was used as the hemispheric mean value: mCBF and mCMRO$_2$.

Statistical Analysis of EEG and PET Data

The Student's paired t-test was employed to determine whether the hemispheric mean values between the unaffected and affected hemispheres differed. Linear regression analysis

was used to establish the relationship between the EEG quotients and CBF or CMRO$_2$.

1) The relationship between mCBF and mCMRO$_2$ was analyzed according to the stages of cerebral infarction.
2) Hemispheric mean values of EEG quotients were compared between the two hemispheres.
3) Hemispheric mean values of EEG quotients were correlated with mCBF or mCMRO$_2$ according to the stage of cerebral infarction.
4) Regional values of EEG quotients were correlated with rCBF or rCMRO$_2$ at each cortical area.

Results

Laterality of EEG and PET Data

The mCBF was significantly higher on the unaffected hemisphere than on the affected hemisphere in the subacute and chronic stages, and mCMRO$_2$ was significantly higher on the unaffected hemisphere throughout (Table 1). There was always a greater variabil-

Table 1. Mean values, standard deviations (SD) and coefficients of variance (CV) for mCBF, mCMRO$_2$ and EEG quotients according to the stage of cerebral infarction.

Stage		Acute stage n = 17			Subacute stage n = 16			Chronic stage n = 19			Overall n = 52		
Side		Affected		Unaffected	Affected		Unaffected	Affected		Unaffected	Affected		Unaffected
mCBF	mean	30.5	ns	35.1	26.6	**	35.0	29.3	***	36.1	28.9	***	35.5
(ml/100ml/min)	SD	8.9		4.7	10.6		6.5	9.6		7.6	9.5		6.4
	CV	29.4		13.9	39.9		19.0	31.6		21.0	33.1		18.0
mCMRO$_2$	mean	2.0	*	2.4	1.8	**	2.5	2.1	***	2.8	2.0	***	2.6
(ml/100ml/min)	SD	0.5		0.5	0.7		0.6	0.6		0.5	0.6		0.5
	CV	23.0		14.5	41.1		23.0	27.7		19.4	30.5		19.9
delta-PPF	mean	26.1	**	22.3	28.7	***	23.5	23.0	**	20.6	25.8	***	22.0
(%)	SD	5.7		3.8	4.7		3.5	5.8		4.9	5.8		4.2
	CV	21.7		17.0	16.3		15.1	25.2		23.8	22.7		19.2
theta-PPF	mean	29.1	**	26.8	29.0	***	26.5	27.2	***	24.4	28.4	***	25.7
(%)	SD	4.5		5.3	4.7		5.5	4.0		3.9	4.4		4.9
	CV	15.3		19.9	16.2		21.0	14.7		16.0	15.4		19.2
alpha-PPF	mean	26.1	***	29.9	26.2	**	30.6	30.0	***	33.4	27.5	***	31.3
(%)	SD	6.3		5.2	7.4		6.2	7.3		7.4	7.1		6.5
	CV	24.1		17.5	'28.2		20.1	24.4		22.3	25.9		20.6
beta-PPF	mean	18.8	*	20.9	18.1	ns	19.2	19.8	**	21.7	18.9	**	20.7
(%)	SD	3.7		4.5	5.5		3.8	4.5		4.0	4.6		4.2
	CV	19.6		21.5	30.8		19.7	22.9		18.4	24.3		20.2
PRI	mean	134.8	***	103.1	133.5	***	111.9	129.3	***	99.0	132.4	***	104.3
(%)	SD	39.6		25.4	36.1		32.1	52.9		36.0	43.2		31.5
	CV	29.4		24.7	27.0		28.7	40.9		36.4	32.6		30.2

* Results of Student's paired t-tests: * p < 0.01 ** p < 0.005 *** p < 0.0005 ns: statistically not significant

ity in the values of mCBF and mCMRO$_2$ on the affected hemisphere than on the unaffected hemisphere. Delta-PPF, theta-PPF and PRI were always significantly larger on the affected hemisphere than on the unaffected hemisphere in all stages, whereas the alpha-PPF was significantly greater on the unaffected hemisphere throughout. Delta-PPF and alpha-PPF showed a larger variability on the affected hemisphere than on the unaffected hemisphere while that of theta-PPF was greater on the unaffected hemisphere in all stages. By contrast, PRI showed a larger variability on the affected hemisphere in the acute stage but this tendency was reversed in the later stages.

Correlation Between mCBF and mCMRO$_2$

On the affected hemisphere, there was always a positive correlation between mCBF and

mCMRO$_2$, and the correlation coefficient was largest in the chronic stage (Table 2). On the unaffected hemisphere, the correlation was significant except for in the acute stage. The correlation coefficients were in general larger on the affected hemisphere than on the unaffected hemisphere.

Correlations of Hemispheric Mean Values

Table 3 illustrates the correlations between the mean hemispheric values of EEG quotients and mCBF. There was a tendency for the correlation coefficients with mCBF to be larger on the affected hemisphere than on the unaffected hemisphere in all stages of cerebral infarction. In the acute stage, delta-PPF and PRI correlated negatively with mCBF whereas alpha-PPF correlated positively on the affected hemisphere. Only the PRI correlated

Table 2. Correlation coefficients, F-values and significance in the linear regression analysis between mCBF and mCMRO$_2$ according to the stage of cerebral infarction.

Acute stage n = 17		Subacute stage n = 16		Chronic stage n = 19		Overall n = 52	
Affected	Unaffected	Affected	Unaffected	Affected	Unaffected	Affected	Unaffected
r = 0.786	r = 0.257	r = 0.739	r = 0.609	r = 0.923	r = 0.819	r = 0.821	r = 0.643
F = 25.259	F = 1.058	F = 16.845	F = 8.239	F = 98.327	F = 43.643	F = 103.686	F = 35.257
p < 0.005	ns	P < 0.005	p < 0.05	p < 0.0001	p < 0.0001	p < 0.0001	p < 0.0001

ns: statistically not significant

Table 3. Correlation coefficients, F-values and significance in the linear regression analysis between the hemispheric mean values of EEG quotients and mCBF according to the stage of cerebral infarction.

Stage	Acute stage n = 17		Subacute stage n = 16		Chronic stage n = 19		Overall n = 52	
Side	Affected	Unaffected	Affected	Unaffected	Affected	Unaffected	Affected	Unaffected
delta-PPF	r = −0.649	r = −0.374	r = −0.535	r = −0.055	r = −0.669	r = −0.562	r = −0.596	r = −0.382
	F = 10.899	F = 2.445	F = 5.62	F = 0.038	F = 13.781	F = 7.839	F = 27.603	F = 8.553
	p < 0.005	ns	p < 0.05	ns	p < 0.005	p < 0.05	p < 0.0001	p < 0.01
theta-PPF	r = −0.362	r = −0.409	r = −0.192	r = −0.448	r = −0.55	r = −0.653	r = −0.354	r = −0.491
	F = 2.259	F = 3.012	F = 0.531	F = 3.526	F = 7.387	F = 12.682	F = 7.18	F = 15.859
	ns	ns	ns	ns	p < 0.05	p < 0.005	p < 0.01	p < 0.005
alpha-PPF	r = 0.612	r = 0.285	r = 0.622	r = 0.232	r = 0.828	r = 0.691	r = 0.669	r = 0.476
	F = 9.013	F = 1.323	F = 8.832	F = 0.792	F = 37.057	F = 15.526	F = 40.582	F = 14.649
	p < 0.01	ns	p < 0.01	ns	p < 0.0001	p < 0.005	p < 0.0001	p < 0.005
beta-PPF	r = 0.39	r = 0.448	r = 0.006	r = 0.071	r = 0.009	r = 0.032	r = 0.113	r = 0.016
	F = 2.618	F = 3.774	F = 0.0005	F = 0.075	F = 0.001	F = 0.011	F = 0.641	F = 1.293
	ns	ns	ns	ns	ns	ns	ns	ns
PRI	r = −0.625	r = −0.556	r = −0.464	r = −0.436	r = −0.727	r = −0.55	r = −0.606	r = −0.509
	F = 9.644	F = 6.701	F = 3.841	F = 3.276	F = 19.124	F = 7.356	F = 29.015	F = 17.474
	p < 0.01	p < 0.05	ns	ns	p < 0.005	p < 0.05	p < 0.0001	p < 0.005

ns: statistically not significant

significantly with mCBF on the unaffected hemisphere in this stage. In the subacute stage, delta-PPF and alpha-PPF correlated significantly with mCBF on the affected hemisphere. All other EEG parameters failed to correlate with mCBF on either the affected or unaffected hemisphere. In the chronic stage, delta-PPF, theta-PPF and PRI correlated negatively with mCBF and alpha-PPF correlated positively on both hemispheres. Beta-PPF did not correlate with mCBF at any stage of cere-

bral infarction. In the overall comparison, a similar tendency was observed as seen in the chronic stage.

Figure 1 shows scattergrams of delta-PPF, alpha-PPF and PRI in relation to mCBF on the affected and unaffected hemispheres. There was a contrast in the correlations of delta-PPF and alpha-PPF: delta-PPF showed a negative correlation whereas a positive correlation was seen with alpha-PPF. Comparing the distributions of the values between

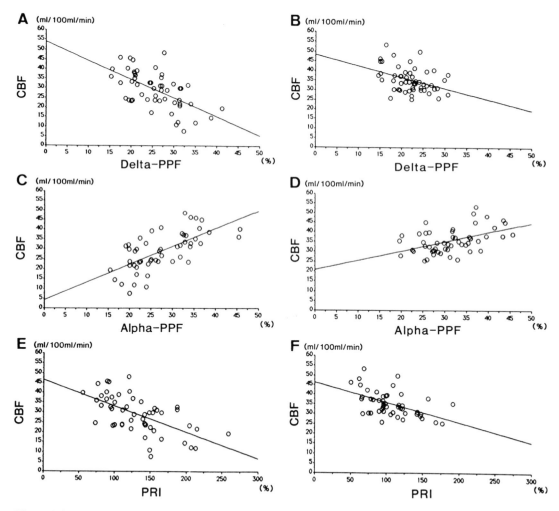

Figure 1. Scatterplots and correlation between the hemispheric mean values of EEG quotients and mCBF in the overall analysis: Delta-PPF correlated negatively with mCBF on the affected (A) and unaffected (B) hemispheres. Alpha-PPF correlated positively with mCBF on the affected (C) and unaffected (D) hemispheres. PRI correlated negatively with mCBF on the affected (E) and unaffected (F) hemispheres. The correlations were, in general, larger on the affected hemisphere than on the unaffected hemisphere.

the two hemispheres, there was a greater variability of the values on the affected hemisphere than on the unaffected hemisphere.

Table 4 summarizes the results of linear regression analysis between EEG quotients and $mCMRO_2$. In the acute stage, only delta-PPF correlated significantly with $mCMRO_2$ on the affected hemisphere. None of the other EEG quotients correlated significantly with $mCMRO_2$ on either the affected or unaffected hemisphere. In the subacute stage, delta-PPF and PRI correlated negatively with $mCMRO_2$ while alpha-PPF showed a positive correlation on the affected hemisphere, but, on the unaffected hemisphere, none of these EEG quotients correlated significantly with $mCMRO_2$. In the chronic stage, delta-PPF, theta-PPF and PRI correlated negatively with $mCMRO_2$ whereas alpha-PPF correlated positively on both hemispheres. No significant correlation was found between beta-PPF and $mCMRO_2$ throughout. In the overall analysis, delta-PPF, theta-PPF and PRI showed a negative correlation whereas alpha-PPF correlated positively.

The correlations were always larger on the affected hemisphere than on the unaffected hemisphere. A striking contrast was noted between the behavior of the slow-wave activity and that of the alpha activity in relation to the reduction of blood flow and oxygen metabolism in cerebral infarction.

Correlations of the Regional Values

Figure 2 shows a scalp distribution of the correlation coefficient for the linear regression analysis between PRI and rCBF. Highly significant correlation was found at the parietal and temporal regions on both hemispheres. A similar pattern was obtained for the correlations between PRI and $rCMRO_2$ (Figure 3).

The comparisons of the hemispheric mean values suggest a tendency that the correlations between EEG parameters and PET data will be larger on the affected hemisphere than on the unaffected hemisphere. Since the present study included 29 patients having a left hemisphere lesion and 18 patients having a right hemisphere lesion, the data from the left hemisphere is expected to show larger correlation than that from the right hemisphere if the EEG quotients and rCBF or $rCMRO_2$ are compared at each region of interest. In order to eliminate this artificial factor, the paired regions of interest at the homotopic areas were pooled: Fp1 and Fp2 as a frontopolar region, F3 and F4 as a frontal region, C3 and C4 as a

Table 4. Correlation coefficients, F-values and significance in the linear regression analysis between the hemispheric mean values of EEG quotients and $mCMRO_2$ according to the stage of cerebral infarction.

Stage	Acute stage n = 17		Subacute stage n = 16		Chronic stage n = 19		Overall n = 52	
Side	Affected	Unaffected	Affected	Unaffected	Affected	Unaffected	Affected	Unaffected
delta-PPF	r = −0.619 F = 9.3 p < 0.01	r = −0.005 F = 0.0003 ns	r = −0.672 F = 11.522 p < 0.005	r = −0.293 F = 1.316 ns	r = −0.543 F = 7.106 p < 0.05	r = −0.528 F = 6.576 p < 0.05	r = −0.609 F = 29.5 p < 0.0001	r = −0.371 F = 8.553 p < 0.01
theta-PPF	r = −0.084 F = 0.1 ns	r = −0.389 F = 2.667 ns	r = −0.008 F = 0.102 ns	r = −0.341 F = 1.841 ns	r = −0.612 F = 10.168 p < 0.01	r = −0.684 F = 14.934 p < 0.005	r = −0.273 F = 4.041 p < 0.05	r = −0.301 F = 5.026 p < 0.05
alpha-PPF	r = 0.448 F = 3.771 ns	r = 0.089 F = 0.129 ns	r = 0.631 F = 9.273 p < 0.01	r = 0.491 F = 4.44 ns	r = 0.624 F = 10.813 p < 0.005	r = 0.505 F = 5.82 p < 0.05	r = 0.587 F = 26.267 p < 0.0001	r = 0.286 F = 11.1 p < 0.005
beta-PPF	r = 0.283 F = 1.333 ns	r = 0.362 F = 2.264 ns	r = 0.293 F = 1.316 ns	r = 0.022 F = 0.007 ns	r = 0.23 F = 0.954 ns	r = 0.361 F = 2.544 ns	r = 0.04 F = 0.08 ns	r = 0.095 F = 0.441 ns
PRI	r = −0.457 F = 3.96 ns	r = −0.063 F = 0.06 ns	r = −0.499 F = 4.633 p < 0.05	r = −0.164 F = 2.74 ns	r = −0.74 F = 20.647 p < 0.005	r = −0.513 F = 6.076 p < 0.05	r = −0.563 F = 23.237 p < 0.0001	r = −0.452 F = 12.875 p < 0.005

ns: statistically not significant

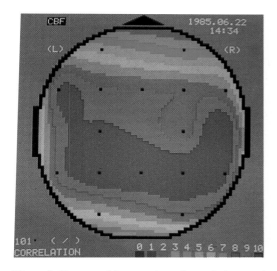

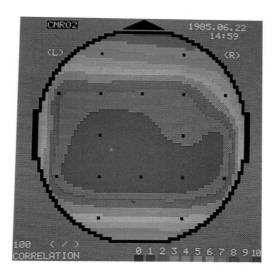

Figure 2. Topographic mapping of correlation coefficients between PRI and rCBF: Red designates the largest correlation coefficient. Highly significant correlation was found at the temporal and parietal regions on both hemispheres.

Figure 3. Topographic mapping of correlation coefficients between PRI and rCMRO$_2$: highly significant correlation was found at the temporal and parietal regions on both hemispheres.

central region, P3 and P4 as a parietal region, O1 and O2 as an occipital region, F7 and F8 as an anterior temporal region, and T5 and T6 as a posterior temporal region.

Table 5 summarizes the results of the linear regression analysis between the regional values of EEG quotients and rCBF at the paired cortical regions. Delta-PPF showed a highly

significant positive correlation with rCBF at all regions except for the frontopolar region. Theta-PPF correlated negatively with rCBF at all seven regions. The correlation coefficients for delta-PPF and theta-PPF were largest at the parietal region. Alpha-PPF correlated positively with rCBF at all regions with the largest correlation coefficient at the posterior

Table 5. Correlation coefficients, F-values and significance between the regional values of EEG quotients and rCBF at the corresponding sites of the EEG electrodes.

	Fp 1, Fp 2	F3, F4	C 3, C 4	P3, P4	O1, O2	F7, F8	T5, T6
	r = −0.11	r = −0.424	r = −0.493	r = −0.588	r = −0.45	r = −0.396	r = −0.536
delta-PPF	F = 1.193	F = 22.462	F = 32.769	F = 54.054	F = 25.961	F = 19.018	F = 41.082
	ns	p < 0.0001	p < 0.0001	p < 0.0001	p < 0.0001	p < 0.0001	p < 0.0001
	r = −0.444	r = −0.383	r = −0.335	r = −0.48	r = −0.352	r = −0.416	r = −0.404
theta-PPF	F = 25.04	F = 17.508	F = 13.776	F = 50.522	F = 14.374	F = 21.318	F = 19.866
	p < 0.0001	p < 0.0001	p < 0.005	p < 0.0001	p < 0.005	p < 0.0001	p < 0.0001
	r = 0.327	r = 0.444	r = 0.485	r = 0.574	r = 0.522	r = 0.517	r = 0.581
alpha-PPF	F = 12.216	F = 25.097	F = 32.244	F = 50.231	F = 38.071	F = 37.141	F = 52.163
	p < 0.005	p < 0.0001	p < 0.0001	p < 0.0001	p < 0.0001	p < 0.0001	p < 0.0001
	r = 0.122	r = 0.247	r = 0.207	r = 0.279	r = 0.19	r = 0.17	r = 0.095
beta-PPF	F = 1.595	F = 6.584	F = 4.587	F = 8.607	F = 0.035	F = 3.036	F = 0.951
	ns	P < 0.05	p < 0.05	p < 0.005	ns	ns	ns
	r = −0.297	r = −0.496	r = −0.506	r = −0.58	r = −0.428	r = −0.514	r = −0.581
PRI	F = 9.834	F = 33.288	F = 35.009	F = 51.667	F = 22.866	F = 36.596	F = 51.756
	p < 0.005	p < 0.0001	p < 0.0001	p < 0.0001	p < 0.0001	p < 0.0001	p < 0.0001

ns: statistically not significant

Table 6. Correlation coefficients, F-values and significance between the regional values of the EEG quotients and $rCMRO_2$ at the corresponding sites of the EEG electrodes.

	Fp1, Fp2	F3, F4	C3, C4	P3, P4	O1, O2	F7, F8	T5, T6
delta-PPF	r = -0.122	r = -0.437	r = -0.507	r = -0.574	r = -0.404	r = -0.362	r = -0.544
	F = 1.595	F = 22.066	F = 38.623	F = 49.522	F = 19.797	F = 15.347	F = 42.816
	ns	p < 0.0001	p < 0.0001	p < 0.0001	p < 0.0001	p < 0.005	p < 0.0001
theta-PPF	r = -0.311	r = -0.307	r = -0.36	r = -0.434	r = -0.263	r = -0.214	r = -0.259
	F = 10.93	F = 10.575	F = 15.186	F = 23.455	F = 7.535	F = 4.868	F = 7.283
	p < 0.005	p < 0.005	p < 0.005	p < 0.0001	p < 0.01	p < 0.05	p < 0.01
alpha-PPF	r = 0.338	r = 0.373	r = 0.479	r = 0.539	r = 0.507	r = 0.418	r = 0.524
	F = 13.175	F = 16.523	F = 30.277	F = 41.247	F = 35.203	F = 21.617	F = 38.768
	p < 0.005	p < 0.005	p < 0.0001	p < 0.0001	p < 0.0001	p < 0.0001	p < 0.0001
beta-PPF	r = 0.032	r = 0.295	r = 0.274	r = 0.266	r = 0.182	r = 0.089	r = 0.089
	F = 0.094	F = 9.727	F = 8.27	F = 7.758	F = 3.427	F = 0.791	F = 0.091
	ns	P < 0.005	p < 0.005	p < 0.01	ns	ns	ns
PRI	r = -0.221	r = -0.474	r = -0.525	r = -0.497	r = -0.351	r = -0.39	r = -0.507
	F = 5.292	F = 29.627	F = 38.827	F = 33.197	F = 14.308	F = 18.254	F = 35.287
	p < 0.05	p < 0.0001	p < 0.0001	p < 0.0001	p < 0.0005	p < 0.0001	p < 0.0001

ns: statistically not significant

temporal region. Beta-PPF correlated positively with rCBF only at the frontal, central and parietal regions. A highly significant negative correlation was obtained between PRI and rCBF at all regions and the correlation coefficient was largest at the parietal and posterior temporal regions.

The same type of analysis was carried out for the correlation with $rCMRO_2$ (Table 6). Delta-PPF correlated significantly with $rCMRO_2$ at all regions except for the frontopolar region. Theta-PPF correlated with $rCMRO_2$ at all regions. Both delta-PPF and theta-PPF showed the largest correlation coefficients at the parietal region. Significant positive correlation was found with alpha-PPF at all regions and the largest correlation coefficient was seen at the posterior temporal region. Beta-PPF correlated significantly with $rCMRO_2$ at 3 regions: frontal, central and parietal regions. PRI showed a significant negative correlation with $rCMRO_2$ at all regions with the largest coefficient at the parietal and posterior temporal regions.

Discussion

The present results show that the slow-wave component including the delta and theta activities correlate negatively with the cortical

blood flow measured at the regions corresponding to the location of the EEG electrodes whereas the alpha activity correlated positively. These results were in accordance with those of previous studies. In addition, it was shown that the slowing of the EEG also correlated with the cortical oxygen metabolism, although the degree of the correlation was weakened or even abolished according to the stage of cerebral infarction.

The presence or absence of delta activity has been included in the discussions of nearly all publications on EEG abnormalities in cerebral ischemia (Jones & Bagchi, 1951; Van Huffelen, 1979). A highly significant correlation was shown between the percentage of delta power and hemispheric mean CBF measured by the two-dimensional method (Tolonen & Sulg, 1981). Delta-PPF correlated negatively with both mCBF and $mCMRO_2$ on the ischemic hemisphere at all stages of cerebral infarction, and it also correlated closely with both rCBF and $rCMRO_2$ at all regions except for the frontopolar region. Delta activity is considered to be a sensitive indicator reflecting the ischemic damages done to the brain tissues during the course of cerebral infarction.

In the literature regarding this type of study, the theta activity was often included in the slow-wave component. Here we considered it separately and found that the theta-

PPF increased in inverse proportion to the reduction of CBF and $CMRO_2$. The behavior of the theta-PPF was similar to that of the delta-PPF in cerebral ischemia even though the degree of correlation was not as large as for the delta-PPF. Thus it seems appropriate to include the theta activity in the slow-wave components together with the delta activity.

In their quantitative analysis, Tölonen and Sulg (1981) concluded that there was no significant correlation between the theta activity and CBF on either the affected or the unaffected hemisphere of the ischemic brain. Here, however, regional values of theta-PPF correlated with rCBF and $rCMRO_2$ at all seven regions. In addition, the hemispheric mean values of theta-PPF correlated significantly with mCBF and $mCMRO_2$ in the chronic stage. The correlation coefficients were larger on the unaffected hemisphere than on the affected hemisphere, whereas the other EEG quotients showed larger correlations on the affected hemisphere than on the unaffected hemisphere. Theta activity, which indicates a slight slowing of the background EEG activity, is considered to correspond to a mild reduction of CBF and $CMRO_2$ on the unaffected hemisphere which might be caused by an indirect process such as a transhemispheric neurogenic effect, increased intracranial pressure and brain edema (Hoedt-Rasmussen & Skinhhoj, 1964; Shishido et al, 1986).

Unlike the slow-wave activities, the alpha-PPF consistently showed a positive correlation with CBF and $CMRO_2$ at all regions and its hemispheric mean values correlated with mCBF and $mCMRO_2$ mainly on the ischemic hemisphere. A decrease of alpha activity along with an increase of the slow-wave activities in patients with cerebral ischemia has been discussed (Strauss & Greenstein, 1948; Farbrot, 1954). Tolonen and Sulg (1981) showed that the relative power of alpha activity correlated positively with the CBF measured by the ^{133}Xe intra-arterial method. The present results confirmed these earlier findings based on the two-dimensional measurements of CBF.

Earlier reports (Lecasble & Farbrot, 1952; Dondey & Gaches, 1958) assumed that the beta activity increased on the hemisphere contralateral to the ischemic lesion. Green and Wilson (1961), however, reported that the beta activity was suppressed on the ischemic hemisphere. In the present results, beta-PPF correlated positively with the rCBF and $rCMRO_2$ at the frontal, central and parietal regions, although the hemispheric mean values did not correlate with mCBF or $mCMRO_2$ at any stage of cerebral infarction. Decrease in the beta activity can be used as a measure of the local cerebral ischemia in the frontal, central or parietal regions that are in the territory of the MCA. Then, the decline of the beta activity could be explained as a part of suppression of the normal background EEG activity.

Highlighting the striking contrast of the behavior of the slow and fast-wave activities in relation to the reduction of CBF and $CMRO_2$, the PRI was calculated to emphasize the slowing of the background EEG activity by dividing the slow-wave component by the fast-wave component. Based on power spectral density analysis, several ratios have been employed to assess brain ischemia clinically and experimentally (Gotman et al., 1973; Gotman et al., 1975; Sotaneimi et al., 1980; Mies et al., 1984). Similar to what we found with PRI, there was a good correlation between the frequency index used by those authors and the changes in CBF. As shown in Figures 2 and 3, a significant negative correlation was found with PRI at all regions and highly significant correlation was obtained at the temporal and parietal regions. Thus, the PRI, which indicates the degree of slowing of the background EEG activity, can be used as a measure of cerebral ischemia in patients with cerebral infarction.

Cerebral metabolic processes are considered to be the primary factors that influence neuronal electrical activity. Thus we may expect that EEG activity will be, in general, more closely associated with $CMRO_2$ than with CBF in brain ischemia. In the acute stage of cerebral infarction, delta-PPF and alpha-PPF correlated significantly with mCBF whereas only the delta-PPF correlated significantly with $mCMRO_2$ on the affected hemisphere. The correlation coefficients were slightly larger with mCBF than with $mCMRO_2$. This indicates a tendency that, in the acute stage, the slowing of the background EEG activity might be more closely correlated with the reduction of CBF than with that of $CMRO_2$ on the affected hemisphere. The reduced blood flow and the relatively preserved metabolic demand for oxygen is expressed as a raised OEF on the PET images. This uncoupling of flow and metabolism is known as a misery perfusion phenomenon (Baron et al., 1984). Owing to the uncoupling of flow to metabolism, the alteration of the EEG activities seems to be more closely associated with reduction of cortical blood flow rather than the suppression of oxygen metabolism in the acute stage of cerebral infarction.

In contrast, delta-PPF and alpha-PPF showed closer correlations with mCMRO$_2$ than with mCBF on the affected hemisphere in the subacute stage including the phase of luxury perfusion phenomenon in which the blood flow increased relative to the oxygen metabolism (Lassen, 1966). As shown in previous reports utilizing the ^{133}Xe two-dimensional method (Ingvar, 1967; Sulg et al., 1981), the correlation between EEG and CBF was weakened in this phase of luxury-perfusion. The present results with the PET studies confirm such findings.

In the chronic stage, the relationship between CBF and CMRO$_2$ is expected to revert to the situation found in normal cerebral tissues (Ackerman et al., 1981; Lenzi et al., 1982). Although the correlation coefficients of delta-PPF and alpha-PPF were larger with mCBF than with mCMRO$_2$, all EEG parameters except the beta-PPF correlated significantly with both mCBF and mCMRO$_2$ in the chronic stage. Thus, the change in correlations between the EEG parameters and CBF or CMRO$_2$ are considered to reflect the pathophysiological relationship of flow and metabolism during the course of cerebral infarction.

There was a variation in the degree of correlation between the EEG parameters and PET data according to the location of the electrodes. The correlation was highly significant at the parietal and posterior temporal regions, whereas it was poor at the frontopolar regions. Buchsbaum et al. (1984) showed that the correlation between glucose metabolism and EEG power differed according to the sites of the brain. In their results, a significant negative correlation was seen between the alpha power and glucose metabolism at the occiput, whereas both delta and theta activities had negative correlations over the temporal lobe.

Delta-PPF correlated negatively with rCBF and rCMRO$_2$ at all regions except for the frontopolar region, where contamination in the form of artifacts from eye movements and blinks might influence the power density of the slow-wave activity. Visual inspection will be superior to computer analysis in differentiating the peculiar types of slow-wave activity from the artifacts.

Alpha activity is expected to be most prominent at the occipital region in normal subjects. From the view point of the topographical distribution of correlation coefficients, a significant positive correlation was obtained between alpha-PPF and rCBF and rCMRO$_2$, respectively, at all 7 regions. However, the correlation of alpha-PPF was not as large at the occipital region as it was at the parietal and posterior temporal regions although a significant positive correlation existed also at the occipital region. This might be partly because the occipital dominancy of the alpha activity was weakened or lost bilaterally in those patients with brain lesions, and the slow-wave activity was more prominent at the central or parietal regions as compared with the occipital regions. Furthermore, the present study included a much larger number of patients with infarction in the MCA territory than with the infarction of the PCA territory. Since there was a tendency for the ischemic hemisphere to show a larger correlation than the healthy hemisphere, the correlations within the PCA territory may be weaker than those within the MCA territory.

References

Ackerman RH, Correia JA, Alpert NM (1981) Positron imaging in ischemic stroke disease using compounds labeled with oxygen-15. Initial results and clinicopathologic correlations. *Arch Neuro, 38*, 537–543.

Baron JC, Rougemont D, Soussaline F, Bustany P, Crouzel C, Bousser MG, Comar D (1984) Local interrelationship of cerebral oxygen consumption and glucose utilization in normal subjects and in ischemic stroke patients: A positron tomography study. *J Cereb Blood Flow Metab, 4,* 140–149.

Buchsbaum MS, Kessler R, King A, Johnson J, Cappelletti J (1984) Simultaneous cerebral glucography with positron emission tomography and topographic electroencephalography. In Pfurtscheller G, Jonkman, EJ, Lopes da Silva EH (Eds.) *Brain ischemia: Quantitative EEG and imaging techniques* (Progress in Brain Research, Vol. 62). Elsevier, Amsterdam, 263-269.

Dondey M, Gaches J (1958) Remarques a propos du diagnostic E.E.G. dans les accidents vasculaires cerebreaux. *Rev Neurol, 99,* 232–234.

Farbrot O (1954) Electroencephalographic study in cases of cerebrovascular accidents (preliminary report). *Electroenceph clin Neurophysiol 6,* 678–681.

Gotman J, Skuce DR, Thompson CJ, Gloor P, Ives JR, Ray WF (1973) Clinical application of spectral analysis and extraction of features from electroencephalograms with slow waves in adult patients. *Electroenceph clin Neurophysiol, 35,* 225–235.

Gotman J, Gloor P, Ray WF (1975) A quantitative comparison of traditional reading of the EEG and interpretation of computer-extracted features in patients with supratentorial brain lesions. *Electroenceph clin Neurophysiol, 38,* 623–639.

Green RL, Wilson WP (1961) Asymmetries of beta-activity in epilepsy, brain tumor, and cerebrovascular disease. *Electroenceph clin Neurophysiol, 13,* 75–78.

Hoedt-Rasmussen K, Skinhoj E (1964) Transneural depression of the cerebral hemispheric metabolism in man. *Acta Neurol Scand, 40,* 41–46.

Ingvar DH (1967) The pathophysiology of occlusive cerebrovascular disorders related to neuroradiological findings, EEG and measurements of regional cerebral blood flow. *Acta Neurol Scand, 43* (Suppl. 31), 93–107.

Ingvar DH, Sulg IA (1969) Regional cerebral blood flow and EEG frequency content in man. *Scand J Clin Invest, 23* (Suppl. 109), 47–66.

Jones EV, Bagchi BK (1951) Electroencephalographic findings in verified thrombosis of major cerebral arteries (14 cases). *Mich Med Bull, 17,* 295–310.

Kanno I, Uemura K, Miura Y, Miura S (1983) Design concepts and performance of HEADTOME, a multiring hybrid emission tomography for the brain. In Heiss WD, Phelps ME (Eds.) *Positron emission tomography.* Springer-Verlag, Berlin/Heidelberg/New York, 46-50.

Lammertsma AA, Jones T (1983) The correction for the presence of intravascular oxygen-15 in the steady state technique for measuring regional oxygen extraction in the brain. Description of the method. *J Cereb Blood Flow Metab, 3,* 416–424.

Lassen NA (1966) The luxury perfusion syndrome and its possible relation to acute metabolic acidosis localized with in the brain. *Lancet, 2,* 1112–1115.

Lecasble R, Farbrot O (1952) Asymmetries du rhythm de base dans les accidents vascularies cerebraux. *Rev Neurol, 87,* 201.

Lenzi G L, Frackowiak RSJ, Jones T (1982) Cerebral oxygen metabolism and blood flow in human cerebral ischemic infarction. *J Cereb Blood Flow Metab, 2,* 321–335.

Mies G, Hoppe G, Hossmann KA (1984) Limitation of EEG frequency analysis in the diagnosis of intracerebral diseases. In Pfurtscheller G, Jonkman, EJ, Lopes da Silva FH (Eds.) *Brain ischemia: Quantitative EEG and imaging techniques* (Progress in Brain Research, Vol. 62). Elsevier, Amsterdam, 85–103.

Nagata K, Mizukami M, Araki G, Kawase T, Hirano M (1982) Topographic electroencephalographic study of cerebral infarction using computed mapping of the EEG (CME). *J Cereb Blood Flow Metab, 2,* 79–88.

Nagata K, Yunoki M, Araki G, Mizukami M, Hyodo A (1984a) Topographic electroencephalographic study of ischemic cerebrovascular disease. In Pfurtscheller G, Jonkman, EJ, Lopes da Silva FH (Eds.) *Brain ischemia: Quantitative EEG and imaging techniques* (Progress in Brain Research, Vol. 62). Elsevier, Amsterdam, 271–286.

Nagata K, Yunoki K, Araki G, Mizukami M (1984b) Topographic electroencephalographic study of transient ischemic attacks. *Electroenceph clin Neurophysiol, 58,* 291–301.

Nagata K, Gross CE, Kindt GW, Geier JM, Adey GR (1985) Topographic electroencephalographic study with power ratio index mapping in patients with malignant brain tumors. *Neurosurgery, 17,* 613–619.

Nagata K, Tagawa, K, Shishido F, Uemura K (1986a) Topographic EEG correlates of cerebral blood flow and oxygen consumption in patients with neuropsychological disorders. In Duffy FH (Ed.) *Topographic mapping of brain electrical activity.* Butterworth, Boston, 363–377.

Nagata K, Tagawa K, Nara M, Shishido F, Uemura K (1986b) Quantitative EEG correlates of cerebral blood flow and oxygen metabolism in brain ischemia. II. Topography of power ratio index (PRI). In Matsuoka S, Soejima T, Yokota A (Eds.) *Clinical topographic electroencephalography and evoked potential.* Shindan-To-Chiryo, Tokyo, 109–116.

Obrist WD, Sokolof L, Lassen NA, Lane MH, Butler RN, Feinberg I (1963) Relation of EEG to cerebral blood flow and metabolism in old age. *Electroenceph clin Neurophysiol, 15,* 610—619.

Shishido F, Uemura K, Inugami A, Ogawa T, Yamaguchi T, Kanno I, Miura S, IIda H, Murakami M, Takahashi K, Sasaki H, Tagawa K, Yasui N (1986) Cerebral circulation and metabolism in cerebral infarction of middle cerebral artery territory. *Jpn J Nucl Med, 23,* 123—134.

Sotaneimi KA, Sulg IA, Hokkanen TE (1980) Quantitative EEG as a measure of cerebral dysfunction before and after open-heart surgery. *Electroenceph clin Neurophysiol, 50,* 81—95.

Strauss H, Greenstein L (1948) The electroencephalogram in cerebrovascular disease. *Arch Neurol Psychiat, 59,* 395—403.

Sulg IA, Sotaniemi KA, Tolonen U, Hokkanen E (1981) Dependence between cerebral metabolism and blood flow as reflected in the quantitative EEG. In Mendlewics J, Praag van HM (Eds.) *Advance Biol. Psychiat., Vol. 6.* Karger, Basel, 102—108.

Tagawa K, Nagata K, Nara M, Shishido F, Uemura K (1986) Quantitative EEG correlates of cerebral blood flow and oxygen metabolism in brain ischemia. I. Percentage power fraction (PPF). In Matsuoka S, Soejima T, Yokota A (Eds.) *Clinical topographic electroencephalography and evoked potential.* Shindan-To-Chiryo, Tokyo, 100—108.

Tolonen U, Sulg IA (1981) Comparison of quantitative EEG parameters from four different analysis techniques in evaluation of relationship between EEG and rCBF in brain infarction. *Electroenceph clin Neurophysiol, 51,* 177—185.

Uemura K, Kanno I, Miura Y, Miura S, Murakami M, Shishido F (1985) High resolution positron emission tomograph: HEADTOME III: System description and preliminary report on the performances. In Greitz T (Ed.) *The metabolism of the human brain studied with positron emission tomography.* Raven Press, New York, 47-55.

Van Huffelen AC (1979) *Quantitative EEG in cerebral ischemia.* TNO Research Unit for Clinical Neurophysiology, The Hague.

Joint Bereitschaftspotential and SPECT Application in the Functional Mapping of Learning-Related Brain Activity and Imagery

W. Lang, M. Lang, I. Podreka, G. Goldenberg, L. Deecke

Two different methods were employed to establish functional-topographical relations in motor tracking tasks: (1) cortical DC shifts preceding (Bereitschaftspotential, BP) and accompanying motor performance and (2) regional cerebral blood flow (rCBF). In Experiment I, visuomotor learning was investigated using the BP method, in Experiment II, the two techniques were used under virtually identical experimental scenarios involving visuomotor learning as well. Results demonstrated a high degree of congruency between movement-related DC shifts and rCBF patterns: The two different methods well agreed in indicating learning-related activation of the frontal cortex. More precisely, DC potential shifts and rCBF data were qualified to localize the parts of the frontal cortex that were activated during visuomotor learning. In addition, the rCBF method demonstrated learning-related activation of basal ganglia (right < left) and cerebellum (left < right). With its excellent time resolution, the movement-related DC potentials demonstrated temporal contingency between performance and electrophysiological signs of cortical activation. In experiment III, the rCBF method was employed to demonstrate cortical areas activated by different forms of mental imagery. When the subjects merely imagined the movements in their mind's eye without actually executing them, the visual cortical areas showed some activation but not the supplementary motor area (SMA).

In 1978 Deecke and Kornhuber reported that the supplementary motor area (SMA) is activated prior to self-initiated human voluntary movement in addition to the primary (rolandic) motor area (MI). This finding is based on movement-related brain potentials (Bereitschaftspotential, BP, Kornhuber & Deecke, 1964, 1965) Independently, Lassen et al. (1978) confirmed this finding with an entirely different method. They reported an increase of regional cerebral blood flow (rCBF) not only in contralateral MI but also in SMA, when the subjects (Ss) performed voluntary movements with one hand. Agreement between two different methods is very important, since the virtues of one method compensate the shortcomings of the other: EEG has instantaneous time resolution but poor localization, whereas rCBF is good at localization but poor in the time domain. In fact, rCBF alone does not show whether the SMA is active before or after the onset of movement. It needs complementary data from the BP, which as a purely premovement phenomenon clearly solves this problem. Furthermore, in conjunction with the Bereitschaftsmagnetfeld (BM), the BP's magnetoencephalographic (MEG) equivalent, the BP method even allows the conclusion that SMA leads MI activation, i.e., is upstream of MI in the temporal chain of motor preparation prior to self-initiated voluntary movement (Deecke et al., 1985a). We wanted to combine these two techniques to study identical groups of Ss with both methods in exactly the same experimental scenario (Experiment II, below).

Neurological Clinic, University of Vienna, Lazarettgasse 14, A-1097 Vienna, Austria

Results

Experiment I: Movement-Related Potentials in Visuomotor Learning

Continuing experiments employing manual tracking, Lang et al. (1983) studied motor learning. The experimental setup is shown in Figure 1. It provided a moving target stimulus (circle on a TV screen), which the S had to track on a photo-detector plate using a pen in his right hand. The position of the pen was coupled back to the TV screen as a light point. This provided continuous visual feedback and it was the Ss' task to keep the light spot within the circle. The circle was set in motion when the S lowered the pen onto the plate. The circle moved in 3 different random directions with each trajectory lasting 1500 ms. This condition is called normal tracking (T). Two other conditions were incorporated into the same experiment (random order between Ss): (1) In No-Tracking controls (NT), the Ss initiated the stimulus program by touching the pen to the plate, but did not track it. (2) In Inverse Tracking (IT), which was the most important task because it involved learning, the feedback signal was multiplied by −1 and the Ss had to mirror the target's movements. This made the task very difficult.

The results are shown in Figure 2. For NT, only a BP prior to the voluntary act of lowering the pen onto the plate was found; however, no negativity during the moves of the stimulus occurred. This absence of tracking negativity in NT as compared to T (normal tracking with +1 feedback) was statistically significant at the 1% level (see Wilcoxon's paired differences in the centre of Figure 2A). The learning experiment of IT showed the highest negativity: due to the difficulty of operating with −1 feedback, the increase in tracking negativity in IT as compared to T was significant (during the first trajectory on the 1%, during the second on the 5% level). To measure the effect of learning, the difference between target circle and feedback point (average of horizontal and vertical components) was established by computer and was defined as an error (E). Learning the motor performance was described as the reduction of the tracking error in percent (dE%). As the next

step, dE% was correlated with the mean enhancement of cortical negativity (dN), when T and IT were compared for each of the 14 Ss during the first trajectory. Significant correlations were found only for the 3 frontal recordings F3, F4 and FCz (overlying SMA) with correlation coefficients ranging from r = 0.7

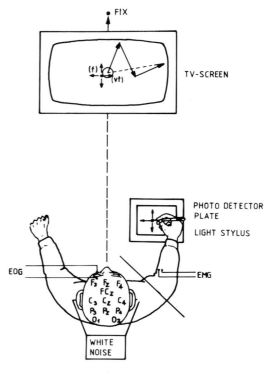

(vt) VISUAL TARGET
(f) FEEDBACK OF HAND TRACKING

Figure 1. Setup for the motor learning experiment (Experiment I). The S is sitting in an EEG chair and fixes his eyes on a fixation point (FIX). He holds a light stylus in his right hand, which he can move on a photo detector plate. When he moves it down to the plate, which is done in a self-initiated voluntary manner, a circle (visual target, vt) starts moving on the TV screen; for 1.5 s in a first random direction, for 1.5 s in a second random direction, and for 1.5 s in a third random direction. The S is to track the stimulus as soon as it moves, and the position of the stylus on the plate is coupled back to the TV screen as a point (feedback, f). It is the S's task to keep the point within the circle. Recordings are done from the electrode positions indicated, EOG and EMG. The ears are masked with white noise, and the S's right arm is kept out of his sight.

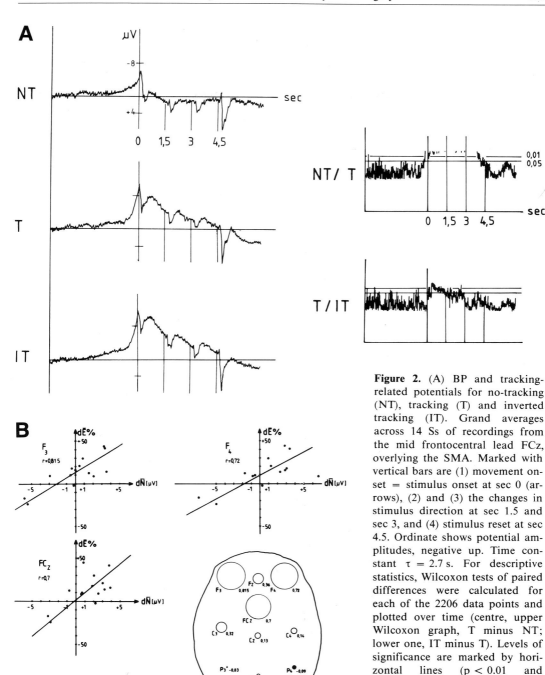

Figure 2. (A) BP and tracking-related potentials for no-tracking (NT), tracking (T) and inverted tracking (IT). Grand averages across 14 Ss of recordings from the mid frontocentral lead FCz, overlying the SMA. Marked with vertical bars are (1) movement onset = stimulus onset at sec 0 (arrows), (2) and (3) the changes in stimulus direction at sec 1.5 and sec 3, and (4) stimulus reset at sec 4.5. Ordinate shows potential amplitudes, negative up. Time constant $\tau = 2.7$ s. For descriptive statistics, Wilcoxon tests of paired differences were calculated for each of the 2206 data points and plotted over time (centre, upper Wilcoxon graph, T minus NT; lower one, IT minus T). Levels of significance are marked by horizontal lines ($p < 0.01$ and $p < 0.05$). (B) In the right section of the Figure, correlations are shown between the reduction of error in motor performance (dE%, ordinate) and the enhancement of cortical negativity (dN, abscissa) when T and IT tasks are compared for every S. There are high and significant positive correlations ($r = 0.7$ to 0.8) only in frontal recordings F3, F4 and FCz. The inset in the lower right illustrates the topographical distribution of these significant correlations. The area of the circle represents the coefficient of determination d ($= r^2$).

(SMA, p < 0.01) to r = 0.82 (left frontal, p < 0.001, Figure 2B). When the coefficients of determination, d (= r^2) were plotted as areas of circles over the 12 recordings, significant positive correlations were seen over the frontal cortex only, in particular over the frontolateral convexity of both hemispheres and the frontomedial SMA region. In view of this functional topographic pattern of the brain (inset at lower part of Figure 2B), we believe that we have found essential electrophysiological evidence in humans for the importance of the frontal cortex for visuomotor learning.

Experiment II: Joint Investigation of Movement-Related Potentials and Tc-99m HMPAO SPECT on Visuomotor Learning

In a recent study carried out by Lang et al. (1988a), the motor learning experiment for horizontal inverted tracking (−1 feedback only in the horizontal plane) was investigated using the regional cerebral blood flow (rCBF) method. rCBF was measured using Single Photon Emission Computer Tomography (SPECT) and a new technetium-labeled compound (Hexa-methyl-propylene-amine-oxime, HMPAO), which crosses the blood brain barrier and becomes trapped in brain cells within about 2 minutes. Tracer concentration correlates well with regional cerebral blood flow shortly after injection (Podreka et al., 1987).

Figure 3 gives the results of the SPECT study in one S (J.B.): in the top row, the tomographic regional emission pattern during horizontally inverted tracking, IT, is shown; in the centre, SPECT during normal tracking, T, is given, and the bottom shows IT minus T. During the more difficult learning task, IT, there is a relative increase in tracer emission as compared to normal tracking, T, in the following brain regions: frontocentral midline including SMA, lateral frontal cortex (i.e., middle and inferior frontal gyri R > L), right occipital cortex, right basal ganglia and cerebellum (L > R). Figure 4 gives the mean differences between IT and T (extra activity of the learning task) of all 17 Ss. There is a significant relative increase in rCBF during IT as compared to T in regions related to frontomedial cortex including SMA (F-M, p < 0.005), lateral frontal cortex, in particular the middle frontal gyrus (MF, left p < 0.005; right p < 0.0001), basal ganglia including caudate nucleus and putamen (BG, right p < 0.05), and cerebellum (CE, left p < 0.005).

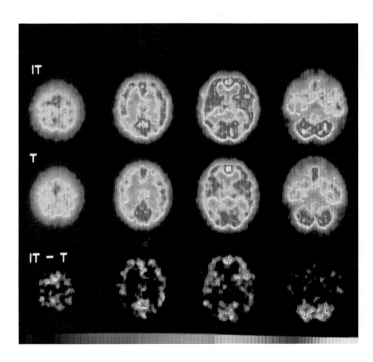

Figure 3. 99 Tc-HMPAO brain SPECT of S J.B. 4 axial slices from high parietal (left) to basal (right). IT (top) inverted tracking with horizontal −1 feedback, T (centre) tracking with +1 feedback, IT−T (bottom) subtraction of IT minus T after normalization of count rates. Relative tracer distribution displayed in colours ranging from blue (low) via yellow and red to white (high concentration, calibration scale on the right side). Note extra activity for the more difficult IT task as compared to T. One region of extra activity is the frontocentral midline (left slice), the other is the striate cortex, particularly the right (2nd and 3rd slice from the left). In addition, note IT-related extra activity in right middle and inferior frontal gyri (3rd slice) and cerebellum (right slice).

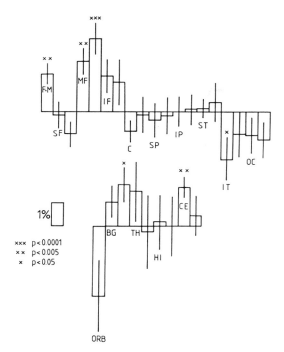

Figure 4. Differences between visuomotor learning (Inverted Tracking, IT) and normal tracking (T) in HMPAO-SPECT across N = 17 Ss. Columns represent means (of the difference in regional indices, dRI, IT minus T), vertical bars indicate double standard error (2SE). Columns above the horizontal line indicate larger relative tracer concentrations in IT as compared to T (extra activity of IT), columns below line indicate lower IT concentrations as compared to T. Regions of interest (ROIs) at corresponding sites of the two hemispheres are represented in adjacent columns, only the one on the left hemisphere (ROI$_l$) is labelled. In the Figure, ROI$_r$ is always on the right side of ROI$_l$ and remained unlabelled. F–M = fronto-medial cortex including SMA, SF = superior, MF = middle, IF = inferior frontal gyrus, C = central region, SP = superior, IP = inferior parietal, ST = superior, IT = inferior temporal, OC = occipital, ORB = orbitofrontal, BG = basal ganglia, TH = thalamus, HI = hippocampus, CE = cerebellum.

vIT vs. T

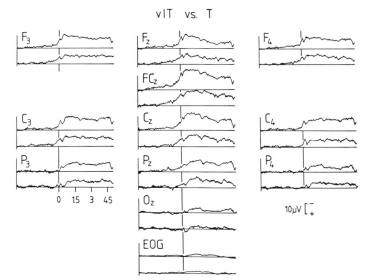

Figure 5. Topographical distribution of performance-related DC-shifts in S J.B. The vertical line indicates self-initiated onset of stimulus movement (t = 0), which changed directions at sec 1.5 and sec 3, reset of stimulus to starting position occurred at sec 4.5. Upper traces, vertical inverted tracking vIT (visuomotor learning due to vertical −1 feedback); lower traces, normal tracking T (no learning, +1 feedback). Negative up. Time constant τ = ∞. The volitional initiation of stimulus onset is preceded by a BP, task performance is accompanied by a long sustained negative DC-shift (tracking potential).

In a second session, movement-related cortical DC shifts were recorded in 15 of the 17 Ss. Experimental design, EEG recording and data analysis were the same as in experiment I except that the frequency band of amplification ranged from real DC to 70 Hz. DC measurements require special equipment (Lang et al., 1987) but have the advantage of not distorting the performance-related DC shift (the decay of negativity during tracking in Figure 2 is a time constant effect!). The other difference was that in order to introduce novelty into the IT learning task, the vertical coordinate was biased by −1 feedback. Figure 5 gives the results of S J.B. The voluntary initiation of the tracking performance is again associated with a BP, the execution of the visuomotor task is accompanied by a slow negative DC shift (tracking potential). Mean amplitudes of the tracking potential as calculated during the 4.5 s of task-performance differed between IT and T. Amplitudes were larger in IT than they were in T. The topographical distribution of this extra IT negativity has a clear frontocentral maximum in S J.B. Significant extra IT negativity was found in frontal and, to a lesser degree, central recordings only.

The good correspondence between SPECT and performance-related cortical DC shifts encourages continuation of parallel investigations of well-defined experimental tasks using the two methods on the same group of Ss. In the tomographic emission study, the maximum relative increase in tracer emission during IT (as compared to T) is found in the right middle frontal gyrus ($p < 0.0001$!). This finding is remarkable and is probably due to the spatial properties of the task involved. Mirror tracking might be a more demanding spatial operation than the noninverted tracking of geometrical structures. Manipulations in conjunction with orientation in space involve the right hemisphere, known to be superior to the left in this respect.

Experiment III: Tc-99m HMPAO SPECT and Motor Imagery

The third experiment was devoted to the distribution of cortical activity when a movement is only imagined but not actually executed. Emission tomography is mandatory for this experiment. BP investigation of a non-executed movement is impossible, since no physical parameter is available as a trigger. To investigate imagined movements, four different tasks were selected and performed by 28 right-handed, paid students: (1) Yes-No, (2) Low imagery, (3) Visual imagery, and (4) Motor imagery. The experiments were done with the eyes closed under a blindfold. An audio tape supplied the Ss via headphones with (1) instructions and (2) the stimuli for the respective experiment. The S held a flashlight in one hand, an intravenous catheter was inserted

into the opposite arm prior to the start of the experiment. Ss were divided into an imagery group and a control group. Within each group, every S performed two experiments at an interval of one week so that within a group the order of tasks and hands (holding the flashlight) was balanced.

(1) Yes-No. Ss heard "Yes" or "No" in random order followed by a 5 s pause and a peeping tone. They were instructed to ignore "Yes" but to actuate the flashlight upon "No." (2) Low imagery. Ss heard 50 sentences, each with a pause of 5 s followed by the peeping tone. They had to judge the correctness of the sentences and actuate the flashlight for incorrect sentences. The sentences tested abstract school und general knowledge thought to be retrievable without imagery. (3) Visual imagery. The procedure was similar to (2); however, the evaluation of the sentences (flashlight for incorrect ones) required visual imagery. (4) Motor imagery. The procedure was similar to (2) and (3); however, the evaluation of the sentences required the imagination of body movements. Ss were strictly requested to avoid executing any movements except gentle pressure to the flashlight button to indicate incorrect. Obedience to this instruction was controlled by EMG in some Ss.

The most salient finding of the experiment concerned the visual imagery condition (cf. V-I in Figure 6). Compared to the control conditions it showed significant elevations of local blood flow in the left inferior occipital region and in inferior temporal regions of both hemispheres. The activation of the left inferior occipital region, in particular, confirms previous findings (Farah, 1984; Goldenberg, 1987; Goldenberg et al., 1987) of a prominent role of this region in visual imagery. It should be considered that the activity of the occipital cortex seen in Figure 6 occurred although the eyes were closed and blindfolded. The results of the motor imagery condition, however, were at first sight less spectacular. Higher local flow rates were generalized over many brain regions. Only in the central regions were the flow rates significantly higher than for visual imagery but inspection of the data suggested that this was rather due to low values for visual imagery than to high ones for motor imagery. These negative findings nonetheless

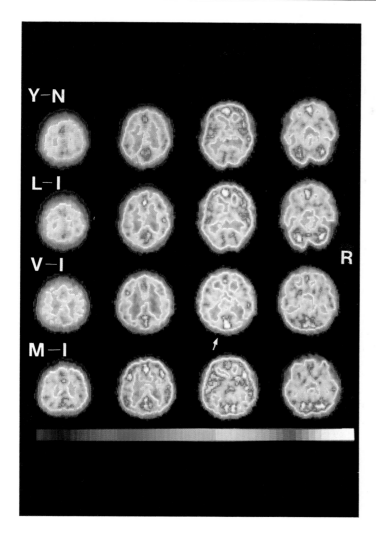

Figure 6. SPECT images obtained in one S in four different paradigms of imagery under eyes-closed and blindfolded conditions: Four adjacent axial sections from high parietal (left) to basal sections (right). Images scaled according to the highest voxel content of the whole brain. Y–N = yes–no; L–I = low imagery sentences; V–I = visual imagery sentences, and M–I = motor imagery sentences. Note maximum local tracer deposition in left inferior occipital region in the V–I condition (arrow), and lack of systematic differences in SMA. Relative tracer distribution displayed in colours ranging from blue (low) via yellow and red to white (high concentration, calibration scale on the bottom).

show that there was no increase of activity in the SMA. Indeed, the numerical values of the flow rates of the SMA were virtually identical across conditions. In contrast, Roland et al. (1980) found increased rCBF in the SMAs of Ss who imagined movements without actually carrying them out. In Roland's experiment Ss had to imagine a sequence of finger movements whereas in the present experiments Ss imagined single, although sometimes quite complex movements. Probably, the SMA is responsible for directing the temporal sequence rather than the spatial structure both in actually executed movements and in motor imagery (Deecke et al., 1985b; Lang et al., 1988b).

Discussion and Some Thoughts on the Function of the SMA

The three experiments showed the value of using two different methods of functional topography of the brain on the same population of Ss performing identical tasks, since one method compensates for the shortcomings of the other. Experiment I, BP study, shows that visuomotor learning involves the frontal cortex; Experiment II, combined BP and SPECT study, proves this by showing an excellent correspondence of the two, and Experiment III, SPECT study, shows that motor imagery alone (without actual execution) involves the occipital cortex but not the SMA. This raises the question as to the function of the SMA. Data given elsewhere (Kornhuber & Deecke, 1985), ascribe a motivational role to the SMA. However, motivation is a complex function with several independent subfunctions concerning what to do, how to do it and when to start. The latter function, finding the right moment for action, is in our view the task of the SMA. This becomes clearer if one compares different motivational situations: in the experimental scenario usually employed in BP investigations, e.g., self-initiated finger or other movements, only the SMA becomes active, not the rest of the frontal lobe. If motivation is required to modify motor programs in motor learning, however, the whole convexity of the frontal lobe shows a large surface-negative potential (Experiments I and II), whose amplitude is significantly positively correlated with learning success (Lang et al., 1983, 1986). On the other hand, in an experimental situation using a manual pursuit movement, which requires attention to an unpredictable stimulus direction but provides a fixed time for the change in direction so that the temporal sequence of events is predictable, the SMA shows anticipatory activity (Deecke et al., 1984; Lang et al., 1984). It gives rise to a large negative potential, which already terminates half a second before the directed attention potential over parieto-occipital areas. The supervision of what to do and how to do it may be provided mainly by the orbital cortex and the frontolateral cortex, respectively (Kleist, 1934). The close temporal association of the BP in SMA with the onset of voluntary movement fits well with the function of governing when to do it, the final "go." Recent experiments employing simultaneous versus sequential movements that require timing showed significantly larger negative DC shifts in SMA for sequential movements than for simultaneous movements of the two index fingers (Lang et al., 1988b).

References

Deecke L, Kornhuber HH (1978) An electrical sign of participation of the mesial "supplementary" motor cortex in human voluntary finger movements. *Brain Res, 159,* 473–476.

Deecke L, Heise B, Kornhuber HH, Lang M, Lang W (1984) Brain potentials associated with voluntary manual tracking: Bereitschaftspotential, conditioned pre-motion positivity, directed attention potential, and relaxation potential. Anticipatory activity of the limbic and frontal cortex. In Karrer, R, Cohen, J, Tueting P (Eds.), *Brain and information: Event-related potentials.* (Ann NY Acad Sci, 425, 450–464).

Deecke L, Boschert J, Brickett P, Weinberg H (1985a) Magnetoencephalographic evidence for possible supplementary motor area participation in human voluntary movement. In Weinberg H, Stroink G, Katila T (Eds.), *Biomagnetism: Applications and theory.* Pergamon Press, New York, 369–372.

Deecke L, Kornhuber HH, Lang W, Lang M, Schreiber H (1985b) Timing function of the frontal cortex in sequential motor and learning tasks. *Human Neurobiol, 4,* 143–154.

Farah MJ (1984) The neurological basis of mental imagery: A componential analysis. *Cognition, 18,* 245–272.

Goldenberg G (1987) *Neurologische Grundlagen bildlicher Vorstellungen.* Springer-Verlag, Wien, New York.

Goldenberg G, Podreka I, Steiner M, Willmes K (1987) Patterns of regional cerebral blood flow related to memorizing of high and low imagery words—An Emission Computer Tomography study. *Neuropsychologia, 25,* 473–485.

Kleist K (1934) *Gehirnpathologie.* J.A. Barth, Leipzig.

Kornhuber HH, Deecke L (1964) Hirnpotentialänderungen beim Menschen vor und nach Willkürbewegungen, dargestellt mit Magnetbandspeicherung und Rückwärtsanalyse. *Pflügers Arch, 281,* 52.

Kornhuber HH, Deecke L (1965) Hirnpotentialänderungen bei Willkürbewegungen und passiven Bewegungen des Menschen: Bereitschaftspotential und reafferente Potentiale. *Pflügers Arch, 284,* 1–17.

Kornhuber HH, Deecke L (1985) The starting function of the SMA. *Behav Brain Sci, 8,* 591–592.

Lang W, Lang M, Kornhuber A, Deecke L, Kornhuber HH (1983) Human cerebral potentials and visuomotor learning. *Pflügers Arch, 399,* 342–344.

Lang W, Lang M, Kornhuber A, Deecke L, Kornhuber HH (1984) Brain potentials related to voluntary hand tracking: Motivation and attention. *Human Neurobiol, 3,* 235–240.

Lang W, Lang M, Kornhuber A, Kornhuber HH (1986) Electrophysiological evidence for right frontal lobe dominance in spatial visuomotor learning. *Arch Ital Biol, 124,* 1–13.

Lang M, Lang W, Uhl F, Kornhuber A, Deecke L, Kornhuber HH (1987) Slow negative potential shifts indicating verbal cognitive learning in a concept formation task. *Human Neurobiol, 6,* 183–190.

Lang W, Lang M, Podreka I, Steiner M, Uhl F, Suess E, Müller CH, Deecke L (1988a, in press) DC-potential shifts and regional cerebral blood flow reveal frontal cortex involvement in human visuomotor learning. *Exp Brain Res.*

Lang W, Lang M, Uhl F, Koska C, Kornhuber A, Deecke L (1988b, in press) Negative DC-shifts of supplementary and motor cortex preceding and accompanying simultaneous and sequential bimanual finger movements. *Exp Brain Res.*

Lassen NA, Ingvar DH, Skinhoj E (1978) Brain function and blood flow. *Sci Amer, 239,* 62–71.

Podreka I, Suess E, Goldenberg G, Steiner M, Brücke T, Müller C, Lang W, Neininckx RD, Deecke L (1987) Initial experience with Technetium-99m-HM-PAO brain SPECT. *J Nucl Med, 28,* 1657–1666.

Roland PE, Larsen B, Lassen NA, Skinhoj E (1980) Supplementary motor area and other cortical areas in the organization of voluntary movements in man. *J Neurophysiol, 43,* 118–136.

Subject Index